EXPLORATIONS IN AGING

ADVANCES IN EXPERIMENTAL MEDICINE AND BIOLOGY

Recent Volumes in this Series

Volume 52
HEPARIN: Structure, Function, and Clinical Implications
Edited by Ralph A. Bradshaw and Stanford Wessler • 1975

Volume 53
CELL IMPAIRMENT IN AGING AND DEVELOPMENT
Edited by Vincent J. Cristofalo and Emma Holečková • 1975

Volume 54
BIOLOGICAL RHYTHMS AND ENDOCRINE FUNCTION
Edited by Laurence W. Hedlund, John M. Franz, and
Alexander D. Kenny   1975

Volume 55
CONCANAVALIN A
Edited by Tushar K. Chowdhury and A. Kurt Weiss • 1975

Volume 56
BIOCHEMICAL PHARMACOLOGY OF ETHANOL
Edited by Edward Majchrowicz • 1975

Volume 57
THE SMOOTH MUSCLE OF THE ARTERY
Edited by Stewart Wolf and Nicholas T. Werthessen • 1975

Volume 58
CYTOCHROMES P-450 and b_5: Structure, Function, and Interaction
Edited by David Y. Cooper, Otto Rosenthal, Robert Snyder,
and Charlotte Witmer • 1975

Volume 59
ALCOHOL INTOXICATION AND WITHDRAWAL: Experimental Studies II
Edited by Milton M. Gross • 1975

Volume 60
DIET AND ATHEROSCLEROSIS
Edited by Cesare Sirtori, Giorgio Ricci, and Sergio Gorini • 1975

Volume 61
EXPLORATIONS IN AGING
Edited by Vincent J. Cristofalo, Jay Roberts, and Richard C.
Adelman • 1975

EXPLORATIONS IN AGING

Edited by

Vincent J. Cristofalo
Wistar Institute of Anatomy and Biology
Philadelphia, Pennsylvania

Jay Roberts
Medical College of Pennsylvania
Philadelphia, Pennsylvania

and

Richard C. Adelman
Fels Research Institute
Temple University School of Medicine
Philadelphia, Pennsylvania

PLENUM PRESS • NEW YORK AND LONDON

Library of Congress Cataloging in Publication Data

Philadelphia Symposium on Aging, 1974.
  Explorations in aging.

  (Advances in experimental medicine and biology; v. 61)
  Includes bibliographical references and index.
  1. Aging—Congresses. I. Cristofalo, Vincent J., 1933-   II. Roberts, Jay. III.
Adelman, Richard C., 1940-   IV. Title. V. Series. [DNLM: 1. Aging—Con-
gresses. W3 AD559 v. 61 1974/ WT104 P544e 1974]
QP86.P55 1974   612.6′7   75-20442
ISBN 978-1-4615-9034-7   ISBN 978-1-4615-9032-3 (eBook)
DOI 10.1007/978-1-4615-9032-3

Proceedings of the Philadelphia Symposium on Aging held in Philadelphia,
Pennsylvania, September 30-October 2, 1974

© 1975 Plenum Press, New York
Softcover reprint of the hardcover 1st edition 1975

A Division of Plenum Publishing Corporation
227 West 17th Street, New York, N.Y. 10011

United Kingdom edition published by Plenum Press, London
A Division of Plenum Publishing Company, Ltd.
Davis House (4th Floor), 8 Scrubs Lane, Harlesden, London, NW10 6SE, England

Preface

The three of us, working in different institutions but in the same city, were very aware of the differences between our diverse approaches to the biology of aging and our perceptions of the subject matter. However, three years ago we began to hold informal meetings to discuss our research. These meetings eventually became more frequent and, with this association, we became increasingly cognizant of the commonality of our research problems despite our separate perspectives.

The idea for this symposium, therefore, grew from our awareness that the underlying problem of the biological basis for aging was a common denominator in our research. The papers presented here represent three areas of active investigation: cell division, biological membranes and hormonal regulation. They are submitted with the expectations that a greater understanding of the role of each of these separate approaches will help clarify, not only the interrelationships between our fields of research, but more importantly, the biology of aging itself.

ACKNOWLEDGEMENTS

We would like to extend our sincere thanks for the interest and contributions of the companies listed below:

Abbott Laboratories
Arthur D. Little
Bristol Laboratories
Burroughs Wellcome Co.
Charles River Breeding Labs.
Dow Chemical Co.
E.R. Squibb & Sons, Inc.
Eli Lilly Research Laboratories
Flow Laboratories

Hoffman-LaRoche
McNeil Laboratories
Mead Johnson & Company
Merck Sharp & Dohme Research Labs.
Rom-Amer Pharmaceuticals
Sandoz Pharmaceuticals
Schering Corp.
Smith Kline Corp.
William H. Rorer

We would also like to express our appreciation to Joan Ashton, Maryellen Farrell and Peggy McGee for their help in the preparation of the final manuscript.

We acknowledge the support of USPHS research grants HD06323, HD05874 and HD06267 from the National Institute of Child Health and Human Development.

Vincent J. Cristofalo
Jay Roberts
Richard C. Adelman

Contents

Regulation of Cell Division in Aging Mouse
    Mammary Epithelium 1
    Charles W. Daniel

Age Dependent Decline in Proliferation of
    Lymphocytes 21
    Gordon Stoltzner and Takashi Makinodan

The Regulation of Cellular Aging by Nuclear Events
    in Cultured Normal Human Fibroblasts (WI-38) 39
    Woodring E. Wright and Leonard Hayflick

Hydrocortisone as a Modulator of Cell Division
    and Population Life Span 57
    Vincent J. Cristofalo

General Considerations of Membranes 81
    E. J. Masoro

Function of Cardiac Muscle in Aging Rat 95
    Myron L. Weisfeldt

Changes in Cardiac Membranes as a Function of Age
    with Particular Emphasis on Reactivity to Drugs 119
    Jay Roberts and Paula B. Goldberg

Changes in Protein Synthesis in Heart 149
    J. R. Florini, S. Geary, Y. Saito, E. J. Manowitz,
    and R. S. Sorrentino

Senescence and Vascular Disease 163
    George Martin, Charles Ogburn, and Curtis Sprague

Changes in Hormone Binding and Responsiveness in
    Target Cells and Tissues During Aging 195
    George S. Roth

Regulation of Corticosterone Levels and Liver
        Enzyme Activity in Aging Rats 209
    Gary W. Britton, Samuel Rotenberg, Colette Freeman,
    Venera J. Britton, Karen Karoly, Louis Ceci,
    Thomas L. Klug, Andras G. Lacko, and Richard C. Adelman

Aging and the Regulation of Hormones:
        A View in October 1974 229
    C. E. Finch

Aging and the Disposition of Glucose 239
    Reubin Andres and Jordan D. Tobin

BANQUET ADDRESS

The Scientist and Social Policy on Aging 251
    Elias S. Cohen

ABSTRACTS

Cell Types Originating from Young and Old
        Mouse Kidney Explants 263
    J. Lipetz and R. E. Boswell

Alterations in the Growth Rate and Glucose Metabolism
        of Chinese Hamster Cells in Vitro 265
    J. M. Ryan and D. M. Pace

The Cristofalo Indices of Mutant Human Cells 266
    R. A. Vincent, Jr. and P. C. Huang

Altered DNA Metabolism and Aged and Progeric Fibroblasts . . . 268
    J. R. Williams, J. B. Little, J. Epstein,
    and W. Brown

The Survival of Haploid and Diploid Vertebrate
        Cells After Treatment with Mutagens 269
    L. Mezger-Freed

Capacity of Cultured Fibroblasts from Different
        Mammalian Species to Metabolize 7,12-
        Dimethylbenz(a)anthracene to Mutagenic
        Metabolites: A Correlation with Lifespan 270
    A. Schwartz

Extension of the in Vitro Lifespan of Human
        WI-38 Cells in Culture by Vitamin E 271
    L. Packer and J. R. Smith

Diminished Inotropic Response to Catecholamines
   in the Aged Myocardium 272
   E. G. Lakatta, G. Gerstenblith, C. S. Angell,
   N. W. Shock, and M. L. Weisfeldt

Studies in Age-Related Ion Metabolism in Rat Myocardium . . . 275
   S. I. Baskin, P. B. Goldberg, and J. Roberts

The Effects of Isoproterenol Stress on the Hearts
   of Old and Young Rats 276
   M. Venus, W. J. DiBattista, and G. Kaldor

The Effect of Age and Fasting on Serum Cholesterol
   Levels and Cholesterol Esterification in the Rat 280
   A. G. Lacko, K. G. Varma, T. S. K. David, and
   L. A. Soloff

Lipid Metabolism in Aging Rats 281
   J. A. Story, S. A. Tepper, and D. Kritchevsky

Exercise, Thyroid Secretion Rate and Lipid
   Metabolism in Rats 283
   J. A. Story and D. R. Griffith

Accelerated Aging of the Brain: Neuroendocrine
   Studies in Huntingdon's Disease 284
   S. Podolsky and N. A. Leopold

Changes in Brain Adenosine - 3'5' - Monophosphate in
   the Aging Rat 286
   I. D. Zimmerman and A. P. Berg

Evidence Relating the Amount of Albumin mRNA to the
   Increased Albumin Synthetic Activity Observed
   in Old Rats 289
   M. F. Obenrader, A. I. Lansing, and P. Ove

Properties of Catalase Molecules in Rats of
   Different Ages 291
   J. A. Zimmerman, H. V. Samis, M. B. Baird, and
   H. R. Massie

Thermal Denaturation of Biomolecules at Normal
   Body Temperature 293
   H. A. Johnson

Participants 295

Index   303

REGULATION OF CELL DIVISION IN AGING MOUSE MAMMARY EPITHELIUM

Charles W. Daniel

University of California

Santz Cruz, CA 95064

INTRODUCTION

The subject of cellular aging is a matter of considerable importance in comtemporary biology. The characteristics and parameters of these aging processes, as well as the mechanisms which underlie them, are currently investigated by a variety of techniques. At present the most widely used methodology is that of continuous cell culture, in which normal diploid tissue cells, even though provided with every known requirement and stimulus for growth, nevertheless display an inevitable decline in proliferative capacity, followed by senescent changes and eventual loss of the culture.

The techniques of cell culture, which make the design of meaningful aging experiments possible, also introduce substantial difficulties in interpretation. Cell culture necessarily involves the use of an artificial chemical and physical environment, and it is difficult to eliminate the possibility that at least some of the aging changes observed in culture are the result of gradual changes accumulating in cells that are directly related to some aspect or aspects of the cultural situation.

For this reason many workers experimenting _in vitro_ attempt, where possible, to relate their findings to analogous results obtained _in vivo_. This is particularly important with regard to the regulation of DNA synthesis and of subsequent cell proliferation. Cristofalo and Sharf (1) have recently found that the age of human fibroblasts in culture is related to changing patterns of DNA synthesis in the cell population, and the fraction of total cells capable of synthesis may be used as an indicator of _in vitro_ age.

1

In this chapter the available in vivo transplant systems
will be very briefly reviewed, and the role of cell proliferation
in aging, serially transplanted mouse mammary epithelium will
be evaluated in some detail, with emphasis upon those experiments which may be meaningfully compared with cell culture findings.

SERIAL TRANSPLANT SYSTEMS

The most desirable experimental design, in terms of fur-
nishing an in vivo corollary to continuous cell culture, is the
repeated transfer of cells or tissues between animals in such
a manner that they have the maximum opportunity to display their
potential for survival, proliferation, and in certain cases,
function. In order to distinguish between aging changes that
are intrinsic to the cell and those which may be a response to
the deteriorating environment of the senescing organism, transplants may be passaged in young, healthy animals. In order to
avoid the use of immunosuppressive measures, which often have
generalized systemic effects, it is also desirable to conduct
the transfer in isogenic animals, a restriction which severely
limits the number of species available for experimentation.

The principle difficulty that arises in serial transplantation studies is the problem which may arise in identifying
transplanted cells. Cells of fibroblastic phenotype are most
commonly studied in regard to aging in cell culture, and the
serial transplantation of fibroblasts in vivo is therefore clearly
desirable. Because fibroblasts cannot be distinguished from
host cells, unless isolated by a diffusion chamber or some other
mechanical device, such experiments have not been successfully
performed. In order to minimize this difficulty in identification, transplants are occasionally placed in unusual sites,
such as the anterior chamber of the eye (2). It is not known
to what extent such unfamiliar environments may effect cell
activities, but at the least it raises problems of interpretation
of results. A second type of experiment involves the ablation
of competing host cells or tissues; this may be acceptable in
some instances, but may lead to serious secondary effects on
the host in other cases. The use of genotypic markers to provide
for cell identification suggests elegant experimental possibilities, but in long-term serial transplants this has been successfully employed only in the case of hemopoietic cells (3,4).

1.   Skin Transplantation

Krohn (5,6) has conducted a series of long term experiments
in which skin was serially transferred between inbred mice.

By transplanting parental strain skin into F_1 hybrids, hair color could be used as a means of identification. The general finding was that skin could be carried for several transfers, during a time period of several years. With successive transfers the grafts became smaller, more shrunken, and identification by hair color became progressively more difficult. Nevertheless, Krohn obtained one transplant that survived serial passage for 10 1/4 years, seven transplants that survived for more than eight years, and 32 which could still be identified at seven years (7).

These are impressive life spans, for they clearly indicate that serially transplanted skin can survive and function for a period far beyond the maximum life span of the laboratory mouse. A great deal of cell proliferation is involved in this study, for both hair production and epithelial maintenance require extensive cell division. It is not known to what extent the ultimate demise of the transplant lines is the result of reduction in proliferative capacity of the cells, or equally likely, is due to the extensive buildup of scar tissue resulting from the surgical trauma of repeated grafting.

2.   Hemopoeitic Cell Transplants

In the hemopoietic system continuous cell proliferation is required, where undifferentiated progenitor cells give rise to large numbers of terminally differentiated descendants. The progenitor cells must also be self-renewing, and produce successive generations of stem cells. In order to test the proliferative potential of these cells, Siminovitch et al. (8) serially passaged marrow cells in host mice that had been heavily X-irradiated in order to ablate host hemopoietic cells. Using the spleen colony assay of Till and McCulloch (9), it was determined that colony forming ability decreased markedly during serial passage, and the ability of transplanted cells to promote the survival of irradiated recipients also declined (8,10).

Because of the necessity for massive whole-body irradiation, these experiments are clearly not performed under physiological conditions. This is of particular concern in later transplant generations where the life promoting capacity of the transplants has been reduced and the transplants exist in a deteriorating environment.

Harrison (3,4) has avoided the necessity for irradiation by using genetically anemic W/W^v recipients, whose anemias can be cured by successful transplants. The hemoglobin could be identified as that of the donor B6 type by electrophoretic means. Using long transplant intervals, and measuring the ability of transplants to cure recipients, Harrison determined that mouse

marrow could function normally in the production of erythrocytes
for 73 months, or more than twice the maximum life span of the
mice used. Spleen colony assays indicated, however, that the
colony forming ability of the transplants declined slowly with
successive generations, suggesting that the stem cell population
has an extensive, but nevertheless finite, capacity for proliferation.

Using another marker, the production of specific antibody,
Williamson and Askonas (11) studied the fate of antibody-secreting
clones during serial passage. They concluded that these cells
also displayed a finite capacity for division, and suggested
that this system provides another model for clonal senescence.
On the basis of a number of assumptions, the authors calculated
that the proliferative potential of these stem cells is not more
than 90 divisions.

MAMMARY TRANSPLANT SYSTEM

Mouse mammary epithelium, which might at first appear to
be an unlikely tissue to employ in the study of cell aging, has
proved to be very useful. This is largely because certain growth
characteristics of the gland, and the transplantation techniques
which are available, make possible a number of unique experimental
designs.

The method is based upon the technique of mammary transplantation devised by DeOme et al. (12) in connection with studies
on mammary tumors and preneoplastic tissues. Briefly described,
the procedure is based upon the observation that in prepubertal
female mice of approximately three weeks of age, the glandular,
epithelial component of the gland is rudimentary, and consists
only of the nipple and a network of short ductal elements.
The fatty stromal tissue, termed the fat pad, is well developed
however, and by surgically removing the epithelial component
the remaining portion of the fat pad is available and furnishes
a convenient site for the implantation of mammary epithelial
transplants (Fig. 1).

The transplants quickly regenerate recognizable mammary
tissues, and begin to proliferate under conditions which are
completely physiological. The transplants are in their natural
environment, white fat, and in the absence of competing host
gland there is ample opportunity for the transplants to display
their full potential for proliferation, morphogenesis, and function. After the glands are removed from the host they may be
routinely processed by fixation, fat extraction, and staining,
which yields a whole mount preparation in which it is easily
possible to determine that the mammary outgrowth is derived from
the transplant, and not from the host.

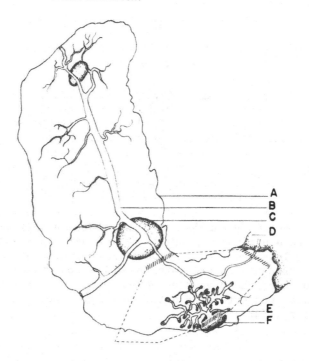

Figure 1. Drawing of a right No. 4 fat pad from a 3 week female mouse. The nipple area, blood vessel, and fat pad are cauterized along the slant lines. The area bounded by the dashed line is removed with fine scissors. A, boundary of fat pad; B, blood vessel; C, lymph node; D, boundary of No. 5 fat pad; E, mammary ducts; F, nipple area. After DeOme et al. (12).

Mammary transplants, after a period of growth, can be distinguished in situ with the aid of trypan blue vital staining (13), making serial transplantation possible (Fig. 2). Using a constant transplant interval of approximately two months, any alterations in growth rate may be detected by estimating the amount of available fat occupied by the glandular outgrowths. This furnishes the mean percent fat pad filled, a figure which may be plotted against either transplant generation or time, and which may be evaluated by conventional statistical techniques.

A. Serial Transplantation

Serial transplantation of normal, non-transformed mouse mammary tissue inevitably leads to a decline in proliferative capacity (14). After a number of serial passages, the mammary

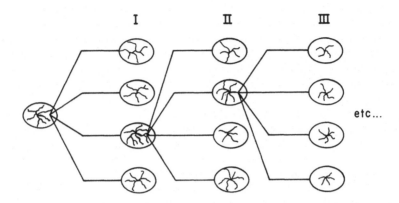

Figure 2. Serial transplantation of mouse mammary tissues. Primary implants are removed from a single donor gland and transplanted into 10–14 gland-free fat pads, which represent generation I. Subsequent transplants are taken from the most vigorously growing outgrowth of the preceding generation. Growth rate is expressed as mean percent fat pad filled at each generation. From Daniel et al. (22).

tissue becomes increasingly unable to fill the available fat (Fig. 3) and the line is eventually lost due to the technical difficulty of identifying and transplanting very minute outgrowths. Data from eight representative transplant lines are summarized in Figure 4, and indicate that the observed decline in growth is approximately linear, and declines at a rate of about 15% in each transfer generation. This loss of growth potential always occurs in response to serial transplantation even though careful selection is exercised for the most vigorously growing tissue, and all conditions are optimal. It is independent of mouse strain and is not related to the presence or absence of Mammary Tumor Virus (14). This phenomenon is interpreted as an expression of aging at the cell and tissue level, when aging is considered exclusively in terms of loss of proliferative potential.

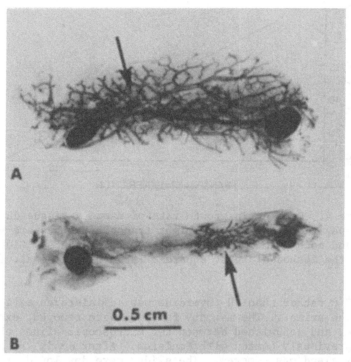

Figure 3. Typical outgrowths of serially transplanted mammary tissues. Darkly staining oval structures are lymph nodes.
Center of outgrowth is indicated by arrows. A. Transplant
generation I, 100% fat pad filled. B. Old outgrowth (transplant
generation VI), 20% fat pad filled. From Daniel and Young (17).

B. Cell Proliferation and Mammary Aging

     The mammary gland, which originates in the foetus as an
epidermal derivative, grows in the non-pregnant female by a
process of ductal elongation. The means by which mammary ducts
are elaborated was described by Bresciani (15), who pulse labeled
the developing gland with ^{3}H-thymidine, disected the various
structures, and performed autoradiography on squash preparations.
Incorporation was found to occur almost exclusively in the tips,
or end buds, of growing ducts, which are composed of several
layers of proliferating mammary epithelial cells.

     This morphogenetic pattern is more clearly visualized using
a recently developed method in which autoradiography is performed
on whole mount preparations, and structural details may be related
to DNA synthetic activity. Because of the thickness of the gland

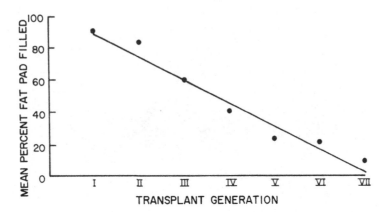

Figure 4. Decline in growth rate of mammary tissue during serial propagation. Results of eight transplant lines are summarized, and each point represents 80-100 transplants. Line fitted by the method of least squares. From Daniel *et al*. (22).

(100 μ), ^{14}C rather than ^{3}H-thymidine was administered as a single pulse to the animal. The mammary fat pads were removed, extracted in acetone, and sandwiched between two microscopic slides that had been previously coated with emulsion. After a six day exposure the gland was removed. The slides were developed, fixed, dried, and the emulsion-coated slide faces were again sandwiched together and cemented with a drop of Permount (see Fig. 5 for further details).

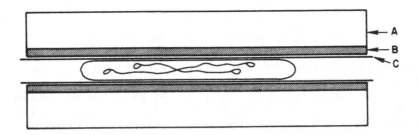

Figure 5. Whole gland autoradiography. Thirty min after a single injection of 25 μC ^{14}C-thymidine, the mammary fat pad was removed, fixed, extracted in acetone, and dried. After gentle compression to a final thickness of 100 μ, the gland was sandwiched between emulsion-coated slides. A, microscope slide; B, Kodak NTB-2 emulsion; C, single layer of Saran Wrap, used to prevent chemical artifacts. After exposure the gland and Saran Wrap were removed. The slides were then developed, fixed, and cemented together with Permount in original alignment.

The reason for employing this somewhat complicated method is
that the mammary ducts frequently grow very close to one side
of the fat pad, and then cross towards the other; this complica-
tion leads to very irregular exposure if only a single layer
of emulsion is employed.

A representative autoradiograph is seen in Figure 6, along-
side its hemotoxylin-stained counterpart. It is apparent that
incorporation is mainly found in the end buds. Further, it is
the large end buds which are most densely labeled, and which
are clearly the most actively growing. The nipple, and the
terminal ducts on which the end buds have regressed, are labeled
very little.

The gland which is visualized in Figure 6

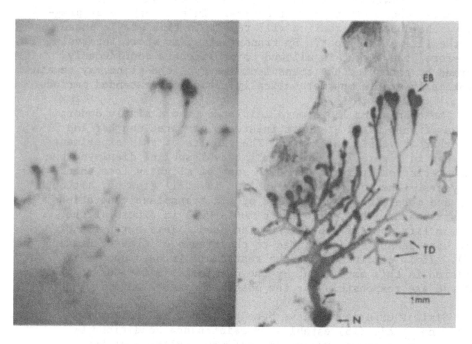

Figure 6. Left, whole gland autoradiograph of rapidly growing mouse mammary gland. Right, same gland stained with hematoxylin. A point by point comparison reveals that the large end
buds (EB) are most intensely labeled. Ducts, terminal ducts
(TD), and the nipple (N), display reduced incorporation.

has not been transplanted, and retains its full growth potential.
Nevertheless certain ducts have ceased proliferation due to the
fact that they have reached the limit of the available fat.
This represents a process of growth regulation operating at the
tissue level, and is the result of normal morphogenetic processes
(16). This regulation apparently proceeds by a simultaneous
reduction in end bud size and a decline in labeling. Final
termination of growth results in the regression of morphologically
distinguished end buds, and the ductal ends are abruptly terminated.

The growth habit previously described permits the design
of experiments which are pertinent to the problems of cellular
aging both in vivo and in vitro. One such problem has to do
with whether the limited life span of somatic cells can be attributed to a finite and specified number of potential cell
doublings, or whether the passage of "metabolic time" can account
for cell senescence. A simple experiment designed to distinguish
between these alternatives takes into account the observation
that a primary mammary transplant requires two to three months
to fill the available fat, after which the end buds regress and
the ducts become mitotically inactive. In the absence of preg-
nancy, the ductal epithelium will remain in this static phase
for the life of the host. By transplanting at short intervals,
therefore, the tissue is allowed to proliferate continuously,
whereas by extending the transplant interval the gland may remain
mitotically static but metabolically active for extended periods.

The transplant lines were initiated from a single donor;
one was transplanted at short intervals of three months, and
the other at yearly intervals. The results of this experiment
are seen in Figure 7. The short interval subline displayed the
characteristically limited growth span of slightly less than
two years. The long interval subline is still growing, although
more and more slowly, at the end of six transplant generations
and six years. This period of time is well in excess of the
maximum life span of the Balb/c mice used. This extension of
life span cannot be attributed to the trauma of transplantation
(17). It is concluded that the restraints imposed upon cell
division in this experiment by the physical limitations of the
fat pad are responsible for the observed tissue longevity.

Similar experiments have been performed in cell culture.
Dell'Orco et al. (18) established maintenance conditions by
reducing serum concentration in confluent cultures of human
fibroblast to 0.5%. They found that cells kept in static phase
for as long as 117 days displayed the same proliferative potential
as controls when returned to growth conditions. McHale et al.
(19), using somewhat different conditions to suppress cell division, found that after a period of time in the non-mitotic

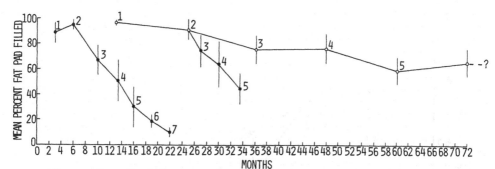

Figure 7. Serial transplants of mouse mammary gland at long and short transplant intervals. Two transplant lines were initiated from a single donor at time 0 and transplanted at intervals of 12 months (0——0) or 3 months (●——●). At 24 months a second short-interval line was split from the 12 month series. Vertical lines represent 95% confidence intervals. Portions of these may have been published previously [Daniel and Young (17,23)].

condition their cells displayed a significantly reduced growth potential. This disparity can perhaps be explained by the differences in methods used. In order to suppress the proliferation of cells in culture, nonphysiological and probably stressful conditions must be used. The results from the mammary transplant experiment may be somewhat more directly interpreted, for the suppression of cell division for long periods of time is accomplished by normal morphogenetic restraints, and homeostatic mechanisms insure that conditions favoring survival are maintained.

The mammary transplant technique is also amenable to the study of the influence of donor age upon the proliferative potential of tissue cells. Transplant lines were initiated from three week and 26 month donors, and were subsequently carried in young hosts. The results (Fig. 8) indicated no difference between the growth span of mammary cells taken from old and young donors (20).

These results appear to be at variance with the findings of Martin et al. (21), who found that skin fibroblasts from donors of increasing age displayed a reduced proliferative potential

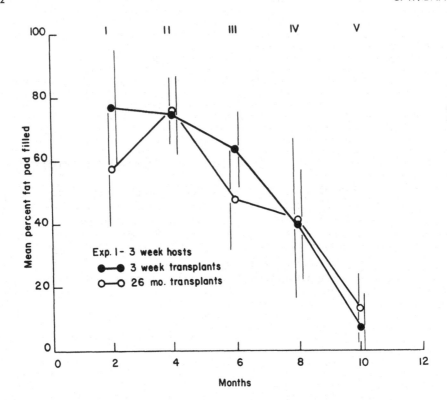

Figure 8. Growth of mammary transplants from young and
old donors serially passaged in young hosts. Each point represents a transplant generation and vertical lines indicate
95% confidence intervals. From Young et al. (20).

in vitro when compared with those from younger donors. This
disparity is probably more apparent than real, for in the case
of the mammary transplants the cells from old donors had not
experienced more cell divisions than cells taken from young
animals, because of growth restrictions imposed by the fat pad.
In the case of human fibroblasts, it is possible that a certain
amount of proliferation continues throughout life, although
evidence is lacking.

C. The End Bud and Mammary Aging

Aging in serially propagated mouse mammary epithelium is
characterized by a progressive loss of growth potential. Because
the end bud represents the proliferative compartment in the virgin
gland, mammary aging may be considered not as a diffuse process
occurring throughout the entire tissue, but as a phenomenon

localized in specific structures -- end buds -- which may be
easily identified by morphological and functional criteria.

The large, actively growing end bud that is characteristic
of young gland is a bulbous structure, several times the diameter
of the subtending duct. Its function, in addition to cell proliferation, is to act as the leading edge of the elongating duct
and to invade, in a very aggressive manner, the fatty stroma.
Certain end bud features may be visualized in a preparation made
for scanning electron microscopy, in which a typical end bud
was dissected away from surrounding fat cells (Fig. 9).

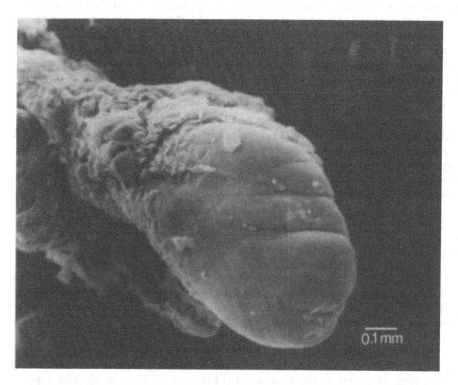

Figure 9. Young mammary end bud dissected from fat pad
and prepared for examination with the scanning electron microscope. Note that the anterior surface of the end bud has separated easily from surrounding tissues, while the subtending
duct is surrounded with adherent fibrous and cellular material.
The smooth surface of the leading edge is the thin basal lamina
overlying end bud epithelium.

Most of the end bud is smooth surfaced, which represents naked
mammary epithelium covered only by a thin basal lamina. It may
be speculated that this foremost region of the structure elab-
orates enzymes which facilitate penetration through surrounding
tissues, but this remains to be demonstrated. Posteriorly the
surface becomes increasingly roughened due to the attachment
of fibrocytes that have been recruited from surrounding host
tissues. These fibrocytes elaborate the dense collagenous tunic
which invests the subtending, differentiated duct.

Additional features of the young end buds are seen in histological section (Fig. 10). The epithelium is multilayered, in
contrast to ducts, which usually consist of a single layer of
differentiated cells. Two layers may be distinguished in the
end bud epithelium. The inner layers consist of tightly packed,
irregularly arranged cells; no intercellular spaces can be distinguished. At the leading edge a monolayer of epithelial cells
is apparent, which is slightly lifted from the underlying cells.
This layer, termed "cap cells", appears to represent the stem
cell population of the end bud. Evidence for this, which will
be presented in detail elsewhere, was obtained by injecting mice
with pulses of ^{3}H-thymidine at six hr intervals over a period
of 30 hr in order to label the entire proliferating pool. Cap
cells were all labeled (99%), and the labeling index progressively
decreased in deeper and more posterior regions. Cap cells have
never been observed in regressing end buds, or at the tip of
terminal ducts, suggesting that the integrity of this stem cell
population is necessarily associated with ductal elongation.

An end bud from very old, serially passaged tissue is seen
in section in Figure 11. The entire structure is much smaller,
and differs only slightly in size from its subtending duct.
The epithelium is thin and somewhat irregular. In addition,
the entire structure is surrounded by abundant fibrous connective
tissue, which is never found at the leading edge of actively
proliferating end buds. Of particular interest is the observation
that cap cells are absent.

The structure of the aged end bud is similar, perhaps identical to that of regressing end buds in young tissue which are
responding to normal regulatory influences. This suggests that
mammary aging is both structurally and functionally related to
normal morphogenetic, regulatory events. The principal distinction between young and old mammary tissue is that while young
end buds regress only when confronted with limitations of the
fat pad or some other obstacle, aged tissue displays a similar
response even in the presence of abundant fat tissue.

Quantitative studies on the rate of cell proliferation in
end buds in relation to mammary aging is currently in progress

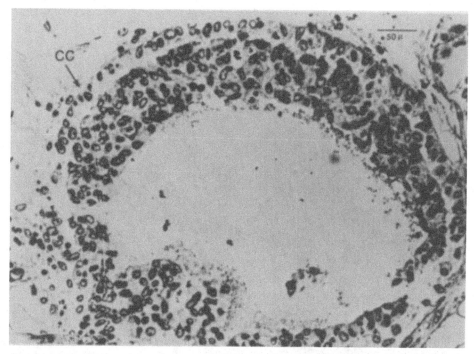

Figure 10. Histological section of young mammary end bud, with the anterior end toward the top of the photograph. Enclosing the large lumen is a thick layer of irregularly arranged epithelial cells. The advancing edge is composed of a monolayer of cap cells.

in this laboratory. At present pulse labeling studies with ^{3}H-thymidine have been successfully carried out with one transplant line. The type of preparation that is obtained is illustrated in Figure 12, in which a first transplant generation end bud is seen to display extensive incorporation. Changes in response to serial propagation are graphed in Figure 13, and an age related decline in labeling is suggested. These experiments are complicated by the large variation between end buds within a single fat pad (e.g., Fig. 6), which is reflected in

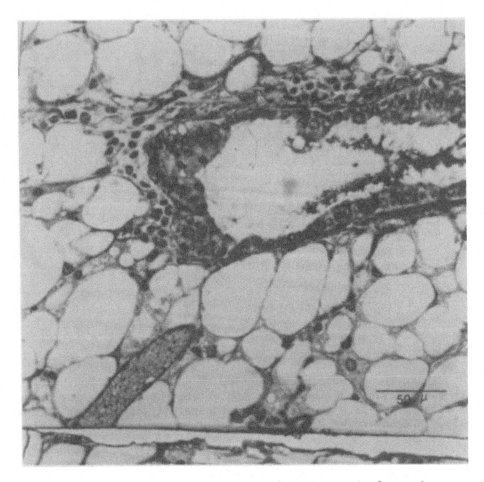

Figure 11. Histological section through terminal portion of a mammary duct from a very old, generation VI mammary outgrowth. End bud structures have largely disappeared, and the duct is capped by epithelial cells surrounded by dense, fibrous connective tissues. Cap cells are no longer apparent.

the large standard errors. It is also possible that age related changes in characteristics of the cell cycle may influence the labeling index. These matters will be pursued; in addition it is anticipated that methods will be developed to allow for extended exposure of end buds to ^{3}H-thymidine, which will provide a means of measuring the size of the proliferating pool in relation to _in vivo_ age -- data which would furnish an interesting

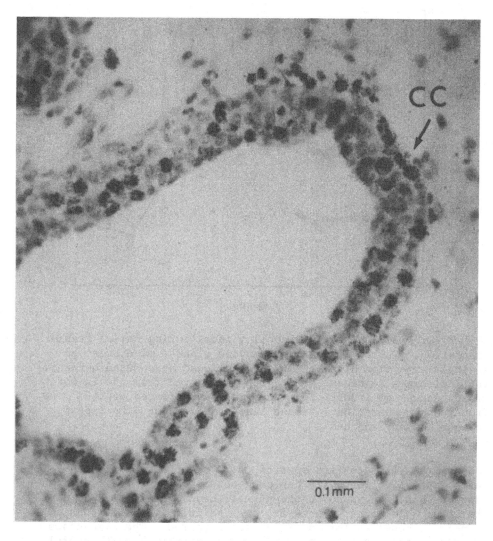

Figure 12. Representative autoradiograph of young (trans-plant generation I) end bud pulse labeled with ^{3}H-thymidine. CC, cap cells.

corollary to parallel cell culture studies of Cristofalo and Sharf (1).

CONCLUSIONS

Several murine serial transplantation techniques have been devised by a number of investigators, which are designed to

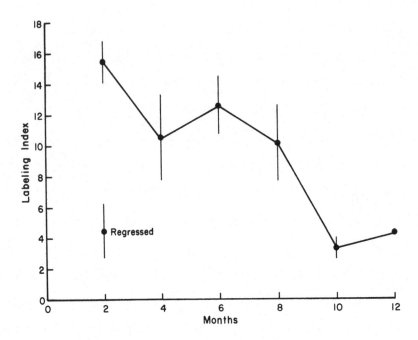

Figure 13. Changes in labeling index during serial transplantation. Thirty min before removing glands, mice received
a single injection of ^{3}H-thymidine, followed by autoradiography.
Vertical lines represent SEM, which is omitted from the 12 month
group because of insufficient numbers. A regressed end bud
from young, generation I tissue has a similar labeling index
to aged mammary end buds.

measure the ultimate life span of cells and tissues. In many
cases impressive longevity has been obtained, in which functional
adequacy has been found to extend well beyond the life span of
the mouse. In no case, however, has the unlimited life span
of normal, non-transformed cells been reported. The mechanisms
underlying these aging processes remain obscure, but in several
instances aging in vivo appears to be associated with limitations
upon cell doubling potential.

With particular reference to the mouse mammary transplant
system, the following is concluded.

1. Mammary tissues serially transplanted in virgin females,
under conditions which are judged to be optimal, inevitably
display a decline in growth rate and the lines are eventually
lost. This decay in growth is linear, and occurs at a rate of
approximately 15% each transfer generation.

2. Aging of mammary cells during continuous propagation is associated only with a decline in growth; further Phase III senescent changes are not observed, and very old, non-proliferating mammary cells may survive in good condition for extended periods.

3. The mechanisms responsible for these aging changes are thought to involve alterations occurring progressively during the course of repeated transplantation to cell regulatory mechanisms which, under usual conditions, direct the course of normal mammary morphogenesis and limit the eventual size of the gland.

REFERENCES

1. Cristofalo, V. J. and B. B. Sharf. Exp. Cell Res. 76:419 (1973).
2. Grobstein, C. J. Exp. Zool. 114:359 (1950).
3. Harrison, D. E. Nature New Biol. 237:220 (1972).
4. Harrison, D. E. Proc. Nat. Acad. Sci. USA 70:3184 (1973).
5. Krohn, P. L. Proc. Roy. Soc. B 157:128 (1962).
6. Krohn, P. L. In: Topics of the Biology of Aging. (Ed.) P. L. Krohn, John Wiley and Sons, New York (1966) p. 125.
7. Krohn, L. P. Personal communication (1972).
8. Siminovitch, L., J. E. Till, and E. A. McCulloch. J. Cell. Comp. Physiol. 64:23 (1964).
9. Till, J. E. and E. A. McCulloch. Radiat. Res. 14:213 (1961).
10. Cudkowicz, G., A. C. Upton, and G. M. Shearer. Nature 201: 165 (1964).
11. Williamson, A. R. and B. A. Askonas. Nature 238:337 (1972).
12. DeOme, K. B., L. J. Faulkin, H. A. Bern, and P. B. Blair. Cancer Res. 19:515 (1959).
13. Hoshino, K. J. Nat. Can. Inst. 30:585 (1963).
14. Daniel, C. W., K. B. DeOme, J. T. Young, P. B. Blair, and L. J. Faulkin. Proc. Nat. Acad. Sci. USA 61:53 (1968).
15. Bresciani, F. Cell Tissue Kinet. 1:51 (1968).
16. Faulkin, L. J., Jr., and K. B. DeOme. J. Nat. Can. Inst. 24:953 (1960).
17. Daniel, C. W. and L. J. T. Young. Exp. Cell Res. 65:27 (1971).
18. Dell'Orco, R. T., J. G. Mertens, and P. F. Kruse, Jr. Exp. Cell Res. 77:356 (1973).
19. McHale, J. S., M. L. Mouton, and J. T. McHale. Exp. Geront. 6:89 (1971).
20. Young, L. J. T., D. Medina, K. B. DeOme, and C. W. Daniel. Exp. Geront. 6:49 (1971).
21. Martin, G. M., C. A. Sprague, and C. J. Epstein. Lab. Invest. 23:86 (1970).
22. Daniel, C. W., B. D. Aidells, D. Medina, and L. J. Faulkin, Jr. FASEB. In press.
23. Daniel, C. W. Experientia 29:1422 (1973).

AGE DEPENDENT DECLINE IN PROLIFERATION OF LYMPHOCYTES

Gordon Stoltzner and Takashi Makinodan
Laboratory of Cellular and Comparative Physiology,
Gerontology Research Center, National Institute of Child
Health & Human Development, NIH, PHS, HEW, Bethesda,
and the Baltimore City Hospitals, Baltimore MD 21224

INTRODUCTION

Only during the past twenty years have attempts been made to
carefully and systematically document declining function of the immunologic system with age. It is now known that senescence of the
immunologic system occurs in all mammalian species studied, as
measured by a variety of immunologic indices. Thus, amongst most
but not all of the cellular components constituting the immune
system, age dependent deficits in proliferation, differentiation
and function have been found. For example, mitogenic responses
of lymphocytes, ability of stem cells to reconstitute irradiated
hosts, recognition of threshold doses of antigen, and maximum
humoral antibody responses are all decreased with aging (Heidrick
and Makinodan, 1972a; Ram, 1967; Lajtha and Schofield, 1971).
The consequences of this immunologic decline are very important
to the organism and have been implicated in increased susceptibility
of old animals to a variety of infectious insults and the increased
incidence of neoplasia. General theories of aging have been postulated linking this decline in immunity, and an associated rise
of autoimmunity, with most of the diseases attributed to the aging
process including cancer and atherosclerosis (Walford, 1969, Robert
and Robert, 1973). Since aging influences the differentiation
and proliferation potential of immunologic cells, the immune system
is an ideal model for the study of aging at the cellular level.
Compelling reasons for this view are listed in Table I.

This paper is arbitrarily divided into two parts and will
initially discuss aging of humoral responses and finally, the cell
mediated reactions. Since much more is known about age changes

21

TABLE I

MERITS FOR INVESTIGATING THE IMMUNE SYSTEM AS A MODEL OF
CELLULAR AGING

---

1. Knowledge of the immune system at the cellular, molecular, genetic,
   developmental and phylogenetic levels is comprehensive.

2. Functional activities of the immune system predictably decline as the
   individual ages.

3. Techniques now available can readily manipulate the immune system at
   cellular and molecular levels permitting maneuvers to slow or reverse
   immunologic decline.

4. Prevention or reversal of the decline in immune activities may modulate
   the severity of age-related diseases.

---

of humoral function, we will explore this area in greater detail.

The discussion will initially deal with a description of
declining humoral activity, and then consider the importance of
alterations intrinsic to the immunocompetent cells and also their
environment. Age dependent variations of macrophage function,
stem cell proliferation, and helper activity mediated by T-lymphocytes (theta antigen bearing) will then be discussed. The paper
will close with an analysis of aging in cell-mediated immunity.

AGING OF HUMORAL ACTIVITY

A. Some Examples of Declining B Lymphocyte Function

Generally, antibody titers to a variety of extrinsic antigens
decline with age, although variations of immune activity among
individuals of the same age increase with age (Makinodan and
Peterson, 1966; Metcalf et al., 1966; Somers and Kuhns, 1972;
Thomsen and Kettel, 1929; Wigzell and Stjernsward, 1966). Primary
responses in older animals are severely affected. For example, in
32-month-old mice injected with sheep red blood cells, the number

of indirect plaque forming units is only about 10% the number
found in young animals; secondary responses to the same antigen
are much less severely affected (Makinodan et al., 1971). Figure 1

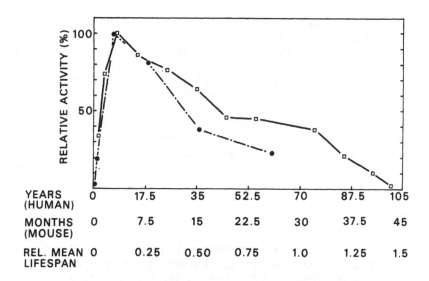

Figure 1. Effect of age on serum agglutinin titers in the
human and mouse. □ natural serum anti-A isoagglutinin titers in
humans (Thomsen and Kettel, 1929). ● peak serum agglutinin response
to sheep red blood cell stimulation by intact mice (Makinodan and
Peterson, 1966).

demonstrates the effect of age on serum agglutinin titers in human
and mouse populations. The life spans of both species are on different scales and are displayed as proportions of total life span.
It is apparent that at a given time of life, the patterns of agglutination activity are similar. The time of maximal response
occurs at puberty when the thymus gland has reached its greatest
size.

Not all investigators report decline of primary antibody response with age, particularly when certain bacterial and viral
vaccines are used (Solomonova and Vizev, 1973; Davenport et al.,
1953; Kishimoto et al., 1969). There are several possible explanations for these observations. It is possible that the recipient
individual had already been exposed to the antigen in question,
and therefore the response is really secondary. In some instances,

the antigen could be one of the so called T-dependent antigens and
therefore the immunologic reaction might be less subject to age
decline.

B.   Mechanisms of Age Dependent Changes in Humoral Activity

1. The Milieu

One can arbitrarily divide potential aging mechanisms into
two broad categories: changes intrinsic to the cells in question
and changes that occur in their environment, that is, the milieu
provided by the host organism. Whether one or both of these categories apply can be tested by a straightforward experimental model,
namely primary response to sheep red blood cells in irradiated young
and old mice, reconstituted with syngeneic spleen cells. This response requires at least three immunologic cellular components:
B-lymphocytes, T-lymphocytes (providing helper function) and macrophages, all three of which are supplied in the spleen suspension.
Table II outlines the possible predictions of such an experiment.

TABLE II

A CELL TRANSFER APPROACH TO RESOLVE
THE ROLE CELLULAR AND ENVIRONMENTAL CHANGES PLAY
IN THE DECLINE WITH AGE IN IMMUNE ACTIVITY[a]

Cause of Decline in Activity	Donors of Cell	Recipients	
		Young	Old
Cellular	Young	High	High
	Old	Low	Low
Environmental	Young	High	Low
	Old	High	Low
Both	Young	High	Low
	Old	Low	Low

[a]A fixed number of donor spleen cells is injected with an optimum dose of
antigen into X-rayed syngeneic recipients and the peak response is assessed
subsequently.

TABLE III

EFFECT OF AGE OF THE RECIPIENT ON THE RELATIVE
HUMORAL IMMUNE RESPONSE OF MOUSE SPLEEN CELLS[a]

DONORS OF SPLEEN CELLS	RECIPIENT	
	YOUNG %	OLD %
YOUNG	100	50
OLD	20	10

[a]From Makinodan and Peterson, (1966); Price and Makinodan, (1972b).

The actual experimental results are summarized in Table III and
clearly show that both environmental and intrinsic mechanisms are
involved. The nature of these environmental mechanisms is presently quite unknown, but it has been shown that the ability of limiting numbers of immunocompetent spleen cells to initiate an immunologic response, and the dose-response relationship to antigen are
both reduced in older animals.

The ability of intact old and young mice to respond to varying
doses of sheep red blood cells is presented in Figure 2. Several
important conclusions can be made. The response slopes to non-
saturation doses of sheep cells differ in old and young (2.7 for
young and 1.2 for old mice) and the younger animals reach their
saturation response at one tenth less antigen than is required by
the old mice. Finally, the maximal response of the old animal
is much less (about 4%) than the young. When dispersed spleen
cells are cultured in vitro there is no antigen dose difference
between the old and young in order to reach a saturation response.
Furthermore, when a primary immunologic reaction is initiated in
vitro, such as in the Mishell-Dutton system, old spleen cells give
poorer responses, on the order of 20% that of the young, but better
than the 4% response of the intact animals (Heidrick and Makinodan,
1972a).

These findings indicate that in addition to declining capacity
of at least some of the cells needed for a humoral response, the
splenic environment is also lacking. The nature of this defi-

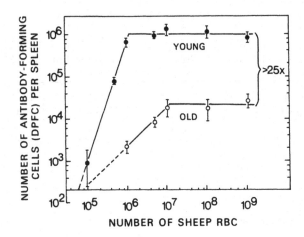

Figure 2. Effect of antigen dose on peak antibody response of young and old mice. Vertical bars indicate 95% confidence limits (Price and Makinodan, 1972a).

ciency is unknown, but is possibly associated with faulty antigen trapping, preventing the optimal interaction of B-lymphocyte, T-lymphocyte and accessory cells. This deficiency might also be correlated with the histologic observation that, with age, germinal follicles disappear.

Although macrophages are important in antigen uptake and processing, two studies have demonstrated no aging decline of in vitro phagocytic activity (Perkins, 1971; Heidrick, 1972b). It is possible that with intact animals some macrophages might sequester or destroy antigen making it relatively inaccessible to immunocompetent units. During dispersion of spleens in preparation for in vitro studies, the large, dendritic macrophages might be selectively disrupted, providing an explanation for the relatively better performance of old spleen cells in vitro than in vivo.

2. Changes Intrinsic to the Immunocompetent Cells

We will assume that the stem cells (S) are the primordial cells of the immune system. These cells may differentiate into more functional states and are classified as thymic derived, T-lymphocytes; bone marrow derived, B-lymphocytes; and accessory cells or macrophages. T- and B-lymphocytes are able to interact specifically with antigen, while macrophages and stem cells probably do not. B and T cells are able to replicate and/or differentiate into functional effector cells producing antibody or participating in delayed hypersensitivity responses.

Hypothetical mechanisms for declining function of these immunocompetent cells could work at several levels. It is possible that the absolute numbers of such cells have decreased through death or inadequate renewal from stem cells. Age acquired new populations of "suppressor cells" analogous to the T-lymphocytic helper cells might impair responses. The ability of immunocompetent cells to interact with antigen or accessory cells might be diminished. The cells could have decreased potential for mitosis, or, once "turned on" have less ability to make antibody or other factors.

Figures 3 and 4 present simplified schemes of conceptual

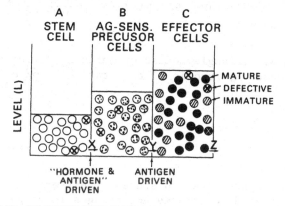

COMPARTMENTS

A
STEM
CELL

B
AG-SENS.
PRECUSOR
CELLS

C
EFFECTOR
CELLS

MATURE
DEFECTIVE
IMMATURE

LEVEL (L)

"HORMONE &
ANTIGEN"
DRIVEN

ANTIGEN
DRIVEN

LEVEL OF COMPARTMENT (L) PER UNIT TIME (T)

a) $\dfrac{dL_A}{dT} = f\left[GT, -\dfrac{dX}{dT} - \dfrac{dF_A}{dT}\right]$

b) $\dfrac{dL_B}{dT} = f\left[\dfrac{dX}{dT} - \dfrac{dY}{dT} - \dfrac{dF_B}{dT}, GT(?)\right]$

c) $\dfrac{dL_C}{dT} = f\left[\dfrac{dY}{dT} - \dfrac{dZ}{dT} - \dfrac{dF_C}{dT}, GT\right]$

where:
GT, generation time; F, functional impairment, X, differentiation of A to B cells; Y, differentiation of B to C cells; Z, cell death.

Figure 3. A three-compartment model of cellular differentiation in an immune response.

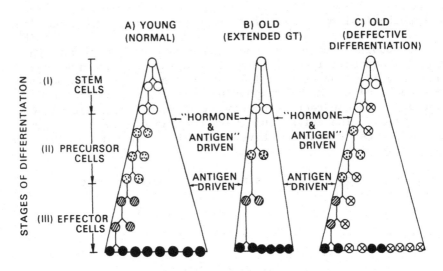

Figure 4. Triangle models of cellular differentiation in an immune response. ● functional effector cell. ⊗ defective cell.

immunologic compartments and stages of differentiation. The compartment diagram demonstrates how changes in compartmental level with time (dL/dT) are dependent on several important variables including differentiation, cell death and generation time. Changes in any of these could profoundly influence the end product, namely the functional effector cell. The triangle diagram (Figure 4) emphasizes how cell division, generation time and differentiation are of critical significance in determining the ultimate clonal size and functional activity.

a. Spleen Cell Density, Number, and Size

Although spleens from mice 25 months or older have a high incidence of neoplasia that can markedly increase cellularity, tumor free spleens remain stable in wt. over most of the adult life. The number of viable cells per unit wet wt. also remains relatively constant. Nevertheless, using Ficoll and albumen discontinuous gradients, we have found the incidence of less dense cell increases at the expense of the denser cells, as illustrated in Figure 5. The significance of this observation is uncertain,

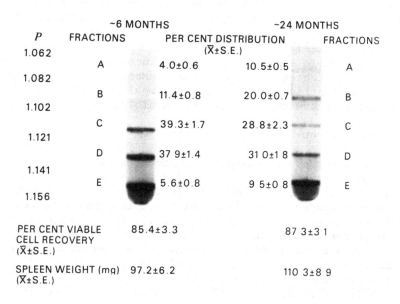

Figure 5. Density distribution of spleen cells of young and old BC3F$_1$ mice. Sample size per group, 6–12 (Halsall et al., 1973).

since there is similar shift to lighter density amongst young animals that have been stimulated by allogeneic lymphocytes or sheep red blood cells, or in mice that are tumor bearing.

b. Stem (S) Cells

Most of the stem cells reside in the bone marrow, and although their concentration declines somewhat during aging, the total cellularity increases. Thus, the number of stem cells remains about constant during life (Chen, 1971; Coggle and Proukakis, 1970; David et al., 1971).

Hematopoietic ability of stem cells does not decline with age (Harrison, 1973; Toya and Davis, 1973), but their ability to generate lymphatic cells might be affected as judged by an impaired capacity to reconstitute irradiated young syngeneic recipients (Price and Makinodan, 1972b) and by a decreased ability to generate B cells in thymectomized irradiated young syngeneic host (Farrar et al., 1974). The capacity of stem cells to recover from fractionated sublethal doses of X-rays and generate hematopoietic

colonies also seems impaired. Neonatal spleen cells bearing the
T_6 chromosome marker were maintained in successive irradiated
hosts for 60 months, but increased loss of recipient mice began
at 40 months (Micklem et al., 1966). This information, when interpreted as a whole suggests that some functional properties of
stem cells are affected by aging. Still uncertain are whether
this decreased function results from an impaired proliferative
response and if these changes are irreversible.

c. Bone Marrow Derived Lymphocyte

The total number of splenic B-lymphocytes does not vary significantly with age (Adler et al., 1971) when measured by indices
utilizing membrane bound immunoglobulin receptors, cells susceptible
to Anti-B cell reagents, or those which are responsive to certain
endotoxin mitogens. It is probable, however that subpopulations
of B-lymphocytes might change over time, dependent in part on extrinsic antigen stimulation. Functionally this might be expressed
in shifts of serum immunoglobulin levels and classes in aging
humans (Buckley and Dorsey, 1971; Haferkamp et al., 1966; Hallgreen
et al., 1973) and a slight fall in the number of B-lymphocytes
responsive to the sheep red cells in mice (Price and Makinodan,
1972a). Although it is uncertain that peripheral blood lymphocytes adequately reflect central lymphoid organ populations, those
studies in humans regarding the proportion of B-lymphocytes and
T-lymphocytes in blood have lead to conflicting results (Immunology
of Aging Workshop, 1974).

d. T-Lymphocyte Helper Activity

This section shall concern itself with the very limited body
of knowledge concerning aging of T-lymphocytes in relation to helper
activity, that is, the requirement of the T cell in modulating
or facilitating a humoral response to a wide number of antigens
including sheep red cells. In a qualitative sense, a small number
of T-lymphocytes will facilitate a humoral response, while many
will suppress it, although it is unknown if this observation
represents one or several subpopulations of lymphocytes. There
seems to be an inverse relationship between T-lymphocyte function,
as measured by in vitro blastogenesis or skin graft rejection,
and autoimmunity manifested by circulating antibodies to nucleo-
proteins, red cells and immune complex disease. Thus amongst
humans, autoantibodies are found in the highest incidence in older
people (Rowley et al., 1968). In the New Zealand Black Mouse there
is a marked decline of T-lymphocyte function and falling levels
of thymosin, a hormone like substance presumably secreted by the
thymus gland (Dauphinee et al., 1974) that is associated with the
appearance of overt autoimmunity. Murine strains that do not develop autoimmunity, such as the C3H maintain T function well into

old age, even at a time when there is an increasing incidence of neoplasia.

e. Accessory Cell

These cells, primarily macrophages, participate in B- and T-lymphocyte immune response in a nonspecific manner, are radio-resistant, adhere to glass, phagocytize opsonized particles effectively and do not give rise to functional effector cells (Mosier and Coppelson, 1969; Hoffman, 1970). Utilizing mouse macrophages, it was found that old cells differed little from macrophages of younger animals in their ability to cooperate with B- and T-lymphocytes as summarized in Table IV. Other studies demonstrated that

TABLE IV

PRIMARY ANTIBODY RESPONSE OF VARIOUS COMBINATIONS OF ADHERENT AND NONADHERENT SPLENIC CELL POPULATIONS FROM YOUNG AND OLD MICE[a]

	Preparation of Interacting Spleen Cells	Relative Antibody-Forming Response (%)	
		Young	Old
Controls	Unseparated	100	20
	Adherent	8	5
	Nonadherent	2	1
	Adherent + Nonadherent	96	18
		Young-Old Combinations	
Experimental	Old Adherent + Young Nonadherent	95	
	Young Adherent + Old Nonadherent	20	

[a]The nonadherent splenic cell fraction (95% lymphocytes) from both young and old mice consisted of approximately 70% of the nucleated cells in the original inoculum,and the adherent cell fraction (70% macrophages) about 30%. Therefore a nonadherent cell to adherent cell proportion of 7 to 3 was used in the 4 reconstituted mixtures, (Heidrick and Makinodan, 1973).

in vitro phagocytic function and certain hydrolytic activities
were also unchanged with age (Perkins, 1971). Therefore, by the
indices measured, macrophages do not seem to acquire aging deficits.

f. Immunocompetent Unit

In the foregoing sections we have dealt with the stem cells
and some of the principles behind their proliferation and differentiation into antigen sensitive precursor cells. The nature of
the three more differentiated cell types, namely B-lymphocytes,
T-lymphocytes and macrophages was then discussed. This last section
will address itself to the interaction of these cells. The response of sheep red cells by mouse spleen is probably a typical
example of an immunologic reaction and requires the interaction
of all three cell types. Unless these cells are assembled in
the correct manner, it is unlikely that an immune response as evidenced by antibody production and plaque formation in a Jerne assay will occur. In order for a detectable reaction to take place,
a required number of each cell type is needed, and this combination of cells we shall call an immunocompetent unit (IU). Thus
an IU is defined as the minimum number of cells necessary to
initiate an immune response. While the number of each cell type
might vary in an IU, it is probable that one of the types will
be rate limiting, either as a result of its numbers per se,
or in a functional sense by virtue of suppressor or
enhancing mechanisms.

Immunocompetent units can be studied in aging by utilizing
the limiting dilution assay (Groves et al., 1970), and will give
an estimate in any given tissue of the number of functional immunocompetent units and/or the number of precursor T- or B-lymphocytes. For example, in a study of antisheep RBC activity in situ,
a 50-fold difference in response per spleen was observed between
young and old mice, but only a 5-fold difference in the number of
IU per spleen (Table V) (Prince and Makinodan, 1972a). An estimate
of the relative efficiency of IU to number of effector cells can
be calculated: (IU/plaque forming units) for young and old.
These estimates, which we call Immunological Burst Size (IBS)
are tabulated in column C, and one can readily appreciate that
the IBS of old animals is only 10% that of the young.

The IBS is, in essence, a quantitative index of differentiation and therefore supports the conclusion of an intrinsic decline in the ability of the aged immunocompetent unit to produce
antibody. The same study, using the limiting dilution assay,
has demonstrated that the numbers of B-lymphocytes and T-lymphocytes constituting the immunocompetent units actually increase
with age. This finding suggests that the proportion of cells
with an ability to prevent antigen-sensitive B cells from re-

TABLE V

EVALUATION OF THE DIFFERENTIATION PROCESS OF
SPLEEN CELLS OF YOUNG AND OLD BC3F$_1$ MICE ON MAXIMAL
RESPONSES TO SHEEP RBC STIMULATION IN SITU

Age of Mice (Months)	(A) Response (DPFC/Spleen)	Ratio of Young/Old	I.U. per Spleen	(B) Ratio of Young/Old	I.B.S. per Spleen (A/B)	(C) Ratio of Young/Old
Young (3-4)	$100 \times 10^{+4}$		1000		1000	
		50X		5X		10X
Old (30-35)	$2 \times 10^{+4}$		200		100	

Abbreviations: DPFC, direct plaque antibody forming cells; I.U., immunocompetent

unit; I.B.S., immunological burst size, (Price and Makinodan, 1972a). See text

for discussion.

sponding to antigenic stimulation is increasing with age. It is
apparent that the B-lymphocyte is highly vulnerable to the aging
process.

AGING OF DELAYED HYPERSENSITIVITY

A.   The Thymus

The thymus is necessary for the development of the T-lymphocyte immune system. Its extirpation in the neonatal period leads
to profound immunosuppression and thymectomy performed in young
adult mice is associated with gradual decline of certain indices
of delayed hypersensitivity as well as decreased longevity in
C57B/6 mice (Jeejeebhoy, 1971). The thymus is the first large
lymphoid organ to atrophy, beginning in the post pubertal period.
Also falling with age, are certain humoral substances, thought to
be thymic hormones (Bach et al., 1973). The mechanism for thymic
atrophy is unknown although considerable evidence indicates that
much of the involution is controlled by factors intrinsic to the

thymus (Metcalf, 1964; Bellamy, 1973). In spite of this atrophy, cell division of thymocytes as measured by the mitotic index seems to persist in older glands, indicating an active cellular turn-over (Bellamy, 1973). Transplantation of thymuses from various aged donors to irradiated and bone marrow reconstituted mice demonstrates that only neonatal thymus can promote peripheraliza-tion of precursor lymphocytes (Hirokawa and Makinodan, 1974). Three-mongh-old thymic transplants can induce bone marrow pre-cursor cells to carry the theta antigen, but are unable to permit these lymphocytes to respond to the T cell mitogens. In the allogeneic mixed lymphocyte reaction, atrophic aged thymus can still enhance responses in irradiated and bone marrow reconstituted mice. It seems that the thymus, with time, loses its ability to modulate differentiation of precursor cells, with peripheralization of lymphocytes being lost first, followed by decreased response to T cell mitogens, helper function, and finally, the most age resistent, the mixed lymphocyte reaction (Hirokawa and Makinodan, 1974).

B. The T-lymphocyte

Although the total number of theta antigen bearing splenic lymphocytes remains constant during the life span in long-lived mice, (Stutman, 1972; Makinodan and Adler, 1974), there seems to be a defect in T-lymphocyte proliferation. The blastogenic response of T cells to phytohemagglutin, concanavalin A, or to the stimulatory effects of allogeneic cells in the mixed lympho-cyte culture are all markedly decreased with age (Adler et al., 1971; Mathies et al., 1973; Hori et al., 1973). Figure 6 demon-strates that the maximal response of splenic lymphocytes to PHA occurs around 8 months, at this age thymic size and serum thymosin level are already falling. A similar age distribution occurs with concanavalin A, but mitogenesis induced by Salmonella typhi lipo-polysaccharide does not fall below 90% the level in 3-month-old mice. It is thought this lipopolysaccharide reacts with receptors present on more mitotically active cells which include B-lympho-cytes, and this material is generally considered a B cell mitogen.

Young lymphocytes, when incubated with mitogen, promptly increase intracellular cyclic 3', 5'-guanosine monophosphate and lower cyclic 3', 5'-adenosine monophosphate. Although old spleen cells have higher basal levels of both nucleotides, upon stimula-tion with concanavalin A only a slight rise in cyclic-GMP was observed (Heidrick, 1973b). Similarly, PHA mitogenic stimula-tion promotes acetylation of histone, an effect that is also de-pressed in aging spleen cells. It seems that age associated deficits of lymphocytic function occur at the earliest stages of a mitogenic reaction, possibly involving changes on the cyto-plasmic membrane and do not solely result for abnormalities in nucleic acid synthesis.

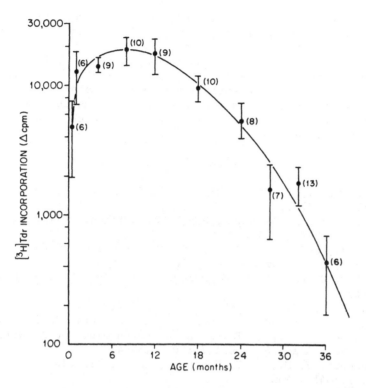

Figure 6. Decline with age in the PHA mitogenic activity of splenic T cells of long-lived mice (Hori et al., 1973).

In vivo estimates of T-lymphocyte function are technically difficult and most assays, such as skin tests and tissue grafting are at best semi-quantitative. The delayed hypersensitivity response associated with a positive skin test is a complicated immunologic reaction dependent on several cell types and is analogous to the interaction necessary for a humoral response to sheep red cells in mice. There does seem to be a somewhat diminished activity in older individuals to contact sensitivity with pentadecylcatechol and dinitrochlorobenzene in guinea pigs and humans (Baer and Bauser, 1963; Gross, 1965).

CONCLUSIONS AND SUMMARY

Immunologic effector cell function is maximal in the young adult mammal, at a time when a portion of the immunologic system, namely the thymus, has already begun a morphological and physio-

logic decline. By old age, many indices of effector cell function
are markedly depressed, although some, such as secondary humoral
responses, are better preserved than others. Immunocompetent
units (i.e. the interactions of macrophages, B- and T-lymphocytes do not vary dramatically with age. Generally both the rate
of proliferation and differentiation of some lymphocytes and their
immunocompetent precursors are impaired. It seems that both environmental factors and changes intrinsic to the cells are involved in this impairment.

REFERENCES

1.   Adler, W. H., T. Takiguchi, and R. T. Smith. J. Immunol.
     107:1357 (1971).
2.   Bach, J. F., M. Dardenne, and J. C. Salomon. Clin. Exp. Im-
     munol. 14:247 (1973).
3.   Baer, H., and R. T. Bowser. Science 140:1211 (1963).
4.   Bellamy, D. Gerontologia 19:162.
5.   Buckley, C. E., and F. C. Dorsey. Ann. Int. Med. 75:673
     (1971).
6.   Chen, M. G. J. Cell. Physiol. 78:225 (1971).
7.   Coggle, J. E., and C. Proukakis. Gerontologia 16:25 (1970).
8.   Dauphinee, M. J., N. Talal, A. L. Goldstein, and A. White.
     Proc. Nat. Acad. Sci. USA 71:2637 (1974).
9.   Davenport, F. M., A. V. Hennessy, and T. Francis. J. Exp.
     Med. 98:641 (1953).
10. Davis, M. L., A. C. Upton, and L. C. Satterfield. Proc. Soc.
     Exp. Biol. Med. 137:1452 (1971).
11. Farrar, J. J., B. E. Loughman, and A. A. Nordin. J. Immunol.
     112:1244 (1974).
12. Gross, L. Cancer 18:201 (1965).
13. Groves, D. L., W. E. Lever, and T. Makinodan. J. Immunol.
     104:148 (1970).
14. Haferkamp, O., D. Schlettwein-Gsell, H. G. Schwick, and K.
     Storiko. Gerontologia 12:30 (1966).
15. Hallgren, H. M., C. E. Buckley, V. A. Gilbersten, and E. J.
     Yunis. J. Immunol. 111:1101 (1973).
16. Halsall, M. H., M. L. Heidrick, J. W. Deitchman, and T. Makinodan.
     Gerontologist 13, No. 3, Part II:46 (1973).
17. Hammar, J. A. Endocrinology 5:543 and 731 (1921).
18. Harrison, D. E. Proc. Nat. Acad. Sci. USA 70:3184 (1973).
19. Heidrick, M. L. and T. Makinodan. Gerontologia 18:305 (1972a).
20. Heidrick, M. L. Gerontologist 12, No. 3, Part II:28 (1972b).
21. Heidrick, M. L. and T. Makinodan. J. Immunol. 111:1502 (1973a).
22. Heidrick, M. L. J. Cell Biol. 59, No. 2, Part 2:139a (1973b).
23. Hirokawa, K., and T. Makinodan. Gerontologist 14, No. 5, Part
     II:33 (1974).
24. Hoffman, M. Immunol. 18:791 (1970).
25. Hori, Y., E. H. Perkins, and M. K. Halsall. Proc. Soc. Exp.
     Biol. Med. 144:48 (1973).

26. Immunology of aging workshop, 1974, The second international congress of immunology, Brighton, Sussex, England, Proceeding in press, Plenum Press, London.
27. Jeejeeboy, H. F. Transplantation 12:525 (1971).
28. Kishimoto, S., I. Tsuyuguchi, and Y. Yamamura. Clin. Exp. Immunol. 5:525 (1969).
29. Lajtha, L. G., and R. Schofield. Adv. Gerón. Res. 3:131 (1971).
30. Makinodan, T., and W. J. Peterson. Developmental Biol. 14: 96 (1966).
31. Makinodan, T., F. Chino, W. F. Lever, and B. S. Brewen. J. Geront. 26:515 (1971).
32. Makinodan, T., and W. H. Adler. Fed. Proc. In press.
33. Mathies, M., L. Lipps, G. S. Smith, and R. L. Walford. J. Gerontol. 28:425 (1973).
34. Metcalf, D. Cancer Res. 24:1952 (1964).
35. Metcalf, D., R. Moulds, and B. Pike. Clin. Exp. Immunol. 2:109 (1966).
36. Micklem, H. S., C. E. Ford, E. P. Evans, and J. Gray. Proc. Roy. Soc. (Biol.) 165:78 (1966).
37. Mosier, D. E., and L. W. Coppleson. Proc. Nat. Acad. Sci. 61:542 (1968).
38. Perkins, E. H. J. Reticol. Soc. 9:642 (1971).
39. Price, G. B., and T. Makinodan. J. Immunol. 108:403 (1972a).
40. Price, G. B., and T. Makinodan. J. Immunol. 108:413 (1972b).
41. Ram, J. J. Gerontol. 22:92 (1967).
42. Robert, L., and B. Robert. Gerontologia 19:330 (1973).
43. Rowley, M. J., H. Buchanan, and I. R. Mackay. Lancet 2:24 (1968).
44. Solomonova, K., and St. Vizev. Zeitschrift Immunitatsforschung 146:81 (1973).
45. Somers, H., and W. J. Kuhns. Proc. Soc. Exp. Biol. Med. 141: 1104 (1972).
46. Stutman, O. J. Immunol. 109:602 (1972).
47. Thomsen, O., and K. Kettel. Zeitschrift Immunitatsforschung 63:67 (1929).
48. Toya, R. E., and M. L. Davis. Biomedicine 19:244 (1973).
49. Walford, R. L. In: The Immunologic Theory of Aging, Williams and Wilkins, Baltimore, Md. (1969).
50. Wigzell, H., and J. Stjernsward. J. Nat. Can. Inst. 37:513 (1966).

THE REGULATION OF CELLULAR AGING BY NUCLEAR EVENTS IN CULTURED

NORMAL HUMAN FIBROBLASTS (WI-38)

Woodring E. Wright and Leonard Hayflick

Department of Medical Microbiology
Stanford University School of Medicine
Stanford, California 94305 U.S.A.

INTRODUCTION

Since the development of an in vitro model for aging in 1961, interest in the biology of vertebrate senescence at the cellular level has increased greatly. Previously it had been widely believed that normal vertebrate cells were immortal (1,2), and consequently that biological aging was not the result of fundamental changes in the genome of individual cells. In 1961 we (3) demonstrated that normal human fetal lung fibroblasts have a limited proliferative capacity of 50 $\pm$ 10 population doublings, a finding that has since been confirmed in many laboratories. This limited proliferative capacity, and the physiological decrements that precede it, have been interpreted by us to be the in vitro counterpart of those processes that occur as an organism ages (3-6). Support for this hypothesis has come from many different studies demonstrating such phenomena as 1) an inverse correlation between population doubling potential of cultured cells in vitro and donor age (4,7,8), 2) a possible direct correlation between mean maximun species lifespan and in vitro proliferative capacity (9-15), and 3) a limited proliferative capacity for normal cells serially transplanted in vivo in syngeneic hosts (16-19).

Theories of the mechanism of cellular senescence can be divided into two general classes. The first considers aging as a programmed genetic event, either as the expression of specific "aging genes" or as a final exhaustion of usable genetic information (4,5). The second regards senescence as the result of progressive and cumulative damage to organelles or errors in information containing molecules (20,21). One popular hypothesis

39

of progressive damage considers biological senescence as the result
of an "error catastrophe" caused by the gradual accumulation of
random errors in those proteins responsible for transcription
or translation (21-23). Such proteins, it is surmised, would
themselves produce molecules containing errors at an escalating
rate until a threshold was reached at which time cell function
would cease. Most of the theories in this latter class imply
that cytoplasmic events should play an important part in the
genesis of cellular senescence. If this were so, we postulate
that young cytoplasm should rejuvenate old cells by replacing
damaged components, or, conversely, old cytoplasm should accelerate
aging when introduced into young cells.

The formation of hybrid cells by virus fusion has been a
powerful tool for the study of mechanisms controlling phenotypic
expression and metabolic regulation in eukaryotic cells. The
classic method for the selection of heterokaryons is that of
Littlefield (24), in which parental cell populations lacking
different enzymes [e.g., hypoxanthine-guanine phosphoribosyltrans-
ferase$^{(-)}$ and thymidine kinase$^{(-)}$] are fused and then planted
in a selective medium requiring both enzymes for growth (e.g.,
HAT medium). We and others have described methods recently that
permit the production of mass populations of anucleate cytoplasms
(25-28). The fusion of anucleate cytoplasms, henceforth called
"cytoplasts", to whole cells should prove useful in elucidating
nucleo-cytoplasmic interactions, and many such experiments will
require the selective isolation of cytoplasmic hybrids. Clearly,
a cytoplast cannot contribute the genetic material necessary to
correct the usual type of heritable defect in its fusion partner,
thus the classic selective systems are unsuitable. We have,
therefore, developed a selective system that will allow for the
isolation of cytoplasmic hybrids between whole cells and cytoplasts
(29). We suggest the term "heteroplasmons" to distinguish cytoplasmic hybrids from whole cell hybrids (heterokaryons).

Recent experiments in which young and old whole cells have
been fused indicate that senescence may be dominant, since the
hybrids failed to multiply (30,31). However, such experiments
do not distinguish between nuclear and cytoplasmic control of
the event. The present study describes the techniques of enucleation and heteroplasmon isolation and their use in testing
the role of nuclear and cytoplasmic factors in in vitro cellular
senescence.

TECHNICAL PROCEDURES

A. Cells and Medium

The normal human diploid fibroblast cell strain WI-38, derived
from fetal lung and developed in our laboratory (4), was used

in these experiments. The medium employed for cell cultivation was Eagle's Basal Medium (BME) (32) supplemented with 10% calf serum, 50 µg/ml chlortetracycline and buffered to pH 7.4 with 28 µM Hepes buffer. Because of the difficulty in maintaining sterility throughout the enucleation procedures, the medium used for that purpose was also supplemented with 500 units/ml penicil-lin, 0.2 mg/ml streptomycin, and 2.5 µg/ml amphoterocin B for the three days following enucleation. In order to provide a richer medium for growth after the trauma of fusion and hybrid selection, the cells were cultured for the next five population doublings in BME containing 50% conditioned medium, 20% fetal calf serum, 50 µg/ml gentamycin, and twice the normal amount of Eagle's vita-mins, amino acids and glutamine. Following this, cultures were returned to the regular medium.

B. Reagents

Stock solutions of cytochalasin B (Aldrich Biochemical Co., Inc.), one mg/ml in DMSO, were prepared and diluted with medium to a final concentration of four µg/ml for enucleation. After each enucleation the cytochalasin solution was filtered through a sterile 0.22 µ millipore filter, and was reused five times before being discarded. Stock solutions of rotenone (Sigma Chemical Co.), 10 mg/ml in DMSO, were diluted one:1000 with BME for use. Stock solutions of iodoacetate (Sigma Chemical Co.), eight mg/ml (4×10^{-2} M) in sterile distilled water, were prepared weekly and diluted with BME to a final concentration of $3-9 \times 10^{-4}$ M.

C. Enucleation

Cells were enucleated using methods recently described by us (25-27), with the following modifications: 14 inch long glass "roller tubes" containing two inch X one inch glass cylinders were constructed as in Fig. 1a. A length of cotton string (boiled in four changes of distilled water) with glass beads at either end was placed between the inner cylinders and the outer tube. One end of the roller tube was closed with a silicon stopper, and the entire apparatus was autoclaved as a unit. A second sterile stopper was used to seal the tube after cells and medium had been added.

Two and one-half days before an enucleation, approximately 3×10^6 cells in 100 ml of BME were added to the roller tube. If the cells were incubated longer than 2-1/2 days, they tended to strip off during the subsequent centrifugation, thus resulting in a low yield of anucleate cytoplasms. If the incubation was less than 2-1/2 days, the anucleate cytoplasms tended to be highly resistant to trypsinization, thus also yielding an inadequate harvest. Two and one-half days (late afternoon of day one to

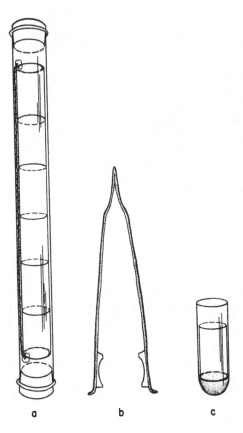

a   b   c

Figure 1. Materials for Cell Enucleation. (a) "Roller
tube" containing enucleation cylinders. (b) Special forceps for
aseptically transferring enucleation cylinders in and out of the
centrifuge tubes. (c) Enucleation cylinder resting on a plastic
hemisphere at the bottom of the centrifuge tube.

the morning of day three) was selected as the optimum time between
these opposing conditions.

The roller tube was rotated overnight at approximately three
rev/min and at 37°C in order to permit the cells to attach to
the inner surface of the small cylinders. Because of the constant
aeration caused by the trapping of air bubbles between the inner
cylinders and the outer tube, increasing amounts of unstable
serum-lipoproteins were precipitated as the tube rotated. In
order to avoid an unmanageable accumulation of this material,
on the following morning the roller tube was completely filled
with medium making further rotation unnecessary.

After 2-1/2 days the inner cylinders were transferred to
sterile cellulose nitrate tubes fitted with a polystyrene plug
that provided a flat surface upon which the cylinders rested (Fig.
1c). This transfer was accomplished by 1) raising the cylinders
to the mouth of the roller tube by pulling the glass bead-string
arrangements with a sterile hemostat, 2) grasping a cylinder with
the rounded surfaces of a specially constructed pair of sterile
forceps (Fig. 1b) (this surface provided a firm grip for manip-
ulating the cylinders), and 3) introducing the two inch cylinders
into the close-fitting centrifuge tubes.

Following a 30 min centrifugation at room temperature and
at $\geq$ 25,000 g in the presence of 4.0 µg/ml cytochalasin B, the
cylinders of anucleate cytoplasms were removed from the centrifuge
tubes and returned to new sterile roller tubes. This was accomplished by 1) tapping one edge of the polystyrene plug until a
space appeared between it and the bottom of the glass cylinder,
2) pulling upward on the cylinder with the bent tip of the special
forceps, 3) removing it entirely from the tube by grasping the
cylinder with the rounded surface of the forceps, and 4) introducing it into the new roller tube.

Approximately 99% of the cells enucleate under these conditions. The cytoplasts were then rotated for 3-1/2 hr in the
presence of 10 µg/ml mitomycin-C in order to render the few cells
that failed to enucleate incapable of further cell division (33).
The cytoplasts were then washed in 20 ml of BME and trypsinized.
It was necessary to use 10 ml of 0.25% trypsin in order to adequately cover the inner surface of the cylinders in the roller
tubes. After suspending the cytoplasts, this trypsin was neu-
tralized with three ml of calf serum. The cytoplasts were then
pelleted, washed once with cold BME, and finally resuspended in
cold BME. Because of their smaller size and absence of a nucleus,
it was assumed that cytoplasts would pellet more slowly than whole
cells. Centrifugation at 760 g for 20 min was arbitrarily selected
to insure adequate pelleting of the cytoplasts.

D. Fusion

Sendai virus, grown in the allantoic fluid of nine-day-old
chick embryos, was inactivated overnight in 0.05% β-propiolactone.
The concentrated virus (HA titer = 16,000) was stored for several
months at -70°C. Immediately before use, the virus was diluted
one:four in cold BME. The cell suspension to be fused was first
diluted with an equal volume of this virus preparation, then
incubated for 10 min in an ice bath, and finally incubated for
30 min in a 37°C water bath. Except for the initial mixing of

cells and virus, the cell suspension was not agitated. The fused cells were then gently aspirated in complete BME and planted in 25 cm^2 flasks (Falcon Plastics, Los Angeles). Heteroplasmons were prepared from all permutations of young and old cytoplasts and whole cells (young/young, old/old, young/old, and old/young). "Young" was defined as population doubling level 20-26, and "old" as population doubling level 49-60.

SELECTION OF HETEROPLASMONS

The fundamental approach in our development of the cytoplasm dependent selective system was to irreversibly inactivate a vital component(s) of the whole cell, then to rescue that cell by fusing it to a cytoplast containing the active component(s). Ideally, an irreversible inhibitor specific for a given enzyme should be used, so that general cellular metabolism would be disturbed as little as possible. Screening studies using ethidium bromide, potassium cyanide, rotenone and streptomycin indicated that these agents were not sufficiently irreversible to produce cell death if the agents were flushed away after a few hours' treatment. Consequently, it was decided to employ an agent that, while not specific for a given cellular component, produced a truly irreversible inactivation. Iodoacetate was chosen because it alkylates sulfhydryl groups and thus irreversibly inactivates a wide variety of enzymes. In order to minimize secondary degenerative effects, the iodoacetate treatment and subsequent BME washes were carried out at 0°-5°C so that the first time the treated cells were returned to physiologic temperatures was during the fusion procedure. A 30 min iodoacetate incubation was selected as a convenient and easily reproducible time of treatment. Under these conditions, 10^{-2} M iodoacetate was found to reliably kill 100% of WI-38 cells.

Preliminary experiments using radioactively labeled whole cells indicated that untreated cells could, in fact, rescue iodoacetate killed cells. ^{3}H-amino acid labeled cells were mixed with ^{14}C-amino acid labeled cells that had just been treated with iodoacetate and divided into two aliquots, one of which was fused with Sendai virus. The ratio of ^{14}C to ^{3}H was significantly greater 24 hr later in those aliquots that were fused, thus indicating an increased survival of the fused ^{14}C-iodoacetate treated cells. However, no rescue was observed when cytoplasts were fused to treated cells. One explanation for this is that enough nuclear enzymes had been inactivated to be lethal, independent of cytoplasmic events, so that only replacing cytoplasmic enzymes would not be sufficient to rescue the cell.

In the early screening experiments, it had been determined that a 24 hr treatment with 10 µg/ml (2.5 X 10^{-5} M) rotenone (an inhibitor of oxidative metabolism) was not lethal to WI-38 cells.

Cells sublethally treated with iodoacetate would, by definition, have enough nuclear enzymes to survive. It was hypothesized that such cells would be much more sensitive to the effects of rotenone than normal cells because of the iodoacetate inactivation of alternate metabolic pathways. It might then be possible to rescue these cells with cytoplasts containing the active enzymes necessary for the alternate pathways.

Cells treated sublethally with iodoacetate were, in fact, found to be much more sensitive to the effects of rotenone. However, in order for the combined treatments to produce 100% killing, the "sublethal" dose of iodoacetate produced approximately 99% killing by itself. Nonetheless, the use of rotenone permitted the concentration of iodoacetate to be decreased by more than an order of magnitude. Under these conditions, cytoplasts were able to rescue iodoacetate treated whole cells (29).

The specific method is as follows: Approximately 3×10^7 cells were trypsinized, pelleted for 10 min at 750 g at 5°C and resuspended in 10 ml of cold BME. Enough of the iodoacetate stock solution was added to yield a final concentration of $3-9 \times 10^{-4}$ M, and the cells were incubated in an ice bath for 30 min. The cells were then pelleted, the supernatant fluid decanted, and the last few drops removed with a Pasteur pipette. Following this, the cells were washed in 10 ml of cold BME, and resuspended in a final volume of 0.4 ml cold BME. Approximately 10^7 mitomycin-C treated anucleate cytoplasms were trypsinized, pelleted, given a cold BME wash to remove traces of serum and trypsin, and resuspended in a final volume of 0.3 ml.

In order to determine if rescue had occurred, the number of cells surviving when cytoplasts and treated cells were mixed and fused was compared to the number surviving when they were only mixed. However, treatment with Sendai virus is a relatively traumatic procedure that can kill a large percentage of previously stressed cells. Thus, the dose of iodoacetate that produces 100% killing with Sendai virus and a subsequent rotenone treatment may not produce a 100% killing if the virus step is eliminated. In order to make the controls truly comparable to the experimental group, the following protocol was adopted (Fig. 2):

The "fusion" consisted of 0.1 ml of the treated cells and 0.1 ml of the cytoplasts mixed in a single tube. The "mixture" consisted of 0.1 ml of the treated cells and 0.1 ml of the cytoplasts in separate tubes. Each was treated separately with Sendai virus, then washed with two ml of BME. Only after the supernatants were discarded were the tubes combined. Because of a concern that there might be some fusion between whole cells and cytoplasts even after the virus was washed away, in some of the later

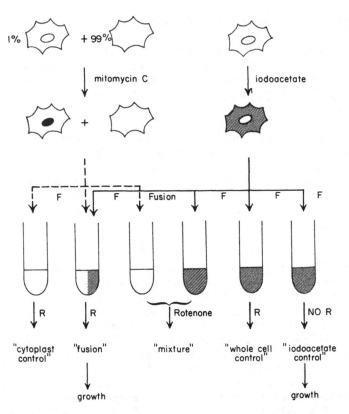

Figure 2.   Experimental Protocol.   The cytoplast control
defines the "background survival" of cells that failed to enucleate, and verifies that they had been rendered unable to divide
by treatment with mitomycin-C.   The whole cell control verifies
adequate killing of the whole cells by iodoacetate.   The iodoacetate control shows the behavior of cells subjected to all the
experimental manipulations except the final killing by rotenone.
The difference in cell density and subsequent growth between the
"fusion" and the "mixture" are the criteria for identifying rescue
of treated cells by untreated cytoplasts.

experiments the cytoplast portion of the "mixture" was not treated
with Sendai virus.   However, there is no evidence indicating that
this precaution was actually necessary.   One drawback of this
modification is that fewer of the mitomycin-C treated cells that
failed to enucleate are killed.   Thus, a greater number of cells
in the "mixture" attach, and the difference in cell density between
the "mixture" and the "fusion" is minimized.

The "whole cell control" contained 0.1 ml of the treated cells alone and the "iodoacetate control" also contained 0.1 ml of the treated cells. This aliquot was not treated with rotenone, thus some of the cells would survive and they could be cultured to assess the effects of the iodoacetate treatment on cell division. Finally, the "cytoplast control" contained 0.1 ml of the cytoplasts alone. All aliquots were diluted 1:2 with a Sendai virus preparation (HA titer of 4000) and incubated in an ice bath for 10 min, then transferred to a 37°C water bath for 30 min. The cells were then planted in BME containing 10 µg/ml rotenone, and the "iodoacetate control" was planted in rotenone-free medium.

Under these conditions, approximately 0.2% of the cytoplasts were able to rescue whole cells. All of the above aliquots were initially cultivated in 25 cm^2 flasks (Falcon Plastics) in order to accomodate the huge excess (> 99%) of cells that were in the process of drying. However, the density of the surviving cells was then much too low to expect significant cell division. Approximately 24 hr after fusion the cells were washed twice with BME, fed with rotenone-free medium, and given one day to recover from these treatments. The cells were then trypsinized, counted, pelleted, and planted in microtiter dishes (Falcon Plastics) with a surface area of only 0.25 cm^2.

Fig. 3 shows the appearance of a typical experiment the day following planting in the microtiter dishes or three days after fusion. The "cytoplast control" (Fig. 3e) illustrates the "background" survival of cells that failed to enucleate, but that had been rendered unable to divide by mitomycin-C. The whole cell control (Fig. 3c) demonstrates the complete killing of the iodoacetate-rotenone treated cells. If the rotenone treatment is eliminated, as in the "iodoacetate control," there is incomplete killing of the cells (Fig. 3d). Even though approximately 99% of the cells have been killed, the cells appear relatively dense since the microtiter dishes have < one percent of the surface area originally covered by these cells. The "mixture" (Fig. 3b) clearly has many fewer cells than the "fusion" (Fig. 3a). This difference in cell density represents the rescue of iodoacetate treated cells by untreated cytoplasts.

Once in the microtiter dishes, the cell densities were scored by comparison to photographs of standard subcultivations at serial two-fold dilutions. In 37 of 41 successful experiments, the "fusion" was at least twice as dense as the "mixture." The cells were then fed twice weekly, and subcultivated at a one:two split ratio when confluent. The cultures were transferred to successively larger vessels until they filled a 75 cm^2 flask (Falcon Plastics), and then were subcultivated at a 1:4 split ratio. While in the microtiter dishes the cells were subcultivated by

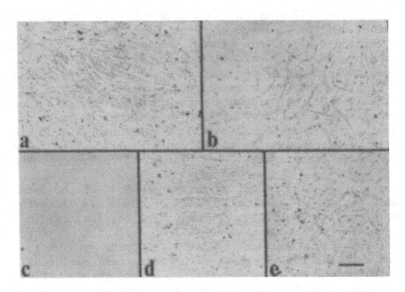

Figure 3. Rescue of Iodoacetate-Rotenone Treated Cells by Fusion to Cytoplasts. Whole cells were treated with 9 X 10^{-4} M iodoacetate for 30 min at 0°-5°C. (a) "Fusion", (b) "mixture", (c) whole cell control, (d) iodoacetate control, (e) cytoplast control. See Figure 2 for definition of these terms. Bar indicates 200 μ.

aspirating the trypsinized cells with a 20 gauge needle. Cells were transferred from one to two and then to four wells in the microtiter dishes. All four wells were then transferred to one 16 mm well of a multi-dish disposo-tray (Linbro Chemical Co., Inc.), then to two and then to four wells. All four wells were then transferred to a 25 cm² flask (Falcon Plastics), and from there to a 75 cm² flask. Since WI-38 cells have a limited proliferative capacity of approximately 50 population doublings, at which time Phase III is reached and the culture deteriorated (3,4), the cultures of heteroplasmons were subcultivated until Phase III.

The "mixture" is by far the most important control, since its failure to multiply simultaneously controls for 1) insufficient iodoacetate killing of the whole cells, 2) insufficient mitomycin-C inactivation of cells that failed to enucleate and 3) any non-specific metabolic rescue that could occur by co-cultivating cytoplasts with iodoacetate treated cells. In many experiments where insufficient cells or cytoplasts were available, the "cytoplast" or "iodoacetate" controls were eliminated.

Experiments were discarded if they met any of the following
criteria: 1) The cells in the "mixture" divided. Clearly, if
the "mixture" grows, cell growth in the "fusion" cannot be interpreted to be due to rescue of iodoacetate treated cells. 2)
An initial cell density in the "fusion" of less than a one:eight
subcultivation ratio. If those cells failed to grow, it could
easily be secondary to density considerations rather than failure
of rescue. 3) The presence of greater than two cells on a high
power search of the entire surface area of the "whole cell control." It was felt that even if the "mixture" did not grow, the
potential of non-fused cells to multiply and take over a culture
was too great to consider an experiment valid if more than a very
few iodoacetate-rotenone treated cells survived. This is to be
compared to an average of approximately 10,000 cells in a typical
"fusion" aliquot.

One purpose of this study was to develop an effective system
for the selection of hybrids between cytoplasts and whole cells.
Only a few common biochemicals were investigated for their ability
to induce an irreversible biochemical lesion that could be overcome
by the addition of fresh, untreated cytoplasm. Once a suitable
agent, iodoacetate, was found, it was used to demonstrate the
feasibility of this approach. An agent with such a non-specific
action as iodoacetate will clearly be of limited usefulness in
many experiments where the biochemical interactions in newly formed
hybrids are to be studied. However, it should prove valuable
in studies of the long-term behavior of hybrid cells, after the
biochemical disturbances of the selection system have stabilized.
Given the almost endless variety of enzyme inhibitors currently
available it should also be possible to tailor selection systems
to the demands of a specific experiment.

Although a completely irreversible specific enzyme inhibitor
is perhaps the most elegant candidate for a biochemical lesion
selection system, there is a wide range of alternate approaches
that may serve as well. For example, even though ethidium bromide
was not sufficiently irreversible to kill cells after a short
treatment, a 24 hr treatment produced enough damage to kill most
of the non-hybrid cells, thus permitting its use as a partially
selective agent (29). Any treatment that has a relatively sharp
time-dependence could be used as a selective system. For example,
if cells could survive four days of treatment but not five, fusion
to untreated cells after four days followed by an additional day
or two of treatment should effectively select for the hybrid cells,
since they would be the only cells receiving replacement in the
form of normal cytoplasm for those substances exhausted by the
prior exposure to the selective agent. Under these conditions

the "agent" could potentially be any lethal stress, from metabolic poisons to vitamin or nutritional deprivations.

The use of iodoacetate provides a system that permits the selection of heteroplasmons between cytoplasts and whole cells of any cell type. Once a second such selective system becomes available it should be possible to select for heterokaryons between any two kinds of whole cells and this will greatly expand the range of questions that can be answered by mammalian hybridization techniques.

HETEROPLASMONS DISPLAY NUCLEAR CONTROL OF IN VITRO AGING

The behavior of the iodoacetate control (young cells treated with iodoacetate but not rotenone and thus able to survive) provides an important baseline for interpreting the behavior of the heteroplasmons. This control not only expresses the effect of iodoacetate on the lifespan of the cells, but also the effect of all the manipulations and trauma experienced by the cell cultures during these experiments. The number of population doublings following treatment for 12 iodoacetate controls is shown in Fig. 4. In four experiments (33%) the cultures were so traumatized that they failed to return to log-phase growth. The average number of subsequent population doublings of the remaining eight cultures was $25 \pm$ six ($\pm$ one standard deviation). Parallel cultures subcultivated under routine conditions without any unusual manipulations traversed $29 \pm$ three subsequent population doublings. This decrease in the total proliferative capacity of four population doublings and the failure of 1/3 of the cultures to grow at all, provide baseline data resulting from the conditions of the experiment.

Even in the cultures that grew, the experimental trauma may have caused the majority of cells to be unable to divide. Those cells that did divide would then have to undergo many more population doublings in order for the culture to become confluent. Thus the difference between the iodoacetate control (or the heteroplasmons) and the routine cultures would be much less in terms of actual cell divisions than the difference in terms of population doublings.

Hybrids between young cytoplasts and young cells behaved similarly to the iodoacetate controls (Fig. 4). A wide range of iodoacetate concentrations was employed in these experiments (29), and whereas 80% of the young/ young cytoplasmic hybrids failed to grow at an iodoacetate concentration of 9×10^{-4} M, only 40% failed to grow at lower doses ($3-7 \times 10^{-4}$ M). The iodoacetate controls described above were in this latter dosage range. The young/young hybrid failure rate of 40% is not suf-

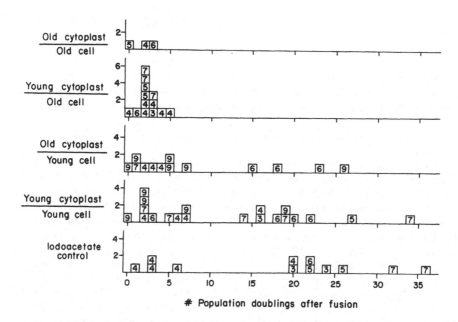

Figure 4. Passage Levels Following Cytoplasmic Hybridization. (a) Old cytoplasts fused to old cells. (b) Young cytoplasts fused to old cells. (c) Old cytoplasts fused to young cells. (d) Young cytoplasts fused to young cells. (e) Young iodoacetate controls. Each square represents one experiment. The number in each square indicates the concentration of iodoacetate (X 10^{-4} M) used in that experiment.

ficiently different from the 33% rate of the controls to be statistically significant. Furthermore, the average subsequent number of population doublings in the 10 young/young experiments that grew, 20 ± six, is comparable to the iodoacetate controls. Hybrids between old cytoplasts and young cells behaved similarly (Fig. 4). Of the four experiments in which the cells grew, the average subsequent proliferative capacity was 20 ± five population doublings. Fifty-seven percent (four of seven) of the lower-dose experiments failed to return to log-phase growth, compared with values of 33% for the iodoacetate control or 44% for young/young hybrids. Although the old cytoplast/young cell failure rate is somewhat higher than control values, it is not statistically significant (p >> .05). Furthermore, since old cells probably have an increased sensitivity to trauma, one might expect a greater proportion of experiments involving old whole cells or cytoplasts to exceed the traumatic threshold from which cells are unable to recover. Although this would be a result of decreased overall

functioning in old cells it would not be a unique manifestation
of aging processes.

In no case did young cytoplast/old cell or old cytoplast/old
cell hybrids grow significantly (Figs. 4a and 4b). This may
represent either a 100% failure rate of a proliferative capacity
insufficient to allow significant subsequent cell multiplication.

ANALYSIS OF NUCLEAR CONTROL OF CELL AGING IN VITRO

In analyzing the results of these experiments it is important
to recognize that possibilities for artifact exist. For example,
if a significant number of young cells managed to survive the
iodoacetate-rotenone treatments, they could potentially overgrow
the culture. It is for this reason that we have discarded any
experiments involving young cells in which the whole cell control
indicated more than $2 \times 10^{-5}\%$ survival. It is also possible
that cytoplasts could rescue treated cells by a form of metabolic
cooperation without any actual cell fusion. This was the rationale
for including the "mixture control" and discarding any experiments
in which the "mixture" grew. However, it might be argued that
this procedure biased the results. We can assume that there is
an element of randomness in the trauma sustained by the "mixture"
and the "fusion." Experiments in which the "mixture" grew but
the "fusion" did not would have been discarded, but not the reverse, thus biasing the results in favor of "fusions" that grew.
Thus, an old cytoplast/young cell experiment that should have
been discarded because of inadequate young cell killing might
have been mistakenly included because the failure of the "mixture"
to grow may have been a random event. By this assumption there
should be a significant number of experiments in which the "mixture" grew but the "fusion" did not. However, this did not occur
in any of the 18 experiments in which the "fusion" failed to grow.
This is to be compared to the "fusion" growing in 18 of the 36
experiments in which the "mixture" failed to grow.

Even the "mixture" control may not be completely adequate.
It is necessary to be extremely critical in the definition of
what is truly a lethal dose to induce biochemical lesions, since
a small variation in the total stress to which a cell is exposed
can make a significant difference in cell survival. For example,
many cell types are stressed at low population densities. Thus,
the dose that just produces total killing in a "control" aliquot
where the final cell density is zero will almost certainly be
less than that necessary to produce total killing in the presence
of significant numbers of viable cells. This consideration is
particularly important if one wishes to use this type of selection
system in conjunction with a HAT medium-type system for the hybridization of whole cells. We have fused iodoacetate-killed

WI-38 cells with Lesch-Nyhan cells (cells deficient in hypoxanthine-guanine phosphoribosyltransferase) followed by cultivation in HAT medium. Since it takes several weeks for Lesch-Nyhan cells to die in HAT medium, the cell density was initially high in both the "mixture" and the "fusion" aliquots. In three of three experiments where "whole cell control" aliquots of the iodoacetate treated cells showed total killing, both the "mixture" and the "fusion" grew, and karyotyping proved the growing cells to be diploid. Thus there had, in fact, been only partial killing of the iodoacetate treated cells in those aliquots not exposed to the additional stress of low population densities. The surviving cells then multiplied and overgrew the cultures. In the experiments reported here we avoided this problem by initially planting all aliquots at low densities so that the number of surviving cells was approximately equal to a one:200 split ratio. Two days later, after the non-fused cells had died, the cultures were replanted at a cell density compatible with growth. However, this approach does not fully determine the cell density in the immediate environment of the individual cell. Since Sendai virus agglutinates cells, it is possible that some iodoacetate treated cells were non-specifically rescued by agglutination to untreated cytoplasts. This would occur only in the "fusion", and thus the "mixture" might not adequately control for this spurious survival of iodoacetate treated cells. Since > 99.5% of the cells and cytoplasts do not survive (29), in order to achieve a surviving density of one:200 it was necessary to add sufficient numbers of cells and cytoplasts to form a confluent layer of dying cells over the bottom of the flask. Thus, there was ample opportunity for adequate whole cell-cytoplast contact even in the "mixture". Although this reduces the possibility for this type of artifact, it clearly does not rule it out.

Because of the absence of adequate cytoplasmic markers, we have been unable to rigorously confirm the hybrid nature of the "fusion" cultures that grew. The evidence that they are truly hybrid is the indirect evidence of increased initial cell survival and subsequent growth in the "fusion" and not in the "mixture." Although we consider the occurrence of these artifacts unlikely, in the absence of direct evidence for the hybrid nature of the "fusion" cultures the possibility of misinterpretation cannot be completely ruled out.

Assuming that our interpretaion is correct, we can draw the following conclusions: If in vitro cell senescence is due to the accumulation of dominant cytoplasmic malfunctions that ultimately cause cell death, then old cytoplasts fused to young cells should cause those cells to undergo fewer population doublings (accelerated aging). The fact that four such cultures grew just as well as young/young cytoplasmic hybrids argues against

this possibility. The number of successful experiments is too
small and the variability too great to allow any conclusions
concerning subtle influences of the effect of old cytoplasm on
the lifespan of young cells. A difference in proliferative capacity of a few population doublings could not be detected in
these experiments. Also, the amount of cytoplasm just necessary
to rescue an iodoacetate treated cell might be less than that
needed to express a cytoplasmic senescence factor.

If in vitro cell senescence is due to a progressive loss
of cytoplasmic function or components, it should be possible to
rejuvenate old cells by replacement with components from young
cytoplasts. In no case was this result obtained. It is always
possible, however, that the failure of any young cytoplast/old
cell hybrids to proliferate is due to non-specific causes. Old
cells might simply be more subject to the trauma of the experimental manipulations, sustaining so much damage that even young
cytoplasm cannot reverse these decrements.

It should be noted that cytoplasts are surrounded by plasma
membranes from the donor cell. Thus, the results of these experiments apply as well to any age related changes in the plasma
membrane.

Our interpretation of these results, therefore, does not
argue in favor of theories of cellular aging which include 1)
accumulation of errors in cytoplasmic macromolecules or 2) degeneration of cytoplasmic organelles. The failure of cytoplasmic
hybridizations to alter the lifespan of young or old cells suggests
that the control of in vitro cellular senescence resides in the
nucleus. Our results, therefore, favor the hypothesis that the
limited proliferative capacity of cultured normal human fibroblasts
is an expression of programmed genetic events.

ACKNOWLEDGEMENTS

We thank Eva Pfendt and Aida Zerrudo for their excellent
technical assistance.

This study was supported, in part, by research grant HD 04004
from the National Institute of Child Health and Human Development,
by contract NIH 69-2053 within the Special Virus Cancer Program
of the National Cancer Institute, and by Medical Scientist Training
Grant No. GM 1922 from the National Institute of General Medical
Sciences, NIH, Bethesda, Maryland.

REFERENCES

1.   Ebeling, A. H. J. Exp. Med. 102:595 (1955).

2.   Parker, R. C. In: Methods of Tissue Culture. Harper and
     Row, New York. (1961).
3.   Hayflick, L. and P. S. Moorhead. Exp. Cell Res. 25:585
     (1961).
4.   Hayflick, L. Exp. Cell Res. 37:614 (1965).
5.   Hayflick, L. Exp. Gerontol. 5:291 (1970).
6.   Hayflick, L. In: Aging and Development. (Eds.) H. Bredt
     and J. W. Rohen. Academy of Science and Literature, Mainz,
     Germany, F. K. Schattauer Verlag, Stuttgart (1972) Band 4,
     p. 1.
7.   Goldstein, S., J. W. Littlefield, and J. S. Soeldner. Proc.
     Nat. Acad. Sci. USA 64:155 (1969).
8.   Martin, G. M., C. A. Sprague, and C. J. Epstein. Lab. Invest.
     23:86 (1970).
9.   Goldstein, S. Exp. Cell Res. 83:297 (1974).
10. Hay, R. J. and B. L. Strehler. Exp. Gerontol. 2:123 (1967).
11. Hayflick, L. J. Amer. Geriatric Soc. 22:1 (1974).
12. Hayflick, L. In: Theoretical Aspects of Aging. (Ed.)
     M. Rockstein, Academic Press, New York (1974) p. 83.
13. Ponten, J. Int. J. Cancer 6:323 (1970).
14. Simons, J. W. I. M. In: Aging in Cell and Tissue Culture.
     (Eds.) E. Holeckova and V. J. Cristofalo, Plenum Press, New
     York (1970) p. 25.
15. Todaro, G. J., and H. Green. J. Cell Biol. 17:299 (1963).
16. Daniel, C. W., K. B. DeOme, J. T. Young, P. B. Blair, and
     L. J. Faulkin, Jr. Proc. Nat. Acad. Sci. USA 61:53 (1968).
17. Krohn, P. L. Proc. Roy. Soc. (London) B 157:128 (1962).
18. Siminovitch, L., J. E. Till, and E. A. McCulloch. J. Cell
     Comp. Physiol. 64:23 (1964).
19. Williamson, A. R., and B. A. Askonas. Nature 238:337 (1972).
20. Harmon, D. J. Geront. 23:476 (1968).
21. Orgel, L. E. Proc. Nat. Acad. Sci. USA 49:517 (1963).
22. Holliday, R. Nature 221:1224 (1969).
23. Orgel, L. E. Nature 243:141 (1973).
24. Littlefield, J. W. Science 135:709 (1964).
25. Wright, W. E. and L. Hayflick. Exp. Cell Res. 74:187 (1972).
26. Wright, W. E. In: Methods in Cell Biology. (Ed.) D. Prescott,
     Academic Press, New York (1973) Vol. VII, p. 203.
27. Wright, W. E. and L. Hayflick. Proc. Soc. Exp. Biol. Med.
     144:587 (1973).
28. Prescott, D., D. Myerson, and J. Wallace. Exp. Cell Res. 71:
     480 (1972).
29. Wright, W. E. and L. Hayflick. Proc. Nat. Acad. Sci. USA.
     In press.
30. Littlefield, J. W. J. Cell Physiol. 82:129 (1973).
31. Norwood, T. H., W. R. Pendergrass, C. A. Sprague, and G.
     M. Martin. Fed. Proc. 33:603 (1974).
32. Eagle, M. J. Exp. MEd. 102:595 (1955).
33. Studzinski, G. P. and L. S. Cohen. Biochem. Biophys. Res.
     Commun. 23:506 (1966).

HYDROCORTISONE AS A MODULATOR OF CELL DIVISION AND POPULATION LIFE SPAN

Vincent J. Cristofalo

The Wistar Institute of Anatomy and Biology
36th Street at Spruce
Philadelphia, Pennsylvania 19104

INTRODUCTION

Previous work in our laboratory on acid phosphatase and β glucuronidase activities in crude homogenates of human diploid cell cultures showed an increase in the specific activity of these enzymes during cellular aging (1). Since these enzymes are typically marker enzymes for lysosomes, the findings implied that older cells contained more lysosomes, a conclusion that has since been documented by electron microscopic studies in our lab and by others (2-4).

Spurred by these findings, we initiated a series of experiments designed to further our understanding of the role of lysosomes in cellular aging in vitro. These included studies to determine the subcellular distribution of lysosomal enzymes, the fraction of enzyme activity that was membrane bound, and the action of a known lysosome stabilizer, hydrocortisone, on both these parameters (5,6).

Although hydrocortisone (cortisol), at a concentration of 5 μg/ml, did retard leakage of acid phosphatase from crude lysosomal preparations (7), the most striking result of these studies was the increase in life span of the cultures in the presence of 5 μg/ml hydrocortisone (14 μM) (6-8). Macieira-Coelho (9) reported a similar finding for human cells treated with cortisone.

This hydrocortisone effect on cell life span represents the action of a chemically defined modulator of cell division and population life span and we have further documented these observations in the hope of using hydrocortisone as a probe for modu-

lating the regulation of cell division and the limitation of
proliferative capacity of these diploid cell cultures (6-8,10).

As a result of our preliminary studies, the principal features
of the hydrocortisone effect can be summarized as follows: 1)
Replicate experiments based on cell counts have shown that the
life span in terms of actual population doublings was extended
30-40% by the continuous inclusion of 5 μg/ml hydrocortisone in
the medium; 2) This effect seemed to be maximal with 5 μg/ml
hydrocortisone; 3) There is no rejuvenation with the hormone,
i.e. once a culture could no longer achieve confluency, hydrocortisone would not reverse this condition; 4) If hydrocortisone
was added at different periods in the life span, the magnitude
of the extension of life span was in direct proportion to the
amount of time the culture was grown in the presence of the hormone; 5) The saturation density of the culture was increased in
the presence of the hormone; 6) The overall effect on proliferative capacity was not due to increased plating efficiency or
an increased fraction of the cells adhering to the glass or plastic
surface.

MATERIALS AND METHODS

Except where noted, all studies were done with human diploid
cell lines WI-38 and WI-26 (11,12). These were obtained either
from frozen stock maintained here at the Wistar Institute or from
Dr. Leonard Hayflick of Stanford University.

The cells were grown as previously described (13) in auto-
clavable Eagle's MEM (Auto-Pow, Flow Laboratories, Rockville,
Md.) modified by the addition of Eagle's BME vitamins. Immediately
before use, the medium was supplemented with L glutamine (2 mM),
$NaHCO_3$ (20 mM) and fetal calf serum (10% v/v). In the earlier
experiments, aureomycin (50 μg/ml) was included in the formulation. In subsequent experiments, no antibiotics were used.
Cultures were grown at 37°C in an atmosphere of 5% CO_2-95% air,
and were monitored for mycoplasma by the method of Levine (14).

Routine subcultivations were carried out when monolayers
were confluent. Briefly, the cells were released from the glass
by treatment with trypsin (0.25%) in Ca^{++}- and Mg^{++}-free phosphate
buffered saline solution. After suspension in medium containing
10% fetal calf serum, the cells were counted and inoculated into
appropriate vessels at a density of 1 X 10^4 cells/cm^2.

Cell population doublings were calculated by comparing the
cell counts/ vessel at seeding and when the cultures reached
confluency. All cell counts were done electronically using a
Coulter Counter.

Autoradiography was carried out by our standard procedures (13). In brief, cells were seeded at a density of 1-1.3 X 10^4 cells/cm^2 either in 60 mm Petri dishes containing 11 X 22 mm coverslips, or in 2-chamber Lab-Tek dishes (Labtech, Inc., Westmont, Ill.) and incubated as described above. Twenty-four hr after seeding, 3H-dT was added to the cultures to a final concentration of 0.1 µCi/ml (spec. act. 2 Ci/mMole). At appropriate time intervals (24-30 hr), the cell monolayers were washed rapidly in a cold buffered balanced salt solution, fixed in Carnoy's solution, hydrated through an alcohol series and air dried overnight. The slides were then dipped in emulsion (Kodak NTB-2). Following the exposure period (4 days), the slides were developed (Kodak D-19 developer, 5 min), fixed (Kodak acid fixer, 5 min), stained lightly with Harris hematoxylin, rinsed in cold running water, and air dried.

The autoradiographs were analyzed microscopically by scoring the percentage of cells with labeled nuclei (5 silver grains or more) in random fields throughout the coverslips. At least 400 cells were counted on each coverslip and all coverslips were prepared in duplicate.

For liquid scintillation counting, coverslips were prepared as for autoradiography, removed at appropriate intervals, dipped in cold 10% trichloroacetic acid and placed directly into scintillation vials and counted in an Intertechnique Liquid Scintillation Spectrometer.

For studies of thymidine kinase activity (ATP: thymidine-5'-phosphotransferase EC 2.7.1.21), WI-38 cells were seeded at a density of 1 X 10^4 cells/cm^2 (13); at appropriate intervals after seeding, the cultures were harvested, washed and suspended in 0.05 M Tris buffer containing 0.01 M dithiothreitol. The cell suspension was sonicated (Branson sonicator 0-4°C), cell debris was removed by low speed centrifugation and the supernatant was assayed immediately according to a method described by Bello (15). The assay depends on measuring the rate of phosphorylation of ^{14}C-dT by adsorbing the phosphorylated product of the reaction to DEAE cellulose. The reaction mixture contained in a final volume of 0.25 ml, 1.5 µmoles dithiothreitol, 0.1 mg BSA, 7 nmoles of ^{14}C-dT (2 X 10^6 cpm/µmole) and 0.02-0.08 ml extract. For all studies, assays were carried out at several concentrations of cell extract and the initial velocity of the reaction was always proportional to the amount of extract used.

For evaluation of the effect of various steroids on DNA synthesis, the hormones were purchased from commercial suppliers at the best grade of purity available. Active hormones were also checked for the presence of impurities by standard thin-layer chromatography. For autoradiographic analysis of their biological activity, the conditions used were identical to those described above. All hormones were used at a concentration of 5 μg/ml. Where solubility was limiting, the hormones were dissolved in 100% ethanol. Subsequent dilution was carried out in medium to give a final concentration of ethanol of no more than 0.5%. Paired controls were always run with an identical concentration of ethanol in the medium. For all active hormones the change in the labeling index was correlated with direct cell counts.

DNA was determined chemically by the method of Volkin and Cohn (16).

RESULTS

Thymidine Metabolism. Initially, our studies were designed to determine how the effect of hydrocortisone in extending the life span of a culture was expressed during a single population growth cycle. Figure 1 shows the results of a typical growth curve in which cell number, DNA synthesis determined chemically, and radioactivity incorporated into DNA from ^{3}H-dT were monitored for hydrocortisone-treated and control cells. The zero time point on the figure represents 24 hr after both cultures were seeded with identical numbers of cells. During the growth cycle, the curves diverged and by 72 hr, there was a clear and consistent difference between the treated and control cultures. The DNA content of the culture followed the same pattern with the hormone-treated cultures having a higher rate of DNA synthesis. Finally, the kinetics of radioactivity incorporated into DNA from the ^{3}H-dT precursor paralleled the rate of synthesis of DNA. Thus, ^{3}H-dT would seem to be an appropriate probe to follow the hydrocortisone effect on cell proliferation.

We then extended these studies to evaluate the effect of hydrocortisone on thymidine metabolism. To be incorporated, thymidine must be taken up and phosphorylated to the triphosphate before incorporation into DNA. Our autoradiographic studies were carried out at a dT concentration of 5 X 10^{-8} M and at this level, it is probably actively transported into the cell (17).

Figure 2 shows the total cellular uptake of ^{3}H-dT and the incorporation into acid insoluble material for young cells. Essentially, all the ^{3}H-dT taken up at this concentration was incorporated into acid insoluble material. The pool was very small and hydrocortisone had essentially no effect on the uptake or incorporation. Note that in the absence of cell division (0.1% fetal calf serum) very little thymidine was transported and essentially none was incorporated.

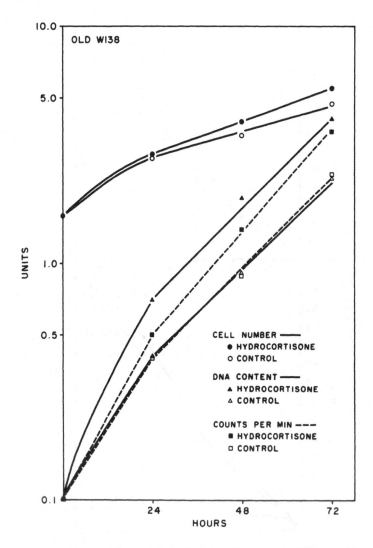

Figure 1.   The effect of hydrocortisone on DNA synthesis and
cell division in WI-38 cells.

Figure 3 shows a similar experimental series for old cells.
Although both uptake and incorporation are much lower here, essentially the same results are evident. Here again, in the presence of cytosyl arabinoside (11 µg/ml) which inhibits cell division
by at least 90%, there was essentially no uptake or incorporation.
Apparently in WI-38 cells, as with other systems (18) thymidine
at 5 X 10^{-8} M is only transported in cells that are synthesizing
DNA.

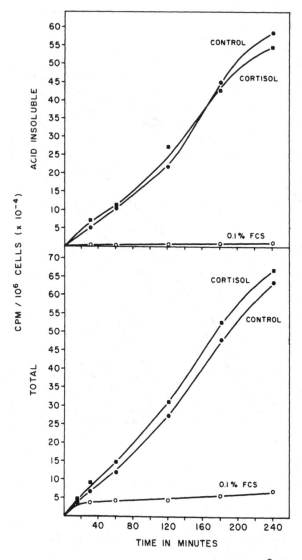

Figure 2.   The effect of hydrocortisone on ^{3}H–dT uptake and incorporation in young cultures of WI–38 cells (FCS = fetal calf serum).

Thymidine uptake is heavily dependent on thymidine phosphorylation which probably traps the thymidine and at the same time may regulate the activity of the thymidine kinase (17,18).   Thus, the characteristics of thymidine kinase and the responsiveness

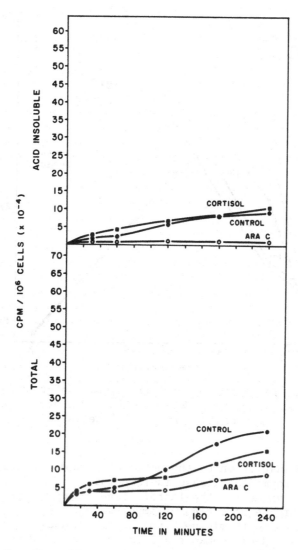

Figure 3. The effect of hydrocortisone on ^{3}H–dT uptake and incorporation by old cultures of WI-38 cells. (Ara C = cytosyl arabinoside, 11 µg/ml).

of this enzyme to hydrocortisone were relevant to these studies. Of additional interest was the fact that thymidine kinase is representative of a class of enzymes involved in DNA synthesis that, like DNA, appear to be synthesized only periodically during the cell cycle. A variety of studies with synchronized, permanently proliferating cell lines has indicated that the synthesis of these enzymes begins just prior to the onset of DNA synthesis

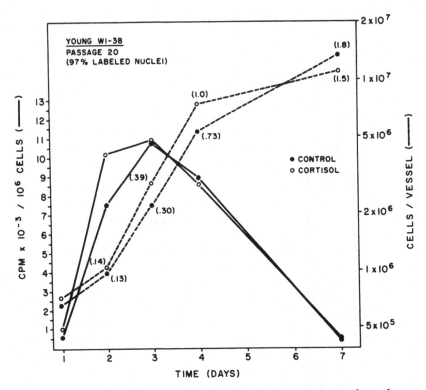

Figure 4. The effect of hydrocortisone on growth and thymidine kinase activity in WI-38 cells. Numbers in parentheses represent cell densities in units of 10^5 cells/cm^2.

and concludes just prior to the onset of mitosis (15,19). Since regulation of thymidine kinase is temporally related to the regulation of DNA synthesis, the factors regulating the synthesis of thymidine kinase were also of importance to our studies. Our observations on thymidine kinase activity during the growth cycle of young and old human cells are summarized below.

Figure 4 shows the fluctuations in dT kinase activity during a single growth cycle of a young, randomly growing population of WI-38 cells. By autoradiographic analysis, almost 100% of the cells were synthesizing DNA. Growth was constant and logarithmic during days 2-4 after which the effects of density dependent inhibition of cell division were apparent in a reduced proliferation rate at a cell density of about 1 X 10^5 cells/cm^2.

As mentioned previously in studies with synchronized cultures of permanently proliferating cell lines, it appears that dT kinase is synthesized just prior to DNA synthesis (15). Our data with

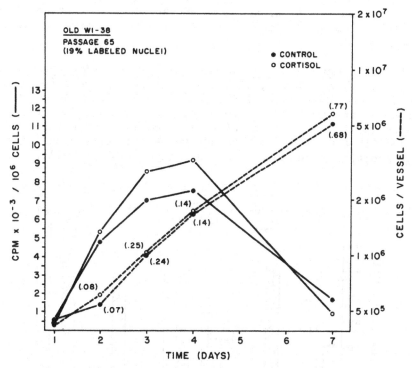

Figure 5. The effect of hydrocortisone on growth and thymidine kinase activity in WI-38 cells. Numbers in parentheses
represent cell densities in units of 10^5 cells/cm^2.

these randomly growing diploid cultures appear to be consistent
with this interpretation.

Figure 5 shows a similar study carried out on an old culture.
Here, by autoradiographic analysis, about 80% of the cells are
unable to synthesize DNA during the period of the experiment.
The reduced growth rate is evidenced by the fact that after 7
days, the cells had still not reached saturation density. The
periodicity of enzyme fluctuation is approximately the same,
however, with the possibility of a slight shift to the right in
the timing of maximum activity. Again, only slight differences
are seen between hydrocortisone-treated and control cultures.
Of significance, however, is the fact that enzyme activity begins
to decline well before the limits imposed on proliferation by
saturation density are reached. In addition, although only about
20% of the cells in the population are in the proliferating pool
(compared to nearly 100% in the young population), the specific
activity of the enzyme is reduced by only 30-50%. This shows
that the decline in labeling index in old cultures is not due

simply to a loss of dT kinase and further suggests that possibly
some cells which are incapable of division still carry out periodic
synthesis of dT kinase.

Hydrocortisone and the Size of the Proliferating Pool of
Cells. The above studies, although establishing the effects of
hydrocortisone directly on DNA synthesis rather than on ^{3}H-dT
metabolism, are directed at the population level. Since there
is a decline in the fraction of cycling cells exponential with
age (13), it was of interest to determine whether the addition
of hydrocortisone increased the fraction of cycling cells.

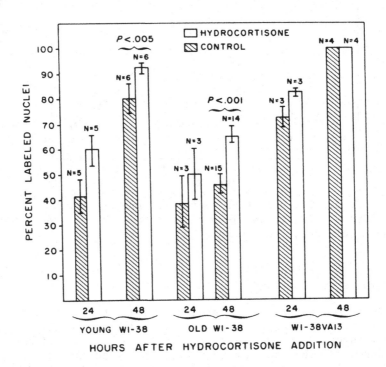

Figure 6. The effect of hydrocortisone on the fraction of
labeled nuclei in cultures not previously exposed to exogenous
hormone.

Figure 6 shows the effect of nuclear labeling of previously
untreated cultures of older cells in which hydrocortisone was
present for either 24 or 48 hr while the ^{3}H-dT was present for
the standard period. There was a statistically significant increase in the percentage of cells in both young and old cultures
incorporating ^{3}H-dT in the presence of hydrocortisone after 48
hr. Here again, the effect is much more striking in older cultures

as the increase in the presence of the hormone was approximately
45% in comparison to only about 15% in young cultures.

As shown above, parallel cultures showed an increase in cell
number in the presence of the hormone and the results are consistent with stimulation of both DNA synthesis and cell division.

Thus, the hydrocortisone mediated increase in DNA synthesis
seems to be due, in part at least, to an increase in the fraction
of cells in the proliferating pool. Hydrocortisone appears to
amplify the stimulus for proliferation. For comparison, we have
included labeling data for the permanently proliferating, SV40-
transformed WI-38 cell line in which, by 48 hr, both treated and
control cultures have essentially 100% labeled nuclei.

Note that in the older group there was a greater difference
between the hydrocortisone-treated and control groups. However,
the responsiveness of the older cells in terms of the fraction
undergoing DNA synthesis was lower.

Specificity of the Hydrocortisone Effect. Initially, the
increase in proliferative capacity seemed enigmatic. Typically,
hydrocortisone has been reported to inhibit cell proliferation
in tissue culture and we were interested in determining whether
our observations were specific for this cell type and whether
under identical conditions, we could duplicate the inhibitory
effects reported by others for other cell types.

Table I shows a partial listing of the results of some experiments that are representative of a larger number of cell
cultures we have screened for their response to hydrocortisone.
In the upper portion of the table are seven human fibroblast-like
populations. These include human fetal lung cell cultures from
four individuals and at comparable passage levels, and cultures
of fetal, infant and adult human skin. The adult skin was received
from Dr. George M. Martin of the University of Washington and
was obtained at autopsy from a patient with Werner's syndrome,
a disease of premature aging. For all of these human cells, both
DNA synthesis and cell division were stimulated by hydrocortisone.

Human fetal kidney cultures of epithelial-like cells, obtained
from Dr. Warren Nichols of the Institute for Medical Research,
Camden, N.J., and studied at passage 5 were unresponsive to hydrocortisone.

In contrast to their normal progenitor strains, the 3 SV40-
transformed cultures (WI-38VA13A, WI-26VA4, W18VA2) showed an
inhibition of cell division of about 30%, but no reduction in
the percentage of cells synthesizing DNA. HeLa cells, on the
other hand, showed an inhibition of both DNA synthesis and cell

Table I. Effect of hydrocortisone on DNA synthesis and cell division in various cell lines.

| Origin | | Designation | Passage | Percent Change With Hydrocortisone | |
Species	Tissue			Cell Count	Percent Labeled Nuclei
human	fetal lung	WI-38	40	+40	+38
human	fetal lung	WI-26	38	--	+33
human	fetal lung	MRC-5	39	--	+51
human	fetal lung	HEL-31	50	+31	+20
human	fetal foreskin	HF	9	+24	+20
human	infant skin	#2	36	--	+27
human	adult skin (Werner's syndrome)	GM-167	5	+60	+47
human	fetal kidney (epith)	HEK-31	5	0	0
human	SV-40 transformed WI-38	WI-38-VA13A	-	-25	0
human	SV-40 transformed WI-26	WI-26-VA4	-	-30	0
human	SV-40 transformed mucosa	W-18-VA2	-	-31	0
human	cervical carcinoma	HeLa	-	-31	-20
monkey	kidney	CV-1	40	-54	-18
hamster	whole embryo	---	2	-61	-15
mouse	areolar tissue	L	-	-34	-24
chick	whole embryo	---	11	-9	-16
lizard	whole embryo	GE-1	33	-20	-35
frog	whole embryo	RP	45	-20	-40
fish	adult minnow tail	FHM	17	-67	-50

division, thus suggesting separate effects of the hormone on cell division and DNA synthesis.

Finally, in the lower portion of the table we show the effect of cortisol on cell lines derived from species representing all the vertebrate classes; three mammalian lines and representatives of lines derived from birds, reptiles, amphibians and fish. For all of these, both DNA synthesis and cell division were inhibited by hydrocortisone. Thus, the hydrocortisone stimulation of proliferation appears to be highly specific for the human diploid fibroblast-like cell lines.

On the other hand, fibroblast-like cells carried in tissue culture would not be expected to respond to glucocorticoids in this way. Indeed, the literature indicates that just the reverse should occur; i.e., that cell growth should be inhibited by glucocorticoids (20). Also to be explained was the requirement for activity of hydrocortisone concentrations on the order of several hundred-fold higher than that found in circulating human blood.

The higher concentration required for response may reflect the absence or low level of specific cytosol receptors for hydrocortisone. Croce et al. (21) have reported that cytosol receptors for glucocorticoids are very low or absent in WI-38 cells. Perhaps the differences in responsiveness of various tissues in vivo and in vitro are concentration dependent. When high affinity cytosol receptors are present, very low concentrations can elicit a response. Alternatively, cells without such receptors appear unresponsive to a given hormone; however, if the concentration is raised to a high enough level, the interaction of the hormone with its target can occur. We are currently studying the nature and subcellular localization of specific protein receptors for hydrocortisone in young and old cells.

To evaluate the effect of hydrocortisone on DNA synthesis further, experiments were designed to determine if the biological activity was specific for this molecular structure or whether it was simply a non-specific effect. To test these alternatives, various steroids were assayed for their biological activity with WI-38 cells as determined by the increase in the percentage of labeled nuclei in the culture. Three groups of compounds were tested: those that were very active, hydrocortisone being the most active in stimulating DNA synthesis; those that were clearly inhibitory to DNA synthesis, testosterone being the most inhibitory; and a third group in which there may have been moderate borderline effects but which were not significantly different from the control.

Figure 7 shows a comparison of the molecular structures of hydrocortisone and the other five stimulatory steroids. Note that all have the 3 keto, $\Delta 4$ configuration in Ring A, an 11β-hydroxy group and a keto group at C-20. Other functional groups such as the 17α and the 21-hydroxy groups, present in hydrocortisone but not in some of the others, or the C-18 methyl group present in all but aldosterone and 18-hydroxycorticosterone seemed of minor and variable significance to the action of the hormone.

Figure 8 shows the results of experiments designed to test the effect of variations in these three functional groups on the biological activity of these hormones. In the first row are shown examples of variations in the structure of the A ring. Prednisolone, which has a structure identical with hydrocortisone except for one additional double bond in the A ring, was a mild inhibitor of DNA synthesis. Similar synthetic steroids such as dexamethasone and triamcinolone (not shown) are either inhibitory or without effect on DNA synthesis. Reduction of the double bond in ring A resulted in compounds which were ineffective in stimulating cell division and this was true for both the cis and trans configurations (5β-dihydrocortisol and 5α-pregnane, 11β, 17α, 21-triol, 3, 20-dione, respectively).

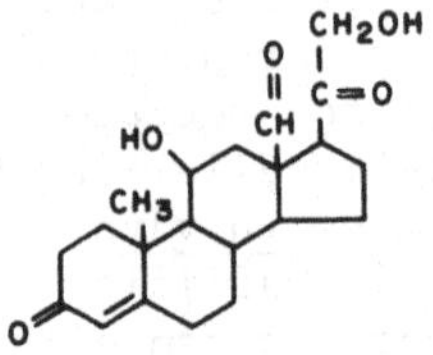

Aldosterone
(+26)

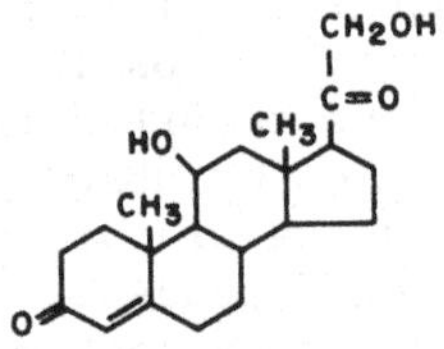

Corticosterone
(+25)

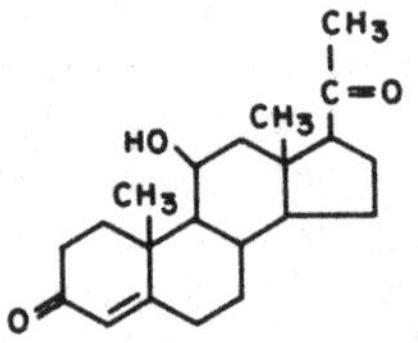

11 β Hydroxyprogesterone
(+21)

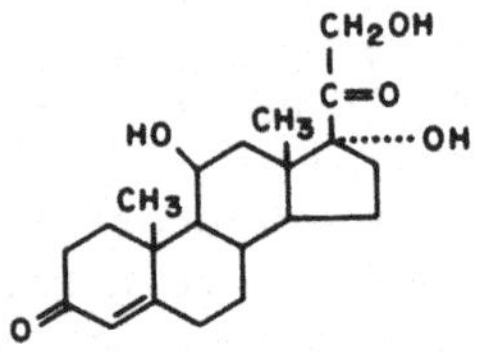

Hydrocortisone
(+41)

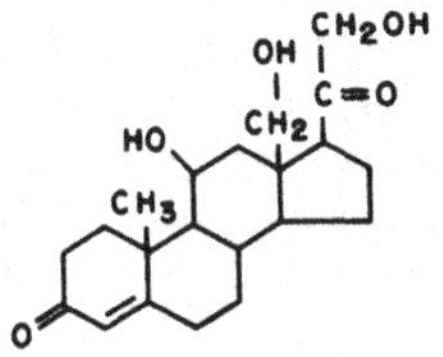

18 Hydroxycorticosterone
(+13)

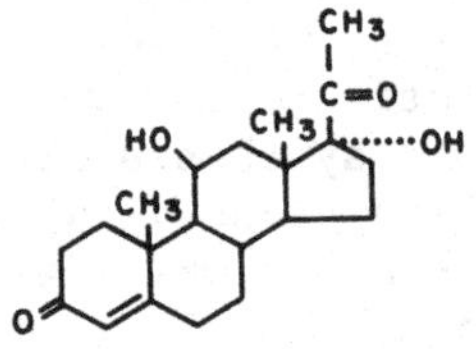

21 Desoxycortisol
(+12)

Figure 7. Molecular structure of steroids active in stimulating DNA synthesis.

In the second row of Fig. 8 are shown two compounds in which the 11β-hydroxy configuration was altered. Cortisone (11 keto) increased DNA synthesis to such a small extent that the data were not statistically significant.

Also shown in Fig. 8 is 11-epicortisol, an inhibitor of DNA synthesis. This compound differs from hydrocortisone in having the 11-OH group in the α position. Thus, the recognition sites in the cell can distinguish between 11α- and β-hydroxy steroids.

In the last row are shown compounds in which reduction of the C-20 keto group (4 pregnene 11β, 17α, 20α, 21-tetrol-3-one) caused loss of activity. Removal of the side chain leaving a carboxylic acid group in the C-20 position (11β-hydroxy-3-keto-etio -4- cholenic acid) also caused loss of activity. Finally, re-

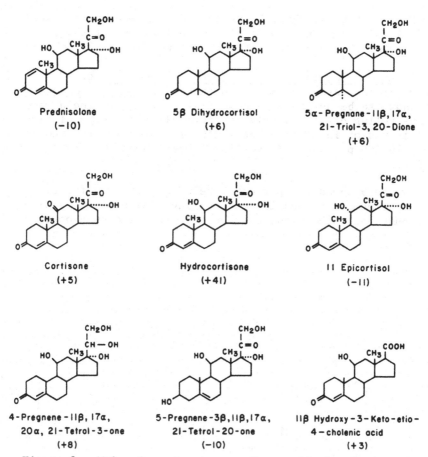

Figure 8. Molecular structures of steroids in which key functional groups of hydrocortisone have been varied.

duction of the 3 keto group resulted in a compound with inhibitory effects. This compound however also has a shift in the position of the double bond from the 4 to the 5 position so that interpretation of this result is not clear. Cortol (5β-pregnane, 3α, 11β, 17, 20α, 21-pentol), a 3-OH structure in which both the A and B rings are saturated (not shown), is also a mild inhibitor of DNA synthesis.

In general the specificity is very similar to that reported for stimulation of cell division in confluent 3T3 mouse fibroblasts by Thrash and Cunningham (22). The major exception is the lack of activity with the synthetic glucocorticoids prednisolone, dexamethasone and triamcinolone, all of which were effective in the mouse system but not in the human system. We have compared

the effects of these three hormones over concentrations ranging
from 5 X 10^{-3} μg/ml to 100 μg/ml. None were stimulating. In
fact at the highest concentrations they were slightly inhibitory.

Effect of Continuous Exposure to Hydrocortisone. Since the
loss of proliferative capacity in these diploid populations has
been shown to be due to an exponential increase in the number
of non-cycling or very slowly cycling cells in the population
(13), it was of interest to determine if cultures grown continuously in the presence of hydrocortisone showed the same heterogeneity.

Figure 9 shows the percent labeled nuclei as a function of
cumulative number of population doublings (determined by direct
cell count) at each subcultivation over the life span of the

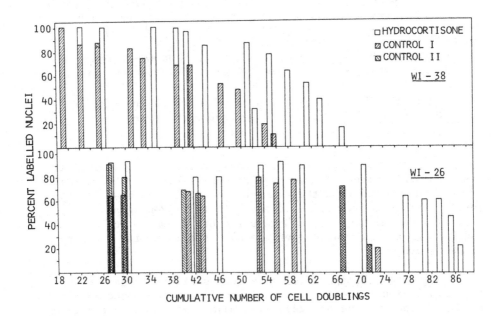

Figure 9. The effect of hydrocortisone on the fraction of
labeled nuclei in the culture after 30 hr continuous exposure to
^{3}H-dT (0.1 μCi/ml).

culture. Both the female-derived (WI-38) and the male-derived
(WI-26) cell cultures were studied. The control and hormone-
treated cultures were started together. Initially, nearly 100%
of the cells were labeled in both cases. As the life span pro-
gressed, however, the accelerated rate of proliferation of the
hormone-treated population was evidenced by the more rapid traverse
of the clear bars (representing the hormone-treated cultures)
across the abcissa; i.e., the hormone-treated cultures were doubling more rapidly.

The decline in the fraction of labeled cells was more rapid
in the control cultures and they phased out well before the hydrocortisone-treated cultures; however, the pattern of decline in
labeling was the same in both cases. Hydrocortisone seemed to
retain the cells in the actively proliferating pool for longer
periods.

Finally, it is important to note that, just as with the short
term autoradiographic experiment, the differences between hydrocortisone and control were greater as the culture aged. However,
the percentage of cells responding to the stimulus for division
declined with age. The rate of decline was slower in the hydrocortisone-treated culture. Thus, it appears from these experiments
as well, that the hydrocortisone amplifies the primary signal
for division. Further evidence for this interpretation is provided
in Figure 10. Here, in the absence of serum there was essentially
no division; the primary signal for division was clearly serum.
With graded increases in serum there was a graded response in
the fraction of cells incorporating labeled precursor. Note that
in the presence of hydrocortisone, 0.3% serum gave a response
higher than 10% serum without hydrocortisone, and 10% serum plus
hydrocortisone was equivalent to or greater than 50% serum.

Similar amplifying effects were found when serum and hydrocortisone were added to confluent, contact-inhibited monolayers
of WI-38 cells (23).

To approach the mechanism of action of this hormone in stimulating cell division, it was of interest to determine the time
course of induction of the effect. For these experiments, cells
were seeded at low density in duplicate so that an equal number
of vessels were available to be used simply for refeeding purposes.
Twenty-four hr after seeding, the medium in half the flasks was
replaced with hydrocortisone-containing medium and the cells were
incubated in this medium for various periods of time. At the
times indicated on the chart, the hydrocortisone-containing medium
was removed and replaced with similarly conditioned medium without
hydrocortisone from the duplicate flasks and then the cells were
fixed after a total incubation of 48 hr. Controls were handled

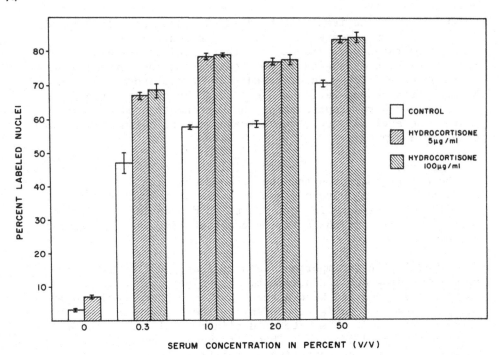

Figure 10.   The effect of serum and hydrocortisone concentration on cell division.

in exactly the same way except the feeding medium did not contain
exogenous hydrocortisone.   The results (Table II)

Table II.   Time course of commitment of hydrocortisone-treated
cultures at increased DNA synthesis.

HC EXPOSURE TIME HOURS	DNA SYNTHESIS (CPM/Coverslip) RATIO HC/CONTROL		
	Experiment I	Experiment II	Experiment III
6	.95	.90	.89
12	1.10	1.06	1.07
18	1.24	1.26	
24	1.28	1.37	1.21
48			1.36

showed that for both experiments, the effect was not a rapid one
and required at least 12 hr. However, when the hormone was present
for more than 12 hr, the cells behaved, qualitatively at least,
as if the hormone had been present continually for the entire
48 hr period. Experiments are now in progress to determine if
the action of hydrocortisone during this 12 hr period is sensitive
to inhibition by actinomycin D and/or cycloheximide.

DISCUSSION

The data presented above show that one: the extension of
the life span of human diploid cells by hydrocortisone is due,
in part at least, to an increase of the fraction of cells synthesizing DNA. We have not ruled out additional effects including
an increase in the rate of transit of the cells through the various
cell cycle periods. This is currently being investigated. Two:
the effect on cell division, however, is not simply mediated
through changes in thymidine metabolism, and three: hydrocortisone
appears to amplify the serum mediated stimulus for division.

We have also shown that the stimulatory effect of hydrocortisone on DNA synthesis was highly specific for certain molecular
configurations in the substituted steroid nucleus. The recognition
sites require unsaturation at the 4-5 position in ring A, the
keto group at position 3, the 11β-hydroxy group and an additional
keto group at position 20. Although some differences exist, this
pattern of molecular structure-function relationship is similar
to that reported for the stimulation of casein synthesis in mammary
organ culture (24), and for glutamine synthetase induction in
embryonic chick retina culture (25,26). Because of the central
role of glutamine in cell culture metabolism and proliferation
in general, we have investigated glutamine synthetase induction
in WI-38 cells and although the enzyme could be induced by glutamine deprivation, hydrocortisone had no effect on this induction
(27).

In addition, since hydrocortisone is generally considered
to be an inhibitor of cell division in tissue culture (20), we
have also tested a number of cultures to determine if the stimulation of cell division is specific for human fetal lung cells
or is a general phenomenon. The results showed that the effect
was highly specific for human diploid cells.

Hydrocortisone, cortisone and other corticosteroids have
been reported to prolong the in vitro survival time of several
cell types (28-30). These studies have been concerned with post-
mitotic maintenance of the cultures. Macieira-Coelho (9) however,
was the first to report the increase in proliferative life span
of diploid, fibroblast-like cells in culture.

Division stimulating effects with hydrocortisone have also been reported by Castor and Prince (31) for cartilage cells and by Smith et al. (32), for human fetal lung cells. Recently, Thrash and Cunningham (33) have shown the stimulation of division by hydrocortisone in density-inhibited 3T3 cells and Armelin (34) and Gospodarowicz (35) have shown that hydrocortisone amplifies the activity of the pituitary and brain-derived polypeptides that stimulate cell division.

In considering possible ways to explain these results, we must consider that although changes in transcription represent the best defined action of glucocorticoids, there is a wide range of other less well understood effects of steroids which must also be considered, many of them involving various membrane effects.

As shown by Absher et al. (36) and Martin et al. (37), there is now ample evidence to indicate that aging of the population is reflected at the cellular level by a transition from a rapidly cycling state to one or a series of more slowly cycling states, and finally, to a sterile state, i.e., a state in which the cells are arrested or are cycling so slowly as to be unable to repopulate the culture vessel. These three transitions are shown in the center portion of Figure 11.

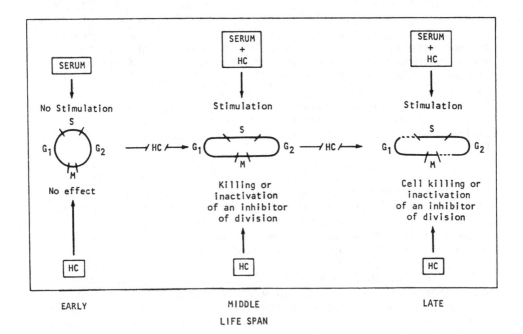

Figure 11. Models for hydrocortisone action.

One simple interpretation of the data is that the steroid delays these transitions.

Another possible interpretation is shown in the upper portion of the figure and is based by analogy with the work of Bresciani (38) in which he showed that as mammary cells differentiate, they lose responsiveness to one hormone but acquire or maintain responsiveness to other hormonal stimuli. Possibly young cells are responsive to 10% serum initially, but eventually lose their responsiveness to this concentration of serum and undergo a transition to a second state where 10% serum plus hydrocortisone are required to elicit a division response. Alternatively, there may be a second population in the culture which succeeds the first and which will only proliferate in the presence of serum plus hydrocortisone.

Finally, a third possibility is shown in the lower portion of the figure and presupposes that slowly cycling or arrested cells inhibit the growth of those cells still capable of division, either simply by the space they occupy or by eliciting an inhibitor or chalone into the environment. In these rapidly dividing cells hydrocortisone has no effect. In the slowly cycling cells, however, hydrocortisone could work either by some inactivation of the hypothetical inhibitor or by killing the cells responsible for its secretion. Thus, the young cells in the population are not inhibited to the same extent. Our current work is designed to clarify these possibilities.

ACKNOWLEDGEMENTS

The expert technical assistance of Barbara Sharf and Joan Kabakjian in various parts of these studies is gratefully acknowledged.

The work reported above was supported by grants HD02721 and HD06323 from the National Institute of Child Health and Human Development.

REFERENCES

1. Cristofalo, V. J., N. Parris, and D. Kritchevsky. J. Cell Physiol. 69:263 (1967).
2. Lipetz, J. and V. J. Cristofalo. J. Ultrastruc. Res. 39: 43 (1972).
3. Robbins, E., E. M. Levine, and H. Eagle. J. Exp. Med. 131: 1211 (1970).
4. Brandes, D., D. G. Murphy, E. Anton, and S. Barnard. J. Ultrastruc. Res. 39:465 (1972).
5. Cristofalo, V. J., J. R. Kabakjian, and D. Kritchevsky. Proc. Soc. Exp. Biol. Med. 126:649 (1967).

6.   Cristofalo, V. J. In: Aging in Cell and Tissue Culture.
     (Eds.) E. Holeckova and V. Cristofalo, Plenum Press, N.Y.,
     p. 83 (1970).
7.   Cristofalo, V. J. and J. R. Kabakjian. Mech. Age Develop.
     (in press).
8.   Cristofalo, V. J. Proc. Eighth Inter. Cong. Gerontol. II,
     6.
9.   Macieira-Coelho, A. Experientia 22:390 (1966).
10. Cristofalo, V. J., D. Kobler, J. Kabakjian, J. Mackessy,
     and B. Baker. In Vitro 6:396 (1971).
11. Hayflick, L. Exp. Cell Res. 37:614 (1965).
12. Hayflick, L. and P. Moorhead. Exp. Cell Res. 25:585 (1961).
13. Cristofalo, V. J. and B. B. Sharf. Exp. Cell Res. 76:419
     (1973).
14. Levine, E. M. Exp. Cell Res. 74:99 (1972).
15. Bello, L. Exp. Cell Res. 89:263 (1974).
16. Volkin, E. and W. E. Cohn. Methods of Biochem. Anal. 1:
     287 (1954).
17. Plagemann, P. G. W. and J. Erbe. J. Cell Biol. 55:161 (1972).
18. Adams, R. L. P. Exp. Cell Res. 56:49 (1969).
19. Littlefield, J. W. Biochim. Biophys. Acta 114:398 (1966).
20. Ruhmann, A. G. and D. L. Berliner. Endocrinol. 76:916 (1965).
21. Croce, C. M., G. Litwack, and H. Koprowski. Proc. Nat.
     Acad. Sci. USA 70:1268 (1973).
22. Thrash, C. R., T. Ho, and D. D. Cunningham. J. Biol. Chem.
     249:6099 (1974).
23. Cristofalo, V. J. In: Impairment of Cellular Functions
     During Aging and Development in Vivo and in Vitro. (Eds.)
     V. J. Cristofalo and E. Holeckova, Plenum Press, N.Y., p.
     7 (1974).
24. Turkington, R. W. and Y. J. Topper. Endocrinol. 80:329
     (1967).
25. Moscona, A. A. and R. Piddington. Biochim. Biophys. Acta
     121:409 (1966).
26. Chader, G. J. and L. Reif-Lehrer. Biochim. Biophys. Acta
     264:186 (1968).
27. Viceps, D. and V. J. Cristofalo. J. Cell Physiol. (in press).
28. Arpels, C., V. J. Babcock, and C. M. Southam. Proc. Soc.
     Exp. Biol. Med. 115:102 (1964).
29. Yuan, G. C. and R. S. Chang. Proc. Soc. Exp. Biol. Med.
     130:934 (1969).
30. Yuan, G. C., R. S. Chang. J. B. Little, and G. Cornil.
     J. Gerontol. 22:174 (1967).
31. Castor, C. W. and R. K. Prince. Biochim. Biophys. Acta 83:
     165 (1964).
32. Smith, B. T., J. S. Torday, and C. J. P. Giroud. Steroids
     22:515 (1973).
33. Thrash, C. R. and D. D. Cunningham. Nature 242:399 (1973).
34. Armelin, H. Proc. Nat. Acad. Sci. USA 70:2702 (1973).

35. Gospodarowicz, D. Nature 249:123 (1974).
36. Absher, P. M., R. G. Absher, and W. D. Barnes. Exp. Cell Res. 88:95 (1974).
37. Martin, G. M., C. A. Sprague, T. H. Norwood, and W. R. Pendergrass. Am. J. Path. 74:137 (1974).
38. Bresciani, F. Cell Tissue Kinet. 1:51 (1968).

GENERAL CONSIDERATIONS OF MEMBRANES

E.J. Masoro

Department of Physiology, The University of Texas Health

Science Center, San Antonio, Texas

It has long been believed that a membrane separates the contents of cells from the extracellular environment. With the advent of electron microscopy, this membrane, called the plasma membrane, was for the first time visualized and in addition it became evident that the internal structure of cells also contained complex systems of membranes (1) which are components of what often are called organelles (e.g., mitochondria, endoplasmic reticulum, Golgi complex, lysosomes, etc.) (Fig. 1). In recent years it has become possible to isolate in relatively pure form many of these membranous organelles from homogenates of tissues by means of differential and density gradient ultracentrifugation. From studies utilizing these isolated membranes the biochemical nature and the functions of many of these organelles have been established.

One of the most important functions of membranes is their role as a barrier (2) preventing rapid diffusion of materials between the intracellular fluid and the extracellular fluid and between the various subcompartments of the cell separated by the membranous organelles. The following are important examples of this barrier function: the ability of the plasma membrane to prevent loss of intracellular ATP and to prevent the rapid entry of Na^+ into most cells; the inability of acetyl-CoA to readily migrate across mitochondrial membranes, an example of the important role played by membranes in compartmentalizing metabolic pathways; the restricting of hydrolytic enzymes by the membrane encapsulating lysosomes.

Another important function of membranes is the transport of needed materials as well as wastes into and out of the cell and between intracellular compartments (3). Examples of this function

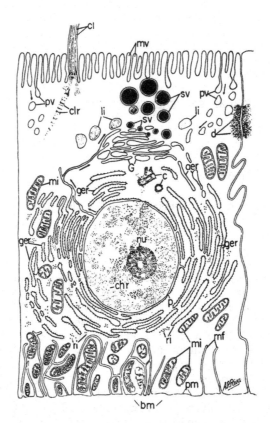

Figure 1. General diagram of ultrastructure of an ideal cell.
aer, agranular endoplasmic reticulum; bm, basal membrane; c,
centriole; chr, chromosome; cl, cilium; clr, cilium root; d,
desmosome; G, Golgi complex; ger, granular endoplasmic reticulum;
li, lysosome; mf, membrane fold; mi, mitochondria; mv, microvilli;
nu, nucleolus; p, pore; pm, plasma membrane; pv, pinocytic vesicle;
ri, ribosome; sv, secretion vesicle [from DeRobertis et al.
(1)].

are the transport of amino acids and glucose across the plasma
membrane and the transport of citrate across the mitochondrial
membrane, a process of great importance in metabolic regulation.

A third function is the role that membranes play as matrices
for the organization of enzyme systems in a spatially appropriate
manner (4). The most obvious example of this is the ability to
generate ATP from ADP and Pi coupled to the oxidation of foodstuffs
which requires enzyme systems present in mitochondrial membranes
in highly organized arrays.

Another important function of membranes, in particular plasma membranes, is their role in information transfer (5). These membranes contain specific receptors that recognize and interact with certain hormones and with the chemical mediators of nervous system activity such as the catecholamines and acetylcholine. In this way, the various effects of the endocrine and nervous systems on their target cells are mediated.

Finally, membranes are involved in many of the immune responses of the organism (Dowben, 1972). The plasma membrane is the major membrane involved in this regard.

Obviously each of the many specific functions carried out by membranes requires the presence of a specialized molecular organization. Unfortunately, the molecular architecture of membranes is still not fully understood even in terms of its general outline. The model of Singer (6) (Figure 2) is compatible with

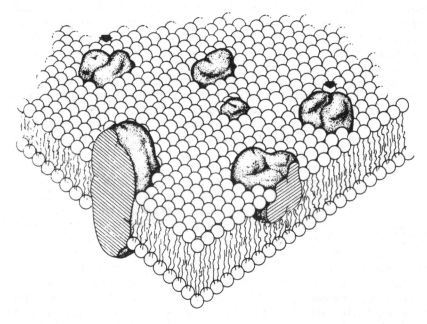

Figure 2. Singer's model of the molecular architecture of biological membranes. The amphipathic lipids are represented by circles indicating polar regions of the molecule and wavy lines indicating the nonpolar regions. The proteins are shown as globular structures floating in the membrane with their polar amino acids protruding from each surface of the membrane and their nonpolar acid residues embedded in the core of the membrane [from Singer (6)].

most of the known facts on membrane structure and function.   In
this model, it is proposed that most of the area of the membrane
is comprised of amphipathic lipids organized in a bilayer fashion
with the polar heads facing the aqueous media on either side of the
membrane and the nonpolar regions of these amphipaths (i.e., the
hydrocarbon regions of phospholipids and the steroid nucleus of
cholesterol) forming the inner core of the membrane. It is further
proposed that globular membrane proteins float in this sea composed of lipid bilayer with some of the proteins passing through
the entire thickness of the membrane, with their polar amino acid
residues interacting with the aqueous media on the two sides of the
membrane along with the nonpolar regions of the lipid. Some of
the membrane proteins do not penetrate the thickness of the membrane
but rather have their nonpolar amino acid residues buried in the
core of the membrane and their polar amino acid residues at one of
the surfaces of the membrane interacting with an aqueous environment.
The lipid bilayer provides most of the barrier function of membranes mentioned above while the proteins are oriented spatially
in such a way as to execute the many other functions of membranes
delineated above. Clearly, the details of this molecular architecture must differ for every different membrane type and must
specifically relate to each of the myriad of functions carried
out by membranes.

It has been theorized (7) that deterioration of membrane
structure may be a basic element for the phenomenon termed aging
and there are many reasons for proposing such a theory. First
of all, there is a deterioration of most of the physiological
activities of a mammal as aging progresses (8). It is likely
that these gross alterations in the function of the various organ
systems of the organism are the result of changes in cell function. Since membranes are key elements in cell physiology, it
is reasonable to suspect that alterations in their molecular
architecture may well be the reason for these alterations in
cell function and it is to be anticipated that aging may involve
deterioration of such a highly organized, complex molecular
architecture. It has also been suggested that lipid peroxidation
is involved in the aging process (9,10). Since the polyunsaturated fatty acids that readily undergo this peroxidation are
components of the membrane lipids, it is to be anticipated that
such peroxidation would occur at the site of the membrane. Such
peroxidation should interfere with both the barrier function
and the other functions of membranes discussed above.

Although there are good reasons to suspect the occurrence of
membrane deterioration as a possible basic cause of aging, there
is little direct experimental evidence in support of this view.
The following is a review of most salient experimental data currently available on the effect of aging on membranes and a con-

TABLE I

ADENYL CYCLASE ACTIVITY ON ADIPOCYTE HOMOGENATES
[modified from Forn et al. (11)]

Age of Rats	Concentration of Norepinephrine Used	Adenyl Cyclase Activity nmoles c-AMP/10^6 cells/min
5-6 weeks	10^{-4}M	~ 4.8
10-12 weeks	10^{-4}M	~ 5.1
18-24 weeks	10^{-4}M	~ 1.7

sideration of certain problems inherent in the interpretation of
some of the data which have been claimed to indicate the occurrence of alterations in membranes with age.

The report of Forn et al. (11) on the adenyl cyclase of
adipocyte plasma membranes is a good example of the later. In this
paper, the authors state "...norepinephrine-stimulated adenyl
cyclase activity was much lower in fat cell homogenates of old rats
than in those of younger rats." This conclusion is based on the
data shown in Table I derived from the graphic presentation of the
data in the original paper. Since all rats used were under 6
months of age, it is clear that these investigators were not studying old rats, but rather were confining their work to a study of
the changes in adenyl cyclase activity in young, developing rats.
Therefore, although the research of Forn and his coworkers is a
good piece of work, it adds nothing to our knowledge in regard
to the activity of adenyl cyclase of the plasma membranes of
adipocytes in senescent rats as claimed by the authors.

Another example of data difficult to interpret in regard to
senescence is the report of Rubin et al (12) that the abundance of
phosphatidylethanolamine relative to other phospholipids in the
plasma membranes of the rat liver (Figure 3) decreases with age.
A fall of phosphatidylethanolamine relative abundance was observed

as rat wt. increases. The difficulty in interpretating these
data and many other pieces of work in which wt. is used as a
criterion of age is that such data provide no really meaningful
index of the age of the animal studied in terms of the total
lifespan of the species. In this case it is quite possible that
the 500g rats were only one-year-old and thus in the first half of
the lifespan of the species.

   Also data of a quite indirect nature have been considered
to be evidence that membrane deterioration is a cause of the aging
phenomenon. An example of this is the work of Hochschild (13)
who was able to increase the lifespan of old mice by administering
to them dimethylaminoethanol (p-acetamidobenzoate salt); on the
basis of these data (shown in Figure 4) the author suggests that
it is the use of the dimethylaminoethanol moiety for the biosynthesis of membrane phosphatidylcholine that may be responsible for

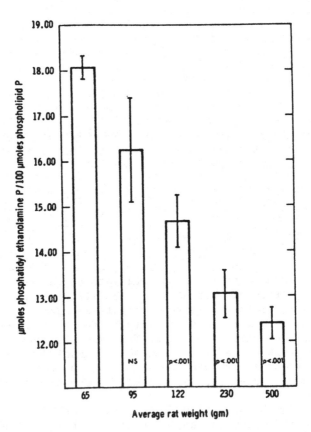

   Figure 3. Changes in the relative abundance of phosphatidylethanolamine in rat liver plasma membranes as a function of rat
wt. [from Rubin et al., (12)].

this increase in life expectancy. In my opinion, these data, although interesting, are too remotely related to membrane biology to be considered as evidence in support of the theory that the deterioration of membrane structure is a basic mechanism in aging.

Important direct data on the effect of age on biological membranes have been reported by Grinna and Barber (14), who have shown that the membranes making up the microsomal fraction of liver and kidney, but not of heart, of six-month-old rats have a higher phospholipid-to-protein mass ratio than do the similar preparations obtained from 24-month-old rats (Table II). There is an interpretational difficulty in regard to this work because microsomes are a mixture of a variety of membrane types; therefore it is possible that the relative abundance of different membrane types isolated is responsible for these findings rather than changes in the composition of a given membrane. In this regard, it is interesting to note that Grinna and Barber did not find any difference in the phospholipid-to-protein mass ratio in the mitochondrial preparations (a much more homogeneous preparation in terms of membrane type) obtained from the young and old rats.

There is a considerable amount of data that alterations in plasma membranes occur with age. O'Bryan and Lowenstein (15) reported changes with age (Table III) in the specific activity of

TABLE II

PHOSPHOLIPID/PROTEIN MASS RATIO OF MICROSOME AND MITOCHONDRIAL
PREPARATIONS FROM SIX AND 24-MONTH-OLD RATS
[From Grinna and Barber (14)]

Membrane Preparation	Age of Rats	
	6 Months	24 Months
	µg lipid P/mg Protein	
Microsomal		
Liver	14.7 ± 1.0	11.6 ± 1.1
Kidney	15.2 ± 1.3	8.8 ± 1.2
Heart	19.0 ± 1.8	18.0 ± 1.1
Mitochondrial		
Liver	8.2 ± 1.3	8.1 ± 1.1
Kidney	8.9 ± 0.8	7.9 ± 0.8
Heart	11.8 ± 1.6	11.0 ± 1.6

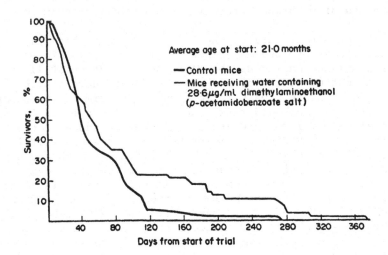

Figure 4. Effect of feeding dimethylaminoethanol (p-acetamida-
benzoate salt) on the length of survival of senile male A/J mice
[from Hochschild, (13)].

TABLE III

EFFECT OF AGE ON RAT RENAL PLASMA MEMBRANE ACTIVITIES
[modified from O'Bryan and Lowenstein (15)].

Enzyme	Ratio of Specific Activities Membranes of 24-mo.old/Membranes of 3-mo.old
Maltase	0.60
Alkaline Phosphatase	0.64
Phosphodiesterase I	0.67

TABLE IV

EFFECT OF AGE ON INSULIN BINDING BY RAT LIVER PLASMA MEMBRANES
[From Freeman et al. (16)]

Age of Rats (mos.)	Insulin Binding Capacity ng/mg Membrane Protein
2	1.17
12	0.57
24	0.50

Barclay et al. (17) have also presented evidence that the plasma membrane changes with age. The most salient aspects of their data are reported in Table V which shows that the amount of

TABLE V

EFFECT OF AGE ON THE % OF RAT HEPATOCYTE PLASMA MEMBRANE PROTEIN
SOLUBLE IN 0.15 M NaCl
[From Barclay et al. (17)]

Age of Rats (weeks)	% Protein Soluble
10	25
52	30
64	34
88	40
116	49

protein extractable with 0.15 M sodium chloride from purified
rat liver hepatocyte plasma membranes increases as the animal
ages. These workers also showed that there are changes in the
relative abundance of various lipoprotein subclasses that can
be isolated from the plasma membranes of rat hepatocytes as the
animal ages, but this study suffers from the following problems:
first, the oldest rats studied were only 64 weeks of age which
means the last half of the lifespan was not being investigated
and second, these so-called lipoprotein subunits of plasma membrane have yet to be well characterized. The work of Detraglia
et al. (18) on the sensitivity of human erythrocytes to hemolysis
(Table VI) provides further evidence that the plasma membrane

TABLE VI

EFFECT OF AGE ON THE FRAGILITY OF HUMAN ERYTHROCYTES
(Modified from Detraglia et al. (18)]

Age of Subjects	Mean Erythrocyte Fragility (moles NaCl/L)
19-36 years old	0.0665 ± 0.0022
64-90 years old	0.0712 ± 0.0039

is probably changing with age since the red cells from older
individuals are more fragile.

Although as just discussed, there are several isolated findings indicating that membranes are altered with age, no really
comprehensive study of a particular membrane has been made in
regard to aging. Since the sarcoplasmic reticulum membrane of
skeletal muscle can be prepared in highly purified form (19)
and since this membrane has only a limited number of functions,
most of which can be explored by in vitro techniques, Drs.
Bertrand, Yu and myself (20) decided to carry out a comprehensive
study of the effect of rat age on this membrane. It should be
noted that Tappel et al. (21) reported that old age in mice did
not influence the calcium transport activity of microsomes isolated from hindleg muscles, a key event in the functional role
of sarcoplasmic reticulum in muscle relaxation, but in those
experiments a crude muscle microsome preparation was used, thus
making it difficult to know if information about sarcoplasmic

reticulum is being obscured by variations in the mixture of membrane types being isolated at different ages.

   In our study, purified sarcoplasmic reticulum membranes were
isolated from skeletal muscle of Fisher 344 strain rats of 1, 2,
3, 6, 12, 24 or 28 months of age and the phospholipid-to-protein
wt. ratio was determined in preparations derived from each of
these ages. This ratio averaged 0.42 and did not change with
age in adult rats. The distribution of lipid phosphorous within
the four subclasses of phospholipid found in sarcoplasmic reticulum membranes (phosphatidylcholine, phosphatidylethanolamine,
phosphatidylinositol and phosphatidylserine) were studied for
each of the age groups (Figure 5). Little change in this dis-

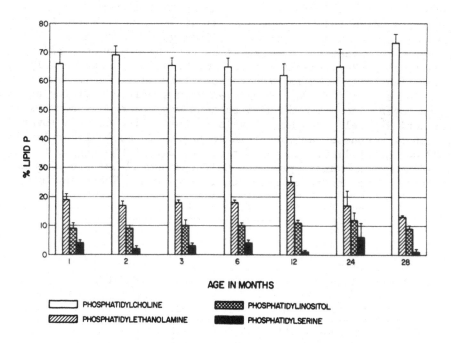

Figure 5. The effect of rat age on the phospholipid composition of skeletal muscle sarcoplasmic reticulum preparations.
The means and standard errors are indicated [from Bertrand et al.
(20)].

tribution occurred with age although membranes from the 28-month-
old rats did have a statistically significant higher fraction of
lipid phosphorous in phosphatidylcholine than did young adults
on a lower fraction in phosphatidylethanolamine.

Isolated sarcoplasmic reticulum are in the form of vesicles than can transport large quantities of Ca^{++} from incubation media into the intravesicular space provided ATP and oxalate are present in such media. This process, called "ATP-dependent, oxalate promoted Ca^{++} transport," is apparently the in vitro counterpart to that occurring in vivo in bringing about the relaxation of contracted muscle. This Ca^{++} transport is energized by a $(Ca^{++} + Mg^{++})$-ATPase energizes Na^+ transport. In addition the functioning of this ATPase involves the generation of a membrane bound phosphorylated intermediate and the steady-state concentration of this intermediate can be measured in in vitro systems.

It was decided to study the effect of age on each of the sarcoplasmic reticulum functions just mentioned. The steady concentration of the phosphorylated intermediate averaged 3.42 nmoles of bound phosphate per mg sarcoplasmic reticulum protein, a value that did not vary significantly with age in adult rats, even in membrane preparations from very old animals. It is of interest that the average value for the phosphorylated intermediate for 2-month-old rats was 6.09, a value considerably higher than that found in preparations from adult rats. The effect of age on the $(Ca^{++} + Mg^{++})$-ATPase specific activity of the sacroplasmic reticulum preparations was remarkably complex. This activity fell from high levels in early life to much lower ones at 12 months of age but then increased to much higher levels by 28 months of life. The effect of the age of the rat on the "ATP-dependent, oxalate promoted Ca^{++} transport" by sarcoplasmic reticulum preparations is recorded in Figure 6. There appears

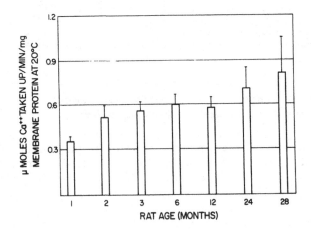

Figure 6. The effect of rat age on the rate of "ATP-dependent, oxalate promoted Ca^{++} transport" by skeletal muscle sarcoplasmic reticulum preparations. The means and standard errors are indicated [from Bertrand et al. (20)].

to be a gradual increase in this transport activity throughout
the period of life studied which is almost the total lifespan
of this strain of rats. Moreover, if the ratio of the rate of
this Ca^{++} transport activity to the rate of $(Ca^{++} + Mg^{++})$-ATPase
activity is used as an index of the efficiency of this Ca^{++}
transport process in terms of energy utilization, it is observed
that this efficiency does not decline with age.

Probably our work on the sarcoplasmic reticulum membrane is
the most extensive yet to have been done on the effect of age on
a specific biological membrane in terms of the span of life studied, the number of ages investigated and extent of analysis of
the chemistry and molecular functioning of the membranes. Although there are some differences between age groups in regard
to basic parameters of sarcoplasmic reticulum composition and
function, the data obtained in our research provide no clear evidence of deterioration of these membranes with age. Since there
is evidence suggesting deterioration of plasma membranes with age
(reviewed above), it is most important that experiments be carried
out at least of as extensive a nature as our research of the sarcoplasmic reticulum membranes on specific plasma membranes, e.g.,
those from hepatocytes, erythrocytes and adipocytes. Indeed,
ideally the kind of research we carried out on the effect of age
on sarcoplasmic reticulum membranes embracing both structure and
function should be extended to all important biological membranes.

REFERENCES

1.   DeRobertis, E. D. P., W. W. Nowinski, and F. A. Saez.
     In: Cell Biology. W. B. Saunders Co., Philadelphia (1970).
2.   Van Deenan, L. L. M. Chem. Physics Lipids 8:366 (1972).
3.   Dowben, R. M. In: General Physiology, a Molecular Approach.
     Harper and Row Publishers, New York (1969).
4.   Packer, L. In: Organization of Energy-Transducing Membranes.
     (Eds.) M. Nakao and L Packer, University Park Press, Baltimore
     (1973) p. 203.
5.   Tepperman, J. In: Metabolic and Endocrine Physiology, 3rd
     ed. Yearbook Medical Publishers, Chicago (1973).
6.   Singer, S. J. Ann. N.Y. Acad. Sci. 195:16 (1972).
7.   Packer, L., D. W. Deamer, and R. L. Heath. Adv. Gerontol.
     Res. 2:77 (1967).
8.   Shock, N. W. J. Amer. Dietetic Assoc. 56:491 (1972).
9.   Tappel, A. L. Geriatrics 23:97 (1968).
10. Pryor, W. A. Chem. Engineering News 49:34 (1971).
11. Forn, J., P. S. Schonhofer, I. F. Skidmore, and G. Kirshna.
     Biochim. Biophys. Acta 203:304 (1970).
12. Rubin, M. S., N. I. Swislocki, and M. Sonnenburg. Proc.
     Soc. Exp. Biol. Med. 142:1008 (1973).
13. Hochschild, R. Exper. Gerontol. 8:185 (1973).

14. Grinna, L. S. and A. A. Barber. Biochim. Biophys. Acta
     288:347 (1972).
15. O'Bryan, D. and L. M. Lowenstein. Biochim. Biophys. Acta
     339:1 (1974).
16. Freeman, C., K. Karoly, and R. C. Adelman. Biochem. Biophys.
     Ress. Comm. 54:1573 (1973).
17. Barclay, M., V. P. Skipski, and O. Terebus-Kekish. Mech.
     Age. Dev. 1:357 (1973).
18. Detraglia, M., F. B. Cook, D. M. Stasiw, and L. C. Cerny.
     Biochim. Biophys. Acta 345:213 (1974).
19. Masoro, E. J. and B. P. Yu. In: Topics in Medicinal
     Chemistry. (Eds.) J. L. Rabinowitz and R. M. Myerson,
     John Wiley & Sons, Inc., New York (1971).
20. Bertrand, H. A., B. P. Yu, and E. J. Masoro. Mech. Age. Dev.
     in press.
21. Tappel, A., B. Fletcher, and D. Deamer. J. Gerontol. 28:
     415 (1973).

FUNCTION OF CARDIAC MUSCLE IN AGING RAT

Myron L. Weisfeldt[+]

Cardiovascular Division and Department of Medicine
John Hopkins University School of Medicine and Hospital
Baltimore, Maryland 21205

INTRODUCTION

The series of studies to be discussed here have attempted to
define the nature and mechanism of age associated alterations in
the function of the heart. I would like to acknowledge the encour-
agement and critical comment of Dr. Nathan Shock and the efforts of
Dr. Edward Lakatta and Dr. Gary Gerstenblith in designing and per-
forming the more recent studies.

Except as noted all the studies involve the use of male rats
from the Gerontology Research Center Aging Rat Colony. These are
Wistar rats which weigh 300 to 600 g as adults. They are fed
Purina Laboratory Chow and live in groups of five or six in wire
bottom suspended cages 24 X 24 X 18 cm. The animal rooms are maintained at a temperature of 24.5°C and a relative humidity of 60%.
Artificial lighting is provided 12 hr continuously each day. Fifty
percent mortality is reached between 24 and 26 months of age. The
most common causes of death are respiratory infection, renal disease,
and tumors.

Rothbaum et al. (1) have demonstrated that these animals are
not hypertensive. These investigators measured intraarterial blood
pressures in the resting state and found no significant difference
between the blood pressures of 12- and 24-month-old rats. Light
microscopic examination of hearts from 12-month-old and 24- to 31-

[+]Dr. Weisfeldt is an Established Investigator of the American
Heart Association. Supported by USPHS Grant No. HL 15565 and
Guest Investigator Program, Gerontology Research Center, NICHD,
NIH, Baltimore, Maryland.

month-old rats from this colony (2) revealed no major coronary
artery lesions aside from coronary arteritis present in one senile
rat. Thus it appears that neither hypertension nor major vessel
coronary artery disease account for the age associated alterations
in function of the hearts from these rats.

     Initial physiological studies performed by Shreiner et al.
(3) and Lee et al. (4) demonstrated distinct deterioration of
overall cardiac function with age in the isolated rat heart and
in the intact open chest rat. Work performance of isolated hearts
from 24-month-old rats was significantly less than that performed
by hearts from 12-month-old rats. In the open chest rat, Lee and
his associates (4) demonstrated that an increase in mean aortic
pressure induced by angiotensin infusion resulted in a significant
decline in aortic blood flow (cardiac output) in older rats, whereas
younger rats showed no change in aortic flow. Also left ventricular
end diastolic pressure which serves here as an index of left ventricular performance was higher in the 24-month-old group than
the 12-month-old group at peak angiotensin response. Thus, it
appears that the functional capabilities of the 24-month-old rat
are distinctly lower than those of the 12-month-old rat.

     There are four broad areas of consideration with regard to the
mechanism of these age associated alterations in overall myocardial
function. The focus of this discussion will be to attempt to clarify which of these mechanisms are physiologically important in the
aging rat heart. The first of these mechanisms is a decrease
in nutrient or oxygen delivery. This might result from either a
decrease in the coronary vascular bed capacity or impeded movement
of nutrients or oxygen from the capillary to the myocardial cell.
The second is altered myocardial structure. If, for example,
aging is associated with extensive replacement of myocardial contractile cells with fibrous tissue, this would obviously have functional importance. The third is a change in ventricular geometry or stiffness. These are changes in the passive properties
of cardiac muscle. Is aging associated with dilation of the left
ventricle such that greater wall tension must be generated at any
level of systolic left ventricular pressure? Are these changes
in the connective tissue or the myocardial cell such that there is
increased stiffness to passive stretch of the myocardium? Such an
increase in stiffness would mean that in order to utilize the Frank-
Starling mechanism to increase cardiac function a higher filling
pressure would be necessary.. Thus a stiffer ventricle would mean
that symptomatic congestive heart failure, as result of a higher
filling pressure, would occur at a lower workload in the heart from
the aged animal. The fourth is change in the intrinsic contractile process or the intrinsic response of the myocardium to
physiological inotropic agents such as catecholamines. Changes in
the intrinsic contractile process might be a result of alterations

in the contractile proteins themselves, the ability to generate or
utilize energy sources for contraction or alterations in excitation-
contraction coupling. The responsiveness of the aging myocardium
to inotropic stimuli is the principe focus of Dr. Lakatta's discussion later in this volume.

CORONARY FLOW AND OXYGEN EXTRACTION

To examine the functional capacity of the coronary artery
vascular bed and oxygen delivery, an isolated non-blood perfused
rat heart preparation was utilized (2). The heart was removed
from the rat and the proximal aorta was tied about a cannula.
The coronary arteries were perfused retrograde from a reservoir
containing Krebs-Ringer bicarbonate solution with 300 mg % glucose
and 3% dextran added. The perfusate was filtered and maintained
at 36°C. The perfusion pressure was maintained at 70 mm Hg. These
hearts were paced at a rate of 220 beats/min. A short piece of poly-
ethylene tubing was placed through the apex of the heart into the
left ventricle so that ejection of perfusate accumulating in this
chamber was performed against essentially no resistance. This
minimized the amount of external work performed by all hearts.
Hearts were placed in a sealed chamber. The outflow from this
chamber was from the aorta via the coronary arteries. Myocardial
oxygen consumption and oxygen extraction were determined from the
coronary flow and the arterio-venous oxygen difference across the
heart. These hearts were subjected to progressive hypoxia. Under
hypoxic conditions the stimulus to coronary vasodilation is considered to be maximal and thus the maximal capacity of the coronary
vascular bed could be measured. Under these conditions the ability
of the heart to extract oxygen from the perfusate could also be
compared. Eleven 12-month- and ten 24- to 27-month-old rat hearts
were examined.

During stepwise lowering of the arterial pO_2 from initial
levels of 650 mm Hg, oxygen consumption (expressed per g dry wt.)
was maintained constant until the arterial pO_2 was lowered to levels
below 350 mm Hg (Fig. 1). Below 300 mm Hg oxygen consumption fell
progressively, as both groups were unable to compensate fully for
the decline in oxygen availability. At 200 and 250 mm Hg a statistically significant age difference was noted (p < .01). This
age difference in the ability to compensate for a lower oxygen
availability was not attributable to decreased ability to extract
oxygen from the perfusate as indicated in Fig. 2. Percent of
oxygen extracted was nearly identical in the two groups at all
levels of perfusate pO_2 examined. The decline in the ability to
maintain oxygen consumption during hypoxia was attributable to a
significant difference in the coronary flow response to hypoxia
(Fig. 3). A significantly lower coronary flow per g dry heart
wt. was noted in the hearts from old animals.

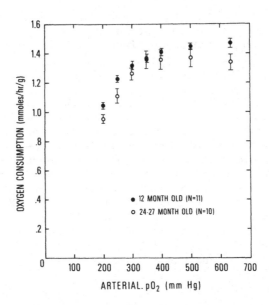

Figure 1. Effect of progressive hypoxia on myocardial oxygen consumption in hearts from 12- and 24-27-month-old male rats. The perfusate oxygen tension was lowered progressively from 635 to 200 mm Hg. Significant age differences were noted at 250 and 200 mm Hg (p < .01). Mean ± S.E. shown. (By permission (2)).

        Shown in Fig. 4 are the coronary flow and coronary flow per g dry wt. at a pO_2 of 250 mm Hg in each group. Although there was a significantly lower maximal coronary flow per g in the 24- to 27-month-old group as seen on the right (amounting to 8.5%), there was no significant difference in the coronary flow per heart when not normalized by heart wt. (shown on the left). This is attributable to the 7.3% greater heart wt. in the older animals. These data suggest that there is some age associated myocardial hypertrophy which is not accompanied by a concomitant increase in the size of the coronary vascular bed. This would be consistent with studies of myocardial capillary-fiber ratios by Rakusan and Poupa (5) and Tomanek (6). It should be noted, though, that the magnitude of this age related change in wt. and coronary flow per g is relatively small and that there is no decrease in the maximal ability to extract oxygen under these conditions.

                            MYOCARDIAL STRUCTURE

        In regard to the possibility that the alterations in myocardial function are attributable to changes in the structure of the aging heart both histologic studies and determination of hydroxyproline

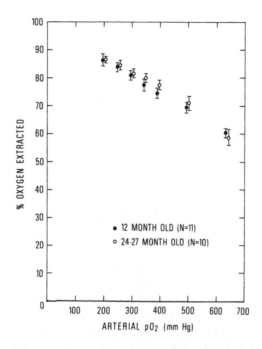

Figure 2. The effect of progressive hypoxia on the percent
of arterial oxygen extracted by the same hearts shown in Figure 1.
The percent of oxygen extracted was not significantly different between these two groups of hearts at any arterial pO_2 examined.
Mean ± S.E. shown. (By permission (2)).

content of the myocardium suggest that even in the subendocardial
zone where fibrosis is maximal there is no more than a 50% increase
in the amount of fibrous tissue present when comparing the two-year-
old heart to the one-year-old heart (7). Thus even in the endo-
cardium, fibrosis could account for a loss of only 2.5% of the total
mass of contractile cells. Electron microscopic studies of myocardium from hearts of rats from the same colony have been performed
by Travis and Travis (8). No major changes were noted in the ultrastructure of the myofilaments. The major age changes were an increase in the number of residual bodies and lipid droplets in the
region of the smooth sarcoplasmic reticulum and an increase in the
number of primary lysosomes in close proximity to mitochondria.
Thus neither the delivery of oxygen or nutrients to the myocardium
nor overwhelming structural myofibrillar changes of fibrosis appear to account for the age associated changes in myocardial function.

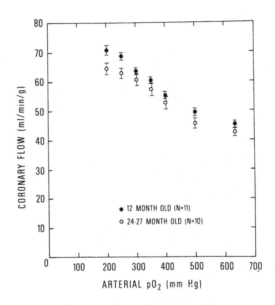

Figure 3. The effect of progressive hypoxia on the coronary
flow of the same hearts shown in Figures 1 and 2. The coronary
flow was expressed in ml/min/g dry heart wt. The coronary flow
was significantly lower in the older hearts at 250 and 200 mm Hg
(p < .01). Mean ± S.E. shown. (By permission (2)).

VENTRICULAR GEOMETRY AND STIFFNESS

To evaluate left ventricular geometry, the left ventricles of
anoxic arrested hearts were rapidly opened and laid flat. The horizontal and vertical dimension of the chamber at its maximal extent
was measured. The maximum vertical dimension was taken as half the
circumference of an ellipse and the horizontal dimension taken as the
circumference of a circle. Both the horizontal and vertical circumference measured in this manner were greater in 24- than 12-month-
old rats. Only the difference in the horizontal circumference was
statistically significant (3). From these measurements left ventricular volume was estimated using a oblate spheroid model of the
left ventricular chamber. Left ventricular wt. was determined by
weighing the septum and the free wall of the left ventricle. There
was a 35% increase in left ventricular volume as estimated in this
manner (p < .001) and a 13% increase in left ventricular wt. p <
.001 (Fig. 5). Left ventricular wall thickness was then estimated
for the ventricular model by evenly distributing the left ventricular muscle mass around the idealized oblate spheroid ventricle.
The average left ventricular wall thickness thus estimated showed
no difference between these two groups (Fig 6). Thus the amount

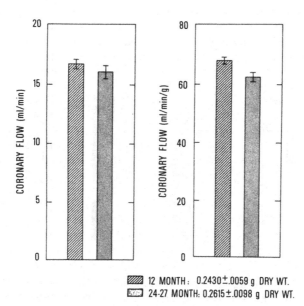

12 MONTH: 0.2430±.0059 g DRY WT.
24-27 MONTH: 0.2615±.0098 g DRY WT.

Figure 4. Coronary flow (left) and coronary flow per g
dry heart wt. (right) for the same hearts shown in Figures 1
through 3. There was no statistically significant difference in
total coronary flow per heart but the coronary flow expressed per
g dry heart wt. was statistically significantly lower in the older
hearts (p < .01). Mean ± S.E. shown.

of left ventricular hypertrophy seems only sufficient to maintain
left ventricular wall thickness constant. In view of the Laplace
relationship, the dilated heart of the old rat with the larger left
ventricular volume would need to generate greater wall tension at
any given level of intraventricular pressure. Since average wall
thickness remained constant, the wall tension per unit cross sectional area would increase. Such an increase in total wall tension
and wall tension per unit area would increase myocardial oxygen
demand and increase the amount of force which must be generated at
any given level of external pump function. In addition, as Burch
(9) has pointed out, the dilated heart has an additional disadvantage during contraction in that the radius decreases less for
any given stroke volume during ejection. Thus the normal decline
in wall tension during ejection of blood from the ventricle would
be less in the old heart than the young. This would again augment contractile and oxygen demands of the heart. Thus these
changes in ventricular geometry may also, at least in part, account for age related changes in pump function.

    Left ventricular stiffness was evaluated in terms of the

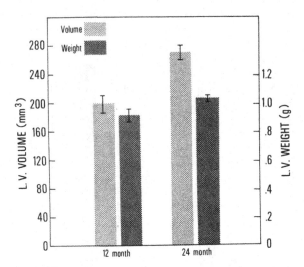

Figure 5. Estimated left ventricular volume and wt. in hearts from 12- and 24-month-old male rats (for methods see text). Both left ventricular wt. and left ventricular volume are greater in the hearts from the older rats (p < .01). The increase in the estimated volume is relatively greater than the increase in estimated wt. in the older group. Mean ± S.E. shown.

resting length-tension curve of trabeculae carneae from the left ventricles of rats of varying age (7). Muscles were mounted between clamps and maintained under isometric conditions. The lower end of the muscle was fixed to the bottom of the bath and the upper end was fixed to the end of the force transducer. The muscles were bathed in Krebs-Ringer bicarbonate solution containing 300 mg % glucose and maintained at 37°C and were paced at a rate of 3 beats/ min. Fig. 7 shows an idealized isometric twitch and reviews the terminology utilized in describing parameters of this isometric twitch. Resting tension to which we will be referring in these studies of muscle stiffness is the force per unit of cross sectional area measured prior to the stimulus and is a function of the length of the muscle. Contractile performance of this preparation and the inotropic responsiveness is indicated by the magnitude of peak de- veloped tension above the resting level during contraction and the maximal rate of rise of tension (dT/dt). Such a twitch is also characterized by the time to peak tension which is the time from the stimulus artifact to peak developed tension and the relaxation time which is the time from peak developed tension to the return of ten- sion to the resting level. RT 1/2 is the time for developed ten- sion to fall from the peak level of 1/2 the peak level.

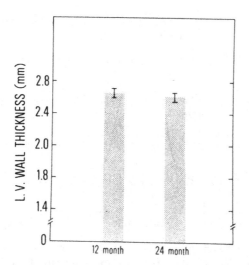

Figure 6. The estimated left ventricular wall thickness in
hearts from 12- and 24-month-old rats (for methods see text).
There was no significant difference in estimated wall thickness
between hearts in these two age groups. Mean $\pm$ S.E. shown.

Figure 8 relates muscle length expressed as a percentage of
L_0. L_0 is the length of the muscle at zero resting tension. The
length of all muscles was increased by increments of 5% at 4 min
intervals. Resting tension was statistically significantly greater
in the muscles from the senile rats at lengths greater than 115%
of L_0. The small numbers indicate the number of muscles at each
point. Thus there is greater resting stiffness in the older muscles.
The simultaneously obtained active length-tension curves are shown
in Fig. 9. Peak developed tension in these trabeculae carneae
paced at a rate of 3 beats/min is related to muscle length. The
increase in active or developed tension with increases in muscle
length reflects the dependence of active tension on muscle length
in cardiac muscle: that is, the Frank-Starling relationship.
The active tension developed did not differ between the age groups
at any point in time. The muscle length at which peak active tension occurred did not differ between the two groups. This suggests
that the differences in resting stiffness noted on the previous
resting length-tension curve is not attributable to an age difference in relative muscle length, when muscle length at zero resting
tension is used as the reference length.

Other studies were performed which examine the stress relaxa-

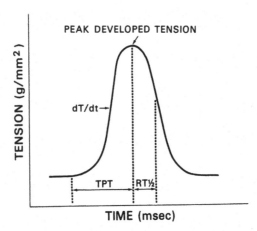

Figure 7. Idealized recording of tension in a rat trabeculae
carneae under isometric conditions. The resting tension is the
tension prior to electrical stimulation or the onset of contraction.
TPT indicates the time from stimulation to the peak developed tension
during contraction. The RT 1/2 is the half relaxation time or the
time taken for tension to fall from the peak value to one half of
the peak value. The total relaxation time (not indicated here) is
the time from the peak developed tension to the return of tension
to the resting level.

tion or time related viscous stiffness changes in resting cardiac
muscle with age using similar preparations. Biological substances
show a fall in tension after a sudden change in length which is
linearly proportional to the logarithm of time. This is similar
to changes in tension that occur with time after rapid stretch in
high molecular wt. rubber polymers. In Fig. 10 is shown tension
versus time after rapid stretch for groups of 11- to 12- and 25-
to 29-month-old muscles. These muscles were stretched so as to
result in the same average tension 4 min after the time of rapid
stretch. The magnitude of the fall in tension of over the 4 min
period was significantly greater in the muscles from young animals
than the muscles from old animals. Thus the muscle from the old
animals exhibits less stress relaxation or change in stiffness with
time. Thus there is less (or at least a slower) adaptation of
cardiac muscle to a change in muscle length in the senile animal.
This decrease in stress relaxation could at least in part account
for the age changes in the resting length-tension curve.

The changes in the resting viscous and elastic stiffness of
cardiac muscle with age would have considerable importance in terms

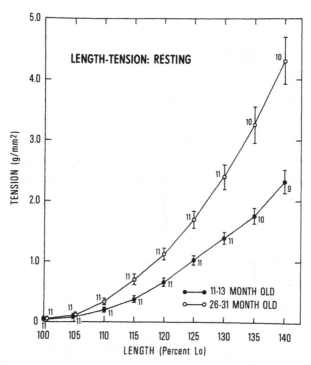

Figure 8. Resting length-tension curves in isometric rat trabeculae carneae from 11- to 13-month- and 26- to 31-month-old male rats. Tension is expressed in g/mm^2 cross-sectional area. Small numbers indicate the number of values at each point. Significant differences are present at lengths greater than 115% of L_0 (p < .01). Mean ± S.E. shown (By permission (7)).

of the overall left ventricular function if similar changes are present across the entire left ventricular wall. Under physiological stress the Frank-Starling mechanism is utilized to augment left ventricular functionn. At any given position along the active length-tension curve a stiffer ventricle would necessarily have a higher filling pressure or left ventricular end diastolic pressure. In addition the reduced stress relaxation of the myocardium of the old rat would mean that with a sudden stress requiring the use of the Frank-Starling mechanism a higher left ventricular filling pressure would be maintained for a longer period of time in the old animal. This longer period of maintenance of an elevated end diastolic pressure would increase the tendency toward symptomatic congestive failure as a result of pulmonary vascular congestion.

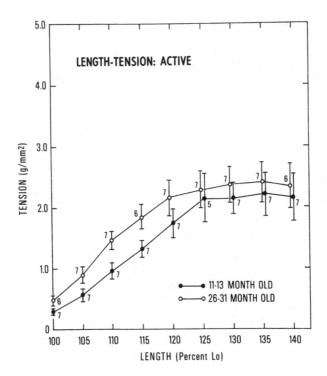

Figure 9. Active length-tension curves from muscles shown in Figure 8. Values from four of the muscles were not included as of spontaneous contractions occurred after increases in muscle length. There is no significant difference in these two groups in active or developed tension at any length examined. Mean ± S.E. shown (By permission (7)).

Studies within the past few years by Templeton and his associates (10) demonstrate very clearly that in isolated muscle preparations and in the intact heart there is a direct relationship between the resting elastic stiffness and the viscous stiffness properties of the myocardium and the elastic and viscous properties of the myocardium during contraction. This is an area of current investigation. If these observations of Templeton are also applicable to the aging heart they may provide a functionally important mechanism which may compensate in part for an age associated decrease in intrinsic contractile ability of the myocardium. If the elastic and viscous stiffness are greater in the old heart during contraction as they are in resting muscle then less energy would be expended by the contractile element of the aging heart in stretching the elastic elements in series with the contractile elements. This may provide an explanation for the apparent discrepancy between the age associated decrease in myosin-ATPase activity noted by Alpert, Gale and Taylor (11) in aging rat and the

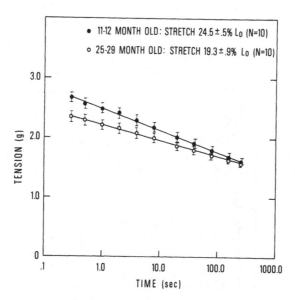

Figure 10. Resting tension after rapid stretch of muscles from 11- to 12-month- and 25- to 29-month-old male rats plotted as a function of the logarithm of time after rapid stretch. Stress relaxation or the magnitude of fall in tension over the four min period of observation was greater in the muscles from the younger animals (p < .01). The experiment was conducted so that muscles from both old and young rats had the same mean resting tension at the end of the four min period. Mean $\pm$ S.E. shown. (By permission (7).

maintenance of the ability to develop tension under isometric conditions. These studies of Alpert were not performed on rats from the same colony. These speculations with regard to the whole heart and the series elasticity point to the need for further studies.

INTRINSIC CONTRACTILE FUNCTION

Alpert et al. (11) and Weisfeldt et al. (7) demonstrated no age associated decrement in the ability of the isolated rat trabeculae carneae to develop force under isometric conditions (Fig. 9). But these two groups of investigators noted that the time for peak tension to be reached after electrical stimulation was significantly prolonged in muscles from older rats (Fig. 11). The latter group also noted that duration of relaxation was longer as is the total duration of systole (the sum of the time to peak tension and the relaxation time, Fig. 11). Investigators utilizing indirect techniques in man have found that the duration of isometric contraction and relaxation is longer in the aged human (12). It has been suggested that this prolongation of relax-

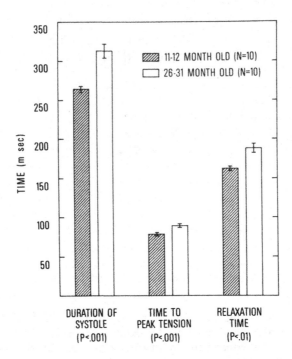

Figure 11. Duration of systole, time to peak tension, and total relaxation time in hearts from 11- to 12- and 26-31-month-old male rats studied at 37°C and the rate of 3 beats/min. Intervals were significantly longer in the muscles from the older rats. Mean ± S.E. shown.

ation is due to changes in the passive visco-elastic properties of cardiac muscle reflecting a slower return of such viscous elements to their original length. Alternatively these changes may be due to alterations in mechanisms which control the duration of tension development and the time course of relaxation of the contractile element. Also, it is well known that depletion of myocardial catecholamines by pharmacologic agents prolongs the duration of contraction. Since it has been shown by a number of groups that aged myocardium is characterized by catecholamine depletion, the prolongation of contraction may be due to catecholamine depletion. Therefore, studies were undertaken to confirm that contraction duration is prolonged in the aged myocardium and to examine whether these changes result from prolongation of the time course of the active state of cardiac muscle during contraction (possibly as a result of catecholamine depletion) or altered passive properties.

The isolated rat left ventricular trabeculae carneae preparation was again utilized (13). All studies were performed at the length

at which contractile tension was maximal (L_{max}). Cross-sectional
area of the trabeculae used averaged 0.9 mm^2 and did not differ
between the age groups examined. The temperature of the bath was
29°C and the Krebs-Ringer bicarbonate solution was modified by
decreasing the calcium concentration to 1.0 mM and the magnesium
concentration to 0.6 mM. These muscles were paced at a rate of 24
beats/min. Fig. 12 shows the active tension at L_{max} measured in

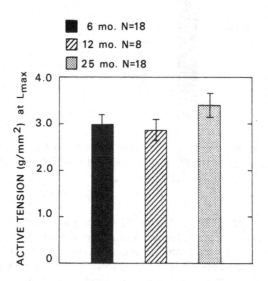

Figure 12. Active tension at L_{max} in muscles from 6-, 12-,
and 25-month-old rats at 29°C and rate of 24 beats/min. There was
no significant difference between any of the age groups. Mean $\pm$
S.E. shown.

g/mm^2 cross-sectional area, for 6-, 12-, and 25-month-old rats
under baseline conditions. There was no statistically significant
difference between these groups. It should be noted that as in
all previous series (most under somewhat differing conditions) the
tension developed by the 25-month-old rats is slightly but statistically significantly greater than that developed by the younger rats. Fig. 13 shows dT/dt, the maximal rate of tension development in the isometric twitch, at L_{max} expressed in units of g/mm^2
cross-sectional area per sec in muscles from the three age groups.
There was no significant age associated change. Contraction duration which is the sum of the time to peak tension and the half relaxation time for the same groups of muscles is presented in Fig. 14.
The prolongation of contraction duration in the 25-month-old group

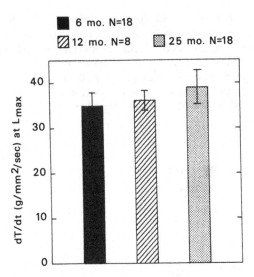

Figure 13.   dT/dt at L$_{max}$ in the same muscles shown in Figure
12. There was no significant difference in dT/dt between any of
the groups studied. Mean ± S.E. shown.

reflects both a prolongation of the time to peak tension and the
half relaxation time. There is no significant difference between
the mature six-month-old rat and 12-month-old rat, but there is
a significant prolongation of contraction in the senile 25-month-
old rat. Thus cardiac muscle from the senile rat shows no deterioration of the ability to generate force or in the peak rate of
force development. But, there is prolongation of the entire time
course of the contraction in the muscle from the old animal.

Total catecholamine content was measured in hearts from 6-,
12-, and 25-month-old rats using a modification of the method of
Von Euler and Lishajko (14). There was little decline in catecholamine content per heart between 6 and 12 months of age (Table 1)
but the content declined substantially between 12 and 25 months
of age. Examined per g heart wt., these differences were statistically significant when comparing the 6- or 12-month-old group
and the 25-month-old group. Thus catecholamine depletion could
at least in part account for the prolonged contraction duration
in the aged myocardium.

To examine this possibility trabeculae carneae were studied
under control conditions and after 1×10^{-6} M dl-propranolol was
added to the bathing fluid. This concentration of propranolol was
sufficient to result in a 50% reduction in the response to 1×10^{-6} M

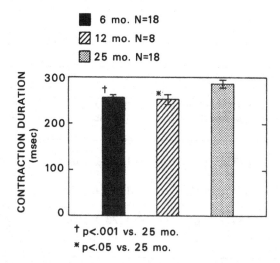

†p<.001 vs. 25 mo.

*p<.05 vs. 25 mo.

Figure 14.   Contraction duration (TPT plus RT 1/2) for the
same muscles shown in Figures 12 and 13. There was stastistically
significant prolongation of contraction duration in the 25-month-
old group and no significant difference between the 6- and 12-
month-old group. Mean ± S.E. is shown.

norepinephrine. The addition of propranolol tended to decrease
contraction duration in both age groups (six and 25 month) but
the decrease was not statistically significant. A statistically
significant prolongation of contraction duration was again present
under the control conditions and after blockade with propranolol
(Fig. 15). To further test the hypothesis that catecholamine
depletion may account for prolongation of contraction duration
in aged myocardium, muscles were studied after depletion of tissue
catecholamines with 6 hydroxydopamine using the technique of
Roberts (15). With this regimen catecholamines were depleted
by 95% in control animals and 97% in the aged animals. The muscles
from 6 hydroxydopamine depleted animals also demonstrated no age
difference in either active tension or dT/dt at L_{max}. Contraction
duration was again significantly prolonged in the older group.
Thus although depletion of myocardial catecholamines appeared
to occur with age, this depletion does not appear to account for
the prolongation of contraction duration in muscles from aged
animals.

We next examined whether the prolongation of contraction duration was due to prolongation of the time course of the active state
or due to changes in the passive visco-elastic properties of the
muscle. Initially, we measured the electrical and mechanical
refractory period of trabeculae carneae to a second electrical

TABLE I

MYOCARDIAL CATECHOLAMINE CONTENT

Age (Mos.)	No.	Total Catecholamine (µg/Heart)	Heart Wt. (grams)	µg Catecholamine Per gm Heart Wt.
6	10	.693 ± .057	1.27 ± .022*	.569 ± .063*
12	11	.687 ± .040	1.50 ± .087	.474 ± .040+
25	10	.555 ± .061	1.73 ± .097	.325 ± .037

* $P < .01$ vs. 25 mo

+ $P < .05$ vs. 25 mo

stimulation. The mechanical refractory period is the shortest interval between electrical stimuli which induces a distinct second
mechanical contraction. In the left panel in Fig. 16 the second
stimulus results in a second mechanical event. If the interval
between stimuli is shortened to below the mechanical refractory
period there is no second mechanical event as in the two panels
on the right. The failure to produce a second mechanical response
may be a function of the electrical refractory period if there is
no second depolarization (as in the center panel) or a function of
the extent of restoration of intracellular calcium release sites
if there is a second depolarization without a second mechanical
event as seen on the far right of this figure. Mainwood and Lee
(16) have suggested that prolongation of the mechanical refractory
period in the absence of prolongation of the electrical refractory
period is a form of electro-mechanical dissociation due to delayed
recovery of calcium release sites. Delayed recovery of mechanical
contractile ability on this basis would likely indicate delayed
calcium removal from the active contractile proteins and thus prolonged active state or delayed relaxation.

The composite results of studies of the mechanical refractory
period of 6-, 12-, and 25-month-old rats are shown in Fig. 17.
All muscles from all groups responded to the second stimulus when

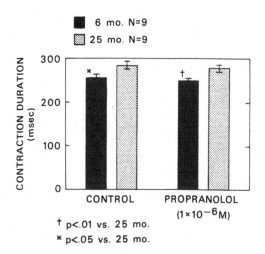

† p<.01 vs. 25 mo.

* p<.05 vs. 25 mo.

Figure 15. Contraction duration of muscles from 6- and 25-month-old male rats before and after blockade with 1 X 10 M dl-propranolol. The prolonged contraction duration persisted after propranolol blockade. Mean + S.E. shown.

the coupling interval was 300 or 400 msec. Coupled at 200 msec, some of the muscles from the 25-month-old group exhibited no second mechanical event. At 160 msec only one 6- or 12-month-old muscle did not respond and the majority of the 25-month-old animals did not respond. At 80 msec none of the muscles responded. The difference between the oldest group and the 6- or 12-month-old group was statistically significant ($p < .01$) using X^2 analysis. This prolongation of the mechanical refractory period of the cardiac muscle in the aged myocardium could either be due to prolongation of the electrical refractoriness or delayed recovery of mechanical contractile ability as previously discussed. The electrical refractory period of muscles under identical conditions was measured utilizing intracellular recording techniques. The effective electrical refractory period of muscles from the two age groups was not significantly different. The refractory period was 83.3 + 5.6 msec in the 6-month-old group (n = 9) and 86.5 + 5.4 msec in the 25-month-old group (n = 10). The failure of mechanical response to impulses 80 msec apart likely represents electrical refractoriness. Age differences in the mechanical refractory period at interstimulus

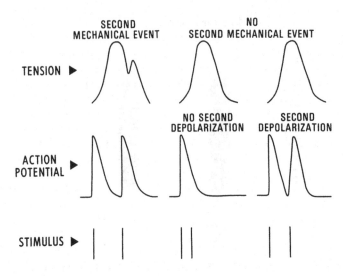

Figure 16. Chart of idealized responses to paired stimulation.
Shown are the isometric tension above, the intracellular action
potential in the center, and the stimulus artifact below. On the
far left, the second stimulus is sufficiently after the first
stimulus to result in a second action potential and a second
mechanical response on the tension trace. In the center the stimulu
occurs early enough to result in is neither an action potential or
a second mechanical event. On the right, is shown paired stimulation with an interval between the stimuli such that there is a
second action potential noted but no second mechanical event. As
shown in Figure 17 findings similar to that on the far right of
this figure occurred at longer interstimulus (coupling) intervals
in the muscles from the oldest rats.

intervals of 120 and 200 msec cannot be attributable to prolongation
of effective electrical refractory period, but appear to be a result
of delayed recovery of calcium release sites in muscles from the
old rats. These studies thus suggest that delayed calcium removal
from the contractile proteins explains delayed relaxation.

Supporting this conclusion are additional data which we obtained during exposure of similar muscles to hypoxia and reoxygenation. The period following hypoxia has been shown to be one characterized by a marked prolongation of the duration of contraction
and particularly prolongation of the duration of relaxation. This
prolongation is felt to be due to inhibition of sarcoplasmic reticulum function and thus delayed calcium removal from the contractile

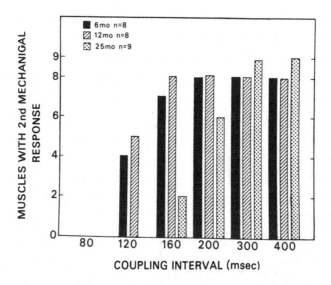

Figure 17. Occurrence of a second mechanical response during
paired pacing with coupling intervals between 400 and 80 msec. As
the coupling interval was shortened, the 25-month-old rats failed
to respond to the second stimulus sooner. For discussion, see text.

element. Measurements of force development during hypoxia and recovery from hypoxia and the rate of tension development under these
conditions of hypoxia and recovery from hypoxia showed no age differences. In contrast there were significant age differences in
the contraction duration during recovery from hypoxia (Fig. 18).
There was no significant age difference in contraction duration expressed as percent control during hypoxia but during reoxygenation
the prolongation of contraction duration above the original control level was significantly greater in the muscles from the older
rats. These differences are expressed as percent of the baseline
values which are longer in the older muscle groups. In terms of
absolute prolongation the age differences are even more striking.

These studies support the notion that cardiac relaxation is
abnormal in the aged heart due to delayed calcium uptake by the
relaxing system. In view of the short duration of the action
potential of the rat and the absence of plateau during phase 2,
it seems very unlikely that the prolongation of contraction duration and the delayed relaxation is due to prolonged calcium entry
or to prolonged calcium release from intracellular sites following electrical stimulation. The electro-mechanical disassociation
at short coupling intervals suggests instead that at short cou-

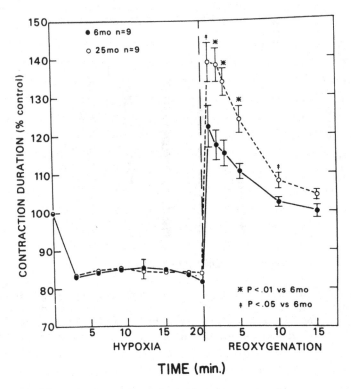

Figure 18. Contraction duration expressed as a percent of
the control value for 6- and 25-month-old rats subjected to
hypoxia and reoxygenation. Expressed as a percent of the control
value, contraction duration was not significantly different between these two groups during hypoxia but during reoxygenation
a significantly greater prolongation of contraction duration was
noted in the muscles from the older rats. Mean ± S.E. shown.

pling intervals there is inadequate time to recharge intracellular
releasing sites for calcium. The prolonged time to recharge these
sites could be due to delayed calcium removal from the contractile
protein or to delayed calcium movement from an intracellular storage
to an intracellular release site. The prolonged contraction duration under baseline conditions in the aged myocardium suggests that
the delay occurs in the removal of calcium from the contractile
proteins itself. These studies thus suggest that delayed relaxation is a result of age changes in the functional capacity of the
cardiac sarcoplasmic reticulum. With the sarcoplasmic reticulum
under the stress of recovery from hypoxia an even greater delay

in relaxation is observed. Another possible but less likely mechanism would be tighter binding of calcium to the contractile proteins.

In summary, we have demonstrated that contraction duration is prolonged in aged myocardium and that this prolongation is due to both prolongation of the tension development and the relaxation time. This prolongation cannot be explained totally by changes in the visco-elastic properties but must reflect some alteration in the active state or the active contractile properties of cardiac muscle. Catecholamines are known to enhance the rate of relaxation of cardiac muscle. Although depletion of catecholamines does occur in the aged myocardium from this colony, it does not appear that catecholamine depletion can account for the prolonged contraction duration of aged myocardium. The results of these studies suggest rather strongly that delayed calcium removal from the contractile proteins in the aged heart accounts for the prolonged contraction duration and relaxation.

Prolonged contraction duration is a disadvantage to the organism since under stress, when the heart rate is rapid, prolonged contraction duration would compromise ventricular filling and may result in incomplete relaxation between beats. Such incomplete relaxation has been shown to occur in animal models (17) under conditions in which contraction duration is prolonged. Incomplete relaxation results in a higher left ventricular end diastolic pressure and a higher pulmonary venous pressure and thus a greater tendency for symptomatic congestive failure in the intact organism. Thus it appears that age changes in the myocardial function are attributable at least in the rat, to specific age changes in ventricular geometry, left ventricular stiffness, and the intrinsic contractile mechanism. The studies of Dr. Lakatta and associates (18) provide additional information to suggest that decreased inotropic response to catecholamines may be another very important, physiologically significant mechanism for the decrease in cardiac performance of the intact heart with age. The applicability of these observations to other species and particularly to man is uncertain and awaits study.

REFERENCES

1. Rothbaum, D. A., D. J. Shaw, C. S. Angell, and N. W. Shock. J. Gerontol. 28:287 (1973).
2. Weisfeldt, M. L., J. R. Wright, D. P. Shreiner, E. Lakatta, and N. W. Shock. J. Applied Physiol. 30:44 (1971).
3. Shreiner, D. P., M. L. Weisfeldt, and N. W. Shock. Am. J. Physiol. 217:176 (1969).
4. Lee, J. C., L. M. Karpeles, and S. E. Downing. Am. J. Physiol. 222:432 (1972).

5.   Rakusan, K. and O. Poupa. Gerontologia 9:107 (1964).
6.   Tomanek, R. J. Anat. Rec. 167:55 (1970).
7.   Weisfeldt, M. L., W. A. Loeven, and N. W. Shock. Am. J.
     Physiol. 220:1921 (1971).
8.   Travis, D. F. and A. Travis. J. Ultrastructure Res. 29:124
     (1972).
9.   Burch, G. E. Arch. Internal Med. 96:571 (1955).
10. Templeton, G. H., T. C. Donald, III, J. H. Mitchell, and L. L.
     Hefner. Am. J. Physiol. 224:692 (1973).
11. Alpert, N. R., H. H. Gale, and N. Taylor. In: Factors In-
     fluencing Myocardial Contractility. (Eds.) F. Kavaler, R. D.
     Tanz, and J. Roberts, Academic Press, New York, p. 127.
12. Harrison, T. R., K. Dixon, R. O. Russell, Jr., P. S. Bidwai,
     and H. N. Coleman. Am. J. Heart 67:189 (1964).
13. Lakatta, E. G., G. Gerstenblith, C. S. Angell, N. W. Shock,
     and M. L. Weisfeldt. J. Clin. Invest. In press.
14. Von Euler, U. S. and F. Lishajko. Acta Physiol. Scand. 51:
     348 (1961).
15. Roberts, J. Fed. Proc. 33:459 (1974).
16. Mainwood, G. W. and S. L. Lee. Science 166:396 (1969).
17. Weisfeldt, M. L., P. Armstrong, H. E. Scully, C. A. Sanders,
     and W. M. Daggett. J. Clin. Invest. 53:1626 (1974).
18. Lakatta, E. G., G. Gerstenblith, C. S. Angell, N. W. Shock,
     and M. L. Weisfeldt. Circulation Res. In press.

CHANGES IN CARDIAC MEMBRANES AS A FUNCTION OF AGE WITH PARTICULAR EMPHASIS ON REACTIVITY TO DRUGS

Jay Roberts and Paula B. Goldberg

Departments of Pharmacology
The Medical College of Pennsylvania
Philadelphia, Pennsylvania 19129

INTRODUCTION

The effects of senescence on the electrophysiological behavior of cardiac tissue have not been studied extensively or
systematically. Yet there is a scattered number of reports indicating that the functioning of the cardiovascular system in
general, and the physiology of the myocardium in particular undergo very subtle yet profound changes with increasing age. The
age effects have been observed both in man and in other mammals.
The normal human myocardium of subjects 50 to 70 years of age
not suffering from degenerative changes or ischemia has been found
to display such electrocardiographic alterations as prolongation
of the P-R interval and QRS complex duration (1). In a group
of normal, healthy humans, the P-R interval was found to increase
progressively from birth through 60 years and over (2). Another
study showed that young adults (mean age for men, 34 years, and
mean age for women, 23.5 years) had shorter left ventricular
ejection times than subjects of 60 years and older (3). Unan-
esthetized Wistar rats have been reported to exhibit increased
heart rates, decreased blood pressures, and decreased cardiac
outputs with increasing age (4). Electrocardiographic changes
and increased incidence of arrhythmias have been reported in aged
rats under control conditions (5,6) and following exercise (7).

That the electrophysiological characteristics of heart muscle
undergo age related alterations is suggested not only by physiological data, but also by observations of striking changes in
reactivity to cardiac and vascular drugs (8). An increase in
the probability of untoward reactions and of cardiotoxicity to

digitalis in elderly patients has been noted (9-11). On the other
hand, the sensitivity to atropine in older patients is apparently
diminished (12). In animals, the lethality of acetylcholine,
epinephrine, and norepinephrine have been reported to increase
with age (13).

In view of the foregoing observations and the paucity of
electrophysiological data regarding the effects of aging on cardiac
membranes and their sensitivity to drugs, the studies herein to
be described were instituted.

METHODS AND RESULTS

A. Characterization of Animals

1. Life Span

Our studies were carried out using CD Fisher strain rats
as the test animals. These rats are bred and supplied by Charles
River Laboratories specifically for research in aging. The maximum
life span of these animals approaches three years. There is 100%
survival up to about 22 months of age; after this time, life
expectancy begins to decrease. The mortality rate increases very
sharply after 24 months, so that only about 50% of the animals
survive 28 months and less than 25% survive 30 months (Gibson,
personal communications). Because of availability and expense,
we decided to use 28-month-old rats as the oldest animals in our
study.

2. Animal Condition

In order to be certain that the changes we observed were
related to the aging process _per se_ rather than to some other
phenomena concomitantly occurring, background data was accumulated
for the rats. Of special interest to us were data on the heart,
vasculature, and kidneys. This consisted of observations of
general appearance of the animal, body wt., organ wt., and pathology and histopathology at all the ages studies.[1] As a consequence we have been able to characterize the CD Fisher rat for
several parameters.

a. Body Weight. Figure 1 shows changes in body wt. of rats
occurring with increasing age. It can be seen that body wt. continues to increase at a rapid pace up to one year of age before

---

[1]Pathology and histopathology studies performed by Drs. Richard
J. Montali and John D. Strandberg of the Department of Pathology,
John Hopkins University Medical School, Baltimore, Maryland.

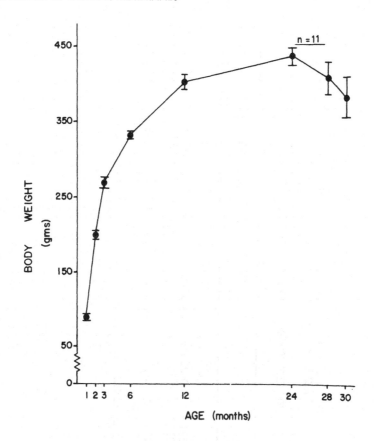

Figure 1. Body wt. of CD Fisher strain rats as a function of age. The ordinate represents the wt. in g and the abscissa the age in months. Each point represents the average of 11 animals. S.E.M. is indicated by the vertical lines.

leveling off and remaining fairly constant thereafter through 30 months. This observation has significance in terms of all studies carried out with rats. For this particular strain of rat, body wt. ranges from about 330 to 430 g for the ages from six through 28 months. Selecting animals on the basis of body wt. alone, therefore, could very well lead to erroneous results by bringing into play an age factor which would be completely masked and unaccounted for.

b. Heart Weight. Because our particular interest is in the function of the heart, we deemed it important to know what happens to the wt. of this organ as the animal ages. The results of our observations are shown in Figure 2. In contrast to total body wt., heart wt. does not change drastically after three months.

TABLE I

RELATIONSHIP OF HEART WEIGHT TO BODY WEIGHT IN THE RAT

AGE (months)	1	2	3	6	12	24	28
Ratio $\dfrac{\text{Heart weight}}{\text{Body weight}}$	0.507 ±0.01	0.321 ±0.01	0.335 ±0.01	0.307 ±0.02	0.297 ±0.02	0.308 ±0.01	0.321 ±0.02
	N = 9*	N = 7	N = 12	N = 9	N = 10	N = 11	N = 7

* $P < 0.05$

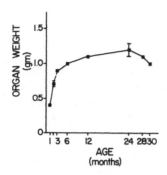

Figure 2. Heart wt. of CD Fisher strain rats as a function
of age. The ordinate represents the wt. of the heart in g and
the abscissa represents the age in months. The values represent
the average of 11 hearts. S.E.M. is indicated by the vertical
lines. The absence of vertical lines indicates values smaller
than the symbol used.

The ratio of heart wt. to total body wt. was also calculated for
all ages of rats. The results appear in Table I, where it can
be seen that although small fluctuations do occur, the ratio does
not change significantly with increasing age; the exception of
a high value at one month being attributable to the extremely
low wt. of the rats at their age.

        c. Abnormalities. The pathology and histopathology studies
on hearts from our animals (unpublished findings) revealed the
following changes: at three months of age, there was a significant
incidence of focal myocarditis which increased with age; by 12
months, evidence of fibrosis appeared, which also increased with
age; necrotic changes appeared in only a few animals.   Hearts
were found to be relatively free of other disease through 24 months
of age. There did appear to be an increase, however, in ventricular collagen as the rats aged. The coronary vasculature did
not show any arteriosclerotic or atherosclerotic lesions.

                    B. Age Effects on Heart Rate

        We then studied cardiac function by several techniques, both
in vivo and in vitro, to determine what changes occur with increasing age, the level at which changes occur, and the effect
of severe pharmacological agents used in cardiovascular therapy
as a function of age.

1. Heart Rate In Vivo

     As a first step, we determined the heart rate of rats in
vivo in all age groups. To do this, an animal was placed in a
holder and two needle electrodes were inserted under the skin.
The electrodes were connected through appropriate amplifiers to
a polygraph. After an interval of acclimitization, a cardiac
electrogram was recorded and heart rate determined. The results
are shown in Figure 3.

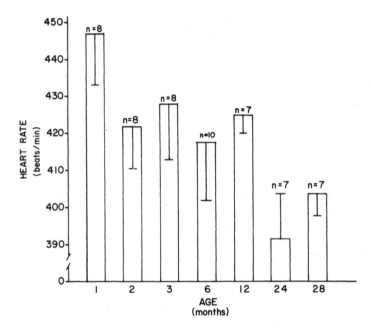

     Figure 3. Heart rate of rats in vivo. The number of ob-
servations are indicated above each bar. The vertical lines
represent the S.E.M. The ordinate is in beats/min and the
abscissa is age in months.

One-month-old rats had the fastest rates, the mean being 447 +
14 beats/min. The two-month-old rats through the 12-month-old
rats had somewhat lower rates, but these were not significantly
different from those in the one-month-old animals (two months
= 422 + 12 beats/min; three months = 428 + 15 beats/min; six months
= 417 + 15 beats/min; 12 months = 425 + five beats/min). The
heart rates of the 24-month-old rats were significantly lower,
as compared to rates of one-month-old rats, being the lowest
of all other age groups (24 months = 391 + 12 beats/min). The
28-month-old animals had a mean heart rate (404 + six beats/min)

that was not significantly different than the mean rate of the one- through 12-month-old animals.

2. Heart Rate In Vitro

In the in vivo situation, the autonomic nervous system, as well as endocrine hormones play a role in modulating cardiac activity. It was thought possible, therefore, that the observed decrease in heart rate in the 24-month-old animals and absence of rate changes at other ages could be caused by alterations in neuro-endocrine activity. To evaluate the effects of age on pacemaker activity in the absence of autonomic and endocrine influences, spontaneous rates were determined in isolated perfused heart preparations. The animals used for this phase of the study were the same as those in which in vivo heart rate was determined. Following the recording of a stable electrogram, the animals were sacrificed by decapitation, their hearts immediately removed, and the latter mounted for retrograde perfusion through the coronary arteries by the method of Langendorff. Stainless steel electrodes were attached to the left ventricle and to each atrium, and the electrogram was recorded on a polygraph.

a. Intact Isolated Heart. The preparation was allowed to stabilize until a constant rate was established (usually 30 min); this was recorded as the intrinsic rate of the preparation. The results of this study are summarized in Figure 4. It can be seen that the spontaneous rate of the isolated Langendorff preparation is lower than the in vivo rate for the corresponding age (compare Figures 3 and 4). The mean initial rates of the isolated hearts were as follows: one month = 355 $\pm$ nine beats/min; two months = 325 $\pm$ eight beats/min; three months = 328 $\pm$ eight beats/min; six months = 291 $\pm$ seven beats/min; 12 months = 278 $\pm$ seven beats/min; 24 months = 232 $\pm$ six beats/min; and 28 months = 225 $\pm$ seven beats/min. Moreover, the spontaneous rate of the isolated heart underwent a progressive diminution with increasing age (except for comparable rates in the two- and three-month-old groups). These data strongly suggest that in the absence of autonomic and hormonal influences there is an age associated decrease in heart rate in the CD Fisher strain rat.

b. A-V Blocked Isolated Heart. In the normal course of events, the myocardium is driven by the sino-atrial pacemaker. However, other cardiac tissue of the conducting system is capable of initiating spontaneous activity when the atrial pacemaker fails. We proceeded, therefore, to evaluate the effects of age on ventricular pacemakers as well. For this purpose, heart block was produced surgically by ligation of the A-V conducting bundle in the Langendorff preparation described above (see Methods and Results, B, 2). In this way, atrial pacemaker activity, as well

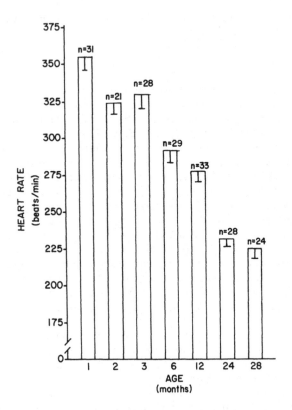

Figure 4.   Initial rate of hearts isolated from rats of
different ages. The ordinate represents beats/min while the
abscissa represents age in months. The number of observations
is indicated above the bar and the S.E.M. is indicated by the
vertical lines.

as that of the ventricular pacemakers could be observed in the
same preparation simultaneously under the same experimental conditions. Perfusion and monitoring of the isolated tissue continued
for 30 min, during which time interval the atrial and ventricular
pacemakers became equilibrated. Figure 5 is a polygraph recording
of the electrogram of a 12-month-old heart in which A-V block
was surgically induced. During the control period (before block),
both the atrial and ventricular rates were 296 beats/min, indicating that the ventricle was following the atrial pacemaker.
After heart block, the atrial rate re-equilibrated at 261 beats/
min. The ventricular rate of 65 beats/min was significantly slower
than that of the atrium, and indicated that the ventricle had
now established its own independent rhythm.

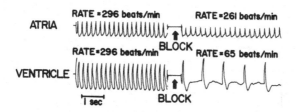

Figure 5. Tracing of recorded electrogram from atrium and
ventricle in an isolated heart with A-V block. The record is
of a heart isolated from a 12-month-old animal. The arrows indicate the point at which A-V dissociation was produced by surgical
means. Note the differences in atrial and ventricular rates.

Hearts with A-V block were perfused for periods of up to
two hr and the atrial and ventricular rates recorded at five-min
intervals. Figure 6 summarizes the results for hearts from three-
month-old rats. The atrial rate was remarkably constant for the
entire two-hr period. Ventricular rate showed somewhat greater
fluctuations, but was not significantly different from 100% (initial ventricular rate immediately following heart block) at
any of the five-min recording periods except at 60 min; the difference here possibly being significant because of the small
standard error. Figure 7 shows the results for hearts from 24-
month-old animals. Similar graphs were obtained for hearts of
rats at all ages. The results indicate that atrial and ventricular
pacemakers remain very stable for extended periods of time regardless of the age of the animal from which the heart is isolated.

As stated previously, the purpose of the A-V block experiments
was to evaluate the effects of age separately on atrial and ventricular pacemakers. Once we determined that the blocked heart
remained stable for long periods of time, we evaluated the data
in terms of initial atrial and ventricular rate after heart block
was induced at all ages studies. These results are shown in
Figures 8 and 9. The initial atrial rate after complete heart
block, shown in Figure 8, was not significantly different among
the one- through three-month-old animals (one month = 309 $\pm$
eight beats/min; two months = 290 $\pm$ eight beats/min; three months
= 285 $\pm$ eight beats/min; $p > 0.05$). The atrial pacemaker rate
decreased significantly in the six month group (270 $\pm$ seven beats/
min). Atrial pacemaker rate showed further progressive and significant decreases in the 12- through 28-month-old groups (12
months = 237 $\pm$ six beats/min; 24 months = 212 $\pm$ five beats/min;

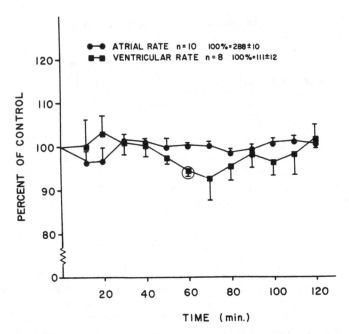

Figure 6. Stability of pacemaker rates during perfusion
of isolated hearts (from three month animals). The ordinate
is pacemaker rate expressed as percent of control; the control
rate is indicated in the upper right hand corner of the graph,
as is the number of observations. The abscissa represents the
time after perfusion with Krebs-Ringer solution was initiated.
The vertical lines represent the S.E.M. The circled value is
significantly different from 100%.

28 months = 203 $\pm$ eight beats/min; p < 0.05). The initial ventricular pacemaker rates (cf Figure 9) followed a somewhat different pattern with increasing age. Ventricular pacemaker rates
were similar for the first six months (one month = 121 $\pm$ eight
beats/min; two months = 115 $\pm$ eight beats/min; three months =
109 $\pm$ seven beats/min; six months = 103 $\pm$ six beats/min; p >
0.05). The rates decreased significantly at 12 months of age
(12 months = 97 $\pm$ five beats/min; p < 0.05), and thereafter showed
a further significant decrease at 24 months (90 $\pm$ four beats/min;
p < 0.05). Ventricular rate at 28 month (89 $\pm$ five beats/min)
was similar to that at 24 months. Comparing ventricular pacemaker
rates to atrial pacemaker rates showed that ventricular rates
were slower than atrial rates in all age groups by some 57 to
75%.

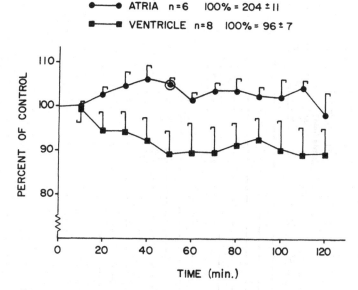

Figure 7. Same as figure 6 except the hearts were isolated
from 24-month-old animals.

3.   Effects of Drugs on Heart Rate

     The above results prompted us to investigate the sensitivity
of the heart to several pharmacological agents, some of which
have clinical usefulness in the geriatric patient suffering from
heart disease.

     a.   Quinidine. First we investigated the effect of quinidine
on atrial and ventricular pacemakers in the Langendorff heart
with A-V block. Quinidine sulfate was perfused in a concentration
of 10 mg/L (expressed as the free base), at a rate of 25 ml/min.
Control atrial and ventricular rates were obtained over a period
of 30 min after A-V block was induced; then quinidine perfusion
was initiated. Quinidine produced a rapidly developing decrease
of both atrial and ventricular rates, the maximum depression of
pacemakers occurring within 50-60 min after the start of perfusion.

     The depressant effects of quinidine were observed in hearts
isolated from animals aged one through 24 months. Results are
presented in Figure 10, with the effect expressed as percent
depression in rate as compared to the period just prior to quinidine
perfusion. The atrial rate was decreased by approximately 40-60%
in the hearts of animals aged one-12 months, with no significance

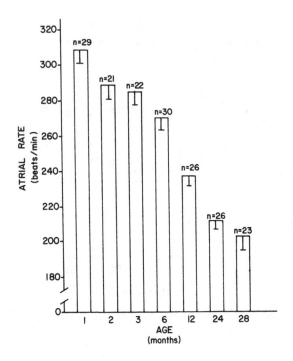

Figure 8. The atrial rate of isolated perfused hearts after
A-V block. The ordinate represents rate in beats/min; the abscissa
the age of the rats from which the hearts were isolated. The
number of observations are noted above each bar and the vertical
lines represent the S.E.M. Rate of six months < at one month,
$p < 0.05$; rates at 24 and 28 months < at 12 months, $p < 0.05$.

in the degree of depression over this age range being apparent.
However, in the older animals, i.e., those aged 24 months, the
degree of depression in atrial rate was not as great, being only
about 30%; this is significantly lower than in the younger groups
($p < 0.05$). Moreover, the depressant effect on atrial rate was
readily reversible, as the rates returned to control values after
washout of drug with Krebs-Ringer solution.

Quinidine also produced a significant depression of ventricular pacemakers in hearts isolated from animals of all age groups
included in this part of the study. This too is shown in Figure
10. Ventricular rates were generally decreased to a greater extent
than atrial rates, the differences being significant in one- and
three-month-old hearts. The greatest depression of ventricular
rate occurred in the younger animals (one month = 83%; two months

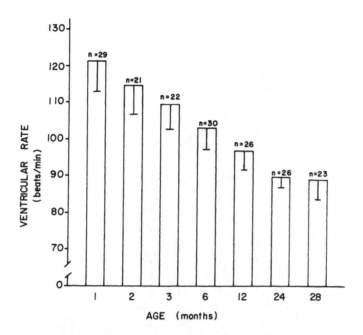

Figure 9.   Same as figure 8 except the rates are those of
the ventricular pacemaker. Rates decreased progressively but
only those at 12, 24, and 28 months were significantly lower
than at one month, $p < 0.05$.

= 69%; three months = 76%). The degree of depression continued
to decrease progressively, reaching a minimum at 24 months, (six
months = 61%; 12 months = 51%; 24 months = 33%), at which point
it was equivalent to that in the atrium.

Another indication of the greater susceptibility of the
ventricle to quinidine was the development of periods of asystole.
In contrast to the effect of quinidine on atrial pacemakers, in
the ventricle asystole did occur during the period of perfusion
with this agent. The incidence of ventricular asystole decreased with increasing age (one month = 5/9; two months = 3/8; three
months = 2/6; six months = 1/6; 12 months = 0/6; 24 months = 0/6)
in a manner similar to the decreased depressant effect on rate.
This effect of quinidine on ventricular pacemakers was found to
be reversible, both in terms of reversal of asystole and in restoration of control rate after removal of drug from the perfusion
medium.

b. 6-Hydroxydopamine. Although it appeared that changes
in pacemaker function per se were responsible for rate changes
related to age, in the intact animal the sympathetics may play

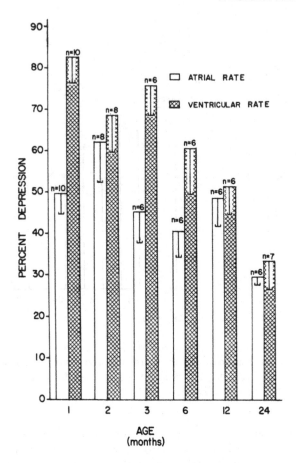

Figure 10. The effect of quinidine on pacemaker rates in
the isolated heart with A-V block. The ordinate represents the
percent depression of the rate due to quinidine (10 mg/L) and
abscissa the age of the animals from which the hearts were isolated. The number of observations are noted above the bar and
the vertical lines represent the S.E.M. Percent depression of
the atrial rate in the 24 month group was lower than in one-12
month groups, $p < 0.05$; percent depression of ventricular rate
in six and 12 month groups was lower than in one-three month
groups, $p < 0.05$, and still lower in the 24 month group, $p <$
0.05. In the one and three month groups, percent depression
of ventricular rate was significantly greater than atrial rate
depression, $p < 0.05$.

a modulating role, especially as evidenced by the observations
that in the isolated heart there were age related changes (see
Methods and Results, B, 2, a). To determine if this occurs,
experiments were carried out with animals of all age groups in

whom chemical sympathectomy had been induced. It is now well
established that 6-hydroxydopamine (6-OHDA) produced a relatively
specific and complete chemical sympathectomy of the heart (14).
To accomplish this in our rats, 6-OHDA was administered subcutaneously in a dose of 20 mg/Kg, 24 hr prior to the experiment.
On the next day, the in vivo heart rate was determined in un-
anesthetized animals as described above (see Methods and Results,
B, 1).

The results of the effect of chemical sympathectomy on heart
rate in vivo are summarized in Figure 11.

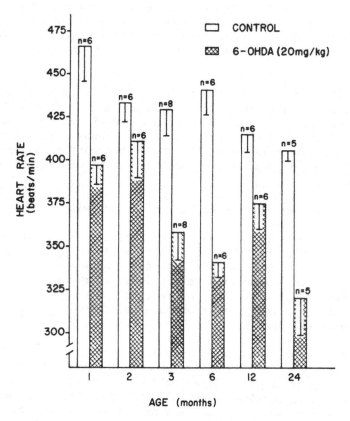

Figure 11. The effect of 6-OHDA pretreatment on the heart
rate of the intact rats. 6-OHDA, 20 mg/Kg, was injected subcutaneously 24 hr prior to the experiments. The ordinate represents the rate in beats/min; the abscissa represents the age of
the rats. The number above each bar is the number of animals
and the vertical line is the S.E.M. Rate after 6-OHDA significantly lower than controls (p < 0.05) at all ages except two and
12 months.

It can be seen, first, that in the control groups of rats in this
study, heart rate was similar at all ages studied, including at
24 months (as opposed to a small, but significantly lower rate
at 24 months in the group depicted in Figure 3). Secondly, the
results show that 6-OHDA pretreatment significantly decreased
heart rate in all the age groups, except at two months. The degree
by which 6-OHDA decreased the heart rate was not the same at all
the ages studied. Depression of rate was least in the two-month-
old animals (5.2%, N.S.[2]) and in the 12-month-old animals (9.9%,
N.S.). At the other ages, the decrease in heart rate due to
6-OHDA-induced sympathectomy was significantly greater (one month
= 15.8%; three months = 16.3%; six months = 22.6%; 24 months =
21.2%). Thus, there appears to be an age related effect on heart
rate produced by chemical sympathectomy. This supports the argument that in the intact animal neuro-endocrine factors may influence the heart rate in such a way as to mask age related differences.

It should also be emphasized that in hearts isolated from
animals pretreated with 6-OHDA, the atrial and ventricular rates
(not shown in Figures) were similar to those of hearts taken from
untreated animals in the corresponding age groups. This indicates
that acute sympathectomy by isolation of the heart or by pretreatment with 6-OHDA are similar, at least in terms of influence on
heart rate.

C. Age Effects on Electrical Activity

Another aspect of the study on the effects of age on cardiac
function involved experiments to determine electrophysiological
properties of the membrane. The objectives here also were two-
fold: firstly, to characterize electrical properties of cardiac
muscle during the life span of the rat; and secondly, to determine
the effect of the aging process on cardiac tissue sensitivity
to pharmacological agents.

In these experiments, right and left atrial preparations
were employed for recording of transmembrane electrical activity.
Conventional intracellular microelectrode recording techniques
were used to obtain action potentials. In addition, the fast
upstroke of the action potential was differentiated to obtain
the rate of rise (dV/dt) of phase 0 and the maximum velocity
(V_{max}).

---

[2]Statistically not significant.

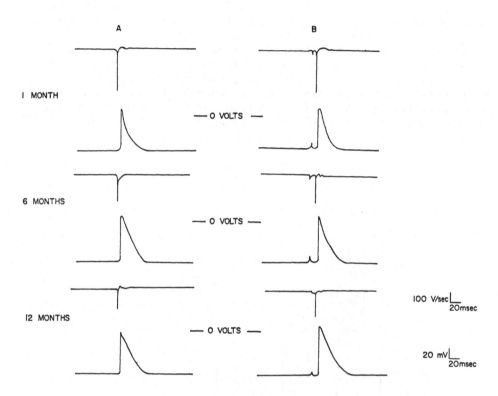

Figure 12. Tracings of transmembrane action potentials recorded in atrial fibers from rats of 1 month, six months, and
one year of age. Tissue used in panel A is driven intrinsically
(SA node) while that in panel B is driven extrinsically (stimu-
lator). Top trace at each age is a recording of rate of rise of
phase 0 of the action potential (dV/dt). Bottom trace in each
panel is a recording of a typical action potential for that age
group. Calibrations are indicated in lower right-hand corner of
figure. Each panel is marked with a zero potential reference
line. Rates of tissues in panel A are one month = 229 beats/min;
six months = 165 beats/min; 12 months = 108 beats/min while tissues
in panel B are paced at 200 beats/min. Stimulus artifact pre-
cedes recording in each trace in panel B. Reproduced by permission of the American Journal of Physiology.

1. Action Potential Configuration

Figure 12 shows characteristic action potentials and their
corresponding rates of rise of phase 0 in spontaneously beating
right atria (column A) and electrically driven left atria (column
B) from a one-, six-, and 12-month-old animal. The points to
be noted are that in both spontaneous and driven preparations,
the maximum rate of rise of phase 0 decreases, the plateau phase
becomes more prominent and prolonged, and repolarization is
delayed with increasing age. On the other hand, the resting
potential, the amplitude of the action potential, and the magnitude
of the overshoot of the action potential are not effected.

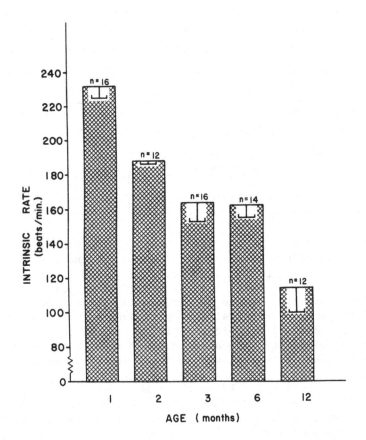

Figure 13. Differences in intrinsic rates of atria isolated
from rats of different ages. Number of animals in each age group
is designated by n. S.E. is indicated with each mean. Reproduced
by permission of the American Journal of Physiology.

Initially, our studies were carried out on right atria, which contracted spontaneously because they contained sino-atrial nodal tissue. In these preparations we noted that spontaneous rate decreased with increasing age. This is shown in Figure 13. Although the spontaneous rates of these preparations, at each age, were lower than the initial atrial rates of the Langendorff preparations at the corresponding ages (compare to Figure 8), the pattern of decline with increasing age was strikingly similar.

It has been shown in atrial tissue that the frequency at which depolarizations occur play a significant role in determining the duration of the action potential (15). Since our spontaneous preparations exhibited a decrease in rate with increasing age, we wanted to determine whether this mechanism was responsible for the increased plateau duration and repolarization time we observed with increasing age. To do this, we isolated left atria, which are devoid of tissue capable of initiating spontaneity, and recorded electrical activity while stimulating at a constant rate of 200 per min. In Figure 12, it can be seen that the action potential configuration change exhibited by the driven tissue underwent changes similar to those exhibited by the spontaneous tissue of the same age. These data would seem to rule out rate effects as being responsible for the prolongation of the action potential and support the contention that it is an age related phenomenon.

A summary of all the data obtained for spontaneous and driven atria appears in Table II.[3] The properties that showed significant change with increasing age were the maximum rate of rise of phase 0 of the action potential, the duration of the plateau, and re-polarization time (measured as the time to 95% repolarization). The values are similar for both spontaneous and driven atria, and the change is in the same direction (i.e., V_{max} decreasing, plateau duration increasing, and repolarization time increasing with increasing age). As indicated earlier, neither the resting potential, the action potential amplitude, nor the overshoot size changed significantly with age in either the driven or spontaneously beating atria. Our observations on driven left atria have now been extended to include those isolated from animals 24- and 28-months-old. The results indicate that electrical properties not affected through 12 months continue to be unaltered in animals 24- and 28-months-old, whereas those that were modified do not appear to show further changes beyond those observed in the animals of 12 months of age.

---

[3] Reproduced by permission of the American Journal of Physiology.

TABLE II

COMPARISON OF MEMBRANE ACTION POTENTIALS FROM RAT ATRIA OF DIFFERENT AGE GROUPS
(Values are given as mean ± standard error)

Age	Heart Rate (beats/min)	Resting Potential (mV)	Amplitude (mV)	Overshoot (mV)	Maximum Rate of Rise (V/sec)	Plateau Duration (msec)	Time to 95% Repolarization (msec)
1 Month (n=8) (I)	232 ± 8	66 ± 3	73 ± 3	9 ± 1	458 ± 10	6 ± 1	52 ± 4
1 Month (n=6) (E)	200	71 ± 2	83 ± 2	11 ± 1	445 ± 9	4 ± 1	51 ± 2
2 Month (n=6) (I)	188 ± 4	80 ± 2	89 ± 2	9 ± 1	412 ± 15	4 ± 1	56 ± 4
2 Month (n=6) (E)	200	78 ± 2	88 ± 2	9 ± 1	401 ± 13	5.3 ± 2	60 ± 2
3 Month (n=8) (I)	164 ± 11	83 ± 1	93 ± 1	10 ± 1	342 ± 11	10.6 ± 1	63 ± 2
3 Month (n=5) (E)	200	82 ± 4	90 ± 4	8 ± 1	308 ± 7	9.5 ± 1	63 ± 1
6 Month (n=7) (I)	162 ± 7	80 ± 2	89 ± 2	10 ± 1	258 ± 13	15 ± 2	73 ± 3
6 Month (n=7) (E)	200	82 ± 3	91 ± 3	9 ± 1	253 ± 10	15 ± 2	72 ± 2
1 Year (n=6) (I)	114 ± 14	73 ± 2	81 ± 2	8 ± 1	226 ± 11	17 ± 2	71 ± 3
1 Year (n=6) (E)	200	73 ± 2	82 ± 2	6 ± 1	221 ± 24	16 ± 1	67 ± 4
* Significance of comparison of mean values: 1 Month vs. 6 Months Probability		N.S.	N.S.	N.S.	$p < .001$	$p < .001$	$p < .001$
* Significance of comparison of mean values: 1 Month vs 1 Year Probability		N.S.	N.S.	N.S.	$p < .001$	$p < .001$	$p < .001$

Symbols: I = intrinsically paced tissue   N.S. = not statistically significant   msec = millisecond
         E = extrinsically paced tissue   mV = millivolt   V/sec = volts per second
         n = number of animals tested   * Refers to either I or E paced tissue

2. Effect of Drugs on Electrical Activity

After having established, as a function of age, the basic physiological patterns of the electrical properties of cardiac muscle, our interest focused on how the action of agents which are used to treat arrhythmias in geriatric patients may be modified by age. We proceeded to determine the alterations of the action potential of left atrial (driven) preparations induced by several pharmacologically active agents. We tested lidocaine, quinidine, and propranolol, all of which are clinically useful antiarrhythmic drugs whose basic actions have been characterized by analyzing their effects on the membrane action potential.

a. Lidocaine. Lidocaine, five mg/L, did not appear to have any effect on the resting membrane potential of atria at any age. It did depress the action potential amplitude by some four-20% over the entire age range (one- to 28-month-old animals); however, this depression did not prove to be significant in terms of relation to age. The maximum rate of rise of phase 0 of the action potential was also depressed (15-33%), but again, this decrease was not age related (see Table III). On the other hand, depression of the size of the overshoot of the action potential and prolongation of the plateau duration and time to 95% repolarization were found to be age related (see Table IV). The action potential overshoot was depressed by lidocaine by 24-77% over the entire age range, the depression being significantly greater in the two-, six-, and 28-month-old atria as compared to the three-month-old group. In many instances, after lidocaine the overshoot was completely abolished. The incidence of the lack of an overshoot was greatest in the 12- and 28-month-old groups. Lidocaine increased the plateau duration by six-120% over the entire age range, the increase being greatest in the six- and 12-month-old groups. The action potential duration was increased by seven-82% over the entire age range, the greatest increases being in the six-, 12-, and 28-month-old animals.

b. Quinidine. With respect to quinidine, (five mg/L), we found it had no effect on the resting potential, action potential amplitude, size of the overshoot or plateau duration (see Table III). Quinidine depressed the maximum rate of rise of phase 0 of the action potential and membrane responsiveness[4] and prolonged repolarization time. Only the effect on membrane responsiveness

---

[4]Membrane responsiveness is a property relating the ability of an excitable cell to propagate a normal action potential at different levels of membrane polarization. It is customarily measured by the size of the maximum rate of rise (V_{max}) of phase 0 of an action potential interposed before a cell is completely repolarized from a previous action potential so that the membrane potential is less negative than resting potential.

TABLE III

EFFECT OF AGE ON MYOCARDIAL SENSITIVITY TO ANTIARRHYTHMIC DRUGS
(Properties not affected by age)

Property (Compared to Control)	Drug	Age of Rat (Months)						
		1	2	3	6	12	24	28
Resting Potential	Lidocaine	0	0	0	0	0	0	0
	Quinidine	0	?	?	0	0	0	?
	Propranolol	0	?	0	0	0	0	?
Action Potential Amplitude	Lidocaine	−	−	−	−	−	−	−
	Quinidine	0	?	?	0	0	0	?
	Propranolol	0	?	0	0	0	0	?
Rate of Rise of Phase 0	Quinidine	−	?	?	−	−	−	?
	Propranolol	−	?	−	−	−	−	?
Action Potential Duration	Quinidine	+	?	?	+	+	+	?
	Propranolol	+	?	+	+	+	+	?
Plateau Duration	Quinidine	+	?	?	+	+	+	?
	Propranolol	+	?	+	+	+	+	?

Legend   Symbols:
  Drug concentrations in perfusate: 0 = no effect
    Lidocaine - 5 mg/L   − = decrease
    Quinidine - 5 mg/L   + = increase
    Propranolol - 1 mg/L   ? = data inconclusive or
                                                      as yet unavailable

appeared to be age related, the depression being greatest in the
younger atria and decreasing with increasing age (see Table IV).

     c. Propranolol. Propranolol was perfused at a concentration
of one mg/L. It increased repolarization time by 85-100% and
decreased maximum rate of rise of phase 0 by 55-70%; however,
these effects did not appear to be age related (see Table IV).
Propranolol had no effect on any other parameters measured.

     Table IV summarizes the changes in reactivity of atria to
lidocaine and quinidine that were age related; Table III summarizes the properties that either were not affected by lidocaine,
quinidine, and propranolol or were affected equally at all ages.
The important implications of this study appear to be that sensitivity to drugs changes with age, and that the changes are not

TABLE IV

EFFECT OF AGE ON MYOCARDIAL SENSITIVITY TO ANTIARRHYTHMIC DRUGS
(Properties affected by age)

Property (Compared to Control)	Drug	Age of Rat (Months)						
		1	2	3	6	12	24	28
Overshoot of Action Potential	Lidocaine	-	---	-	---	--	---	---
Rate of Rise of Phase 0	Lidocaine	-	--	-	-	-	-	-
Action Potential Duration	Lidocaine	0	-	+	++	+++	+	++
Plateau Duration	Lidocaine	0	-	0	++	++	+	+
Membrane Responsiveness	Quinidine	--	?	?	0 to +	-	0	?

Legend
Drug concentrations in perfusate:
   Lidocaine - 5 mg/L
   Quinidine - 5 mg/L

Symbols: 0 = no effect
            - = small decrease
           -- = moderate decrease
          --- = large decrease
            + = small increase
           ++ = moderate increase
          +++ = large increase
            ? = data inconclusive or as
                yet not available

in the same direction for all drugs. In general, of the three
agents tested, lidocaine showed increased activity, quinidine
showed decreased activity, and propranolol showed no change of
activity with increasing age.

DISCUSSION

The results of this study demonstrate that heart rate decreases with increasing age. Furthermore, decreases in heart
rate as animals age is due primarily to some basic change in
pacemaker cells proper rather than to changes in the influence
of chemical mediators. In the intact animal, sympathetic influences may have varying effects on heart rate at different age
levels, which may be manifested in different ways depending on
animal species and conditions of observations. This is borne
out by the divergent findings in some instances of heart rate

increases (4), decreases (1,2), or no significant changes (see
Methods and Results, B, 1; Figure 3). That chemical mediators
play a role in modulating heart rate is also illustrated by our
findings of slower rates in isolated heart preparations (compare
Figures 3 and 4). Furthermore, in the absence of sympathetic
tone produced by isolating the heart or pretreating the animals
with 6-OHDA, a decrease in heart rate with increasing age becomes
apparent (Figure 11). That decreased pacemaker activity is most
likely responsible for decreased heart rate observed with increasing age is further illustrated by the pattern of independent
atrial and ventricular rates (Figures 8 and 9). In the A-V blocked
heart preparations, both the atrium and ventricle showed decreased
rates in the older animals. It may be argued that isolated hearts
are only acutely denervated preparations and may still contain
viable nerve terminals (16), so that spontaneous liberation of
transmitter might occur and thereby influence the basic rate.
However, this would seem unlikely since such nervous activity
would be random and asynchronous, and would therefore not represent
a major rate determinant. Such activity may be linked to miniature
end-plate potentials at the neuromuscular junction, which are
generated by spontaneous random leakage of acetylcholine from
nerve terminals; yet they do not result in action potentials of
muscle cells. Only when a propagated action potential in a motor
nerve leads to synchronous liberation of acetylcholine does a
full size end-plate potential result and a muscle action potential
is generated.

The mechanism for decreasing pacemaker activity as animals
age is as yet not clear. Pacemaker activity in automatic tissue
has been attributed for the most part to a time- and voltage-
dependent decrease in potassium conductance relative to sodium
conductance during the same time period, i.e., during the phase
of slow diastolic depolarization (17-19). If the observed age
related decreases in pacemaker rate are indeed due to direct
changes in membrane function, they are most likely caused by an
enhancement of the factors responsible for the potassium conductance as the animal ages. Further study is required in order
to characterize these factors and their behavior as a function
of age.

Microelectrode techniques for measuring transmembrane electrical activity have revealed several interesting points. We
find, with increasing age, that the maximum rate of rise of phase
0 of the action potential decreases, and the plateau duration
as well as the phase of repolarization become prolonged (Figure
12, Table II). It is believed that the fast upstroke phase of
the action potential is largely due to a very fast inward sodium
current and a somewhat slower calcium current (21,20), whereas
the plateau and repolarization phases are determined to a great

extent by slow calcium and potassium currents (22,23). Our results
suggest that the fast currents (or channels) are somehow reduced
(either in number or in functional activity) as evidenced by
diminishing rates of rise, while the slow currents (or channels)
become enhanced, as indicated by the prolongation of the plateau
and repolarization phases with increasing age of the animal.
The modification of these two properties (decreased V_{max} and
increased plateau and repolarization duration) as the animal ages
would also lead to slower intrinsic pacemaker rates, and our data
bear this out. Perhaps voltage-clamp methods or manipulation
of external ionic environment is needed to aid in describing
the fundamental changes in the membrane as it ages.

It has been observed that the heart becomes more susceptible
to arrhythmia with increasing age (see Methods and Results).
That the heart may become more vulnerable to arrhythmia as an
organism grows older is also suggested by our findings that both
atrial and ventricular pacemakers decreased in activity with
senescence. The capacity of a pacemaker cell to drive the heart
is related to its rate compared to other sites. Generally, the
fastest pacemaker will be dominant. Since the atrial pacemaker
was found to be greatly slowed during the aging process, its
capacity to overdrive latent ventricular pacemakers diminishes,
leading to an increased potential for the development of arrhythmia. Such a mechanism is consistent with the reported propensity
toward the development of rhythm disturbances in older hearts
(5,6).

Another important determinant of cardiac rhythm is impulse
conduction velocity. Conduction velocity is largely determined
by the rate of rise of the action potential. In our study we
found that the maximum rate of rise of the action potential decreased as the animals grew older (Table II). As a consequence,
conduction velocity would also be expected to decrease with increasing age. In such a setting the normal pacemaker, whose rate
has also been found to decrease with age, would be expected to
have even more difficulty in driving the heart. Indeed, with
slowing or blockade of conduction, re-entrant arrhythmias of
various kinds may develop (24-26).

We have studied the effects of age on the sensitivity of
myocardial tissue to drugs for two reasons: one, by using drugs
whose mechanism of action at the cellular level was known to some
extent, we could possibly gain some insight into the changes of
the membrane with increasing age; and two, to gain some information
about the possible usefulness of antiarrhythmic drugs in the
geriatric patient.

Lidocaine is a drug which finds wide clinical applications

in treatment of arrhythmias. Its antiarrhythmic properties are
generally attributed to its ability to increase membrane potassium
conductance in conducting tissue, thus slowing the rate of diastolic depolarization (27). In conducting tissue, it has also
been found to increase the rate of repolarization, and in high
concentrations to decrease the maximum rate of rise of the action
potential (28). Ventricular fibers show an increase in the duration of the refractory periods and a decreased maximum rate of
rise of the action potential, but these effects usually become
apparent with high concentrations of drugs (28). Such actions
would be consistent with an interference with both fast sodium
channels and slow potassium channels. In our study on atrial
tissue, lidocaine was found to affect the maximum rate of rise
of the action potential, the amplitude of the action potential,
the size of the overshoot, the plateau duration and time to 95%
repolarization. The first two properties were decreased equally
at all ages (Table III); however, the effect on the last three
properties appeared to vary with age (Table IV). The increased
degree of depression by lidocaine on the action potential overshoot
would suggest that it has a special depressant effect on calcium
currents which seem to be involved in the latter phase of the
depolarization process (21). Inasmuch as lidocaine also increased
the duration of the plateau and repolarization time with increasing
age, it may be that it prolongs the calcium and potassium currents
responsible for maintaining the plateau, as well as the late
potassium currents responsible for repolarization as the animal
ages.

It is interesting to note that not all drugs whose action
is to produce antiarrhythmic effects are modified by age necessarily in the same way. In contrast to lidocaine, whose effect
on many phases of the action potential increased with increasing
age, quinidine appeared to show decreased effectiveness with age
in altering membrane responsiveness (See Methods and Results,
C, 2, b). Quinidine has been reported to slow the rate of depolarization and conduction velocity of the action potential and
prolong the phase of repolarization (29-31). Such actions are
linked intimately to the sodium carrier activation system and
the activity of Na+K activated ATPase. The reason for the decreased effectiveness of quinidine on membrane responsiveness
with increasing age is obscure; it may be that there is a decrease
in the availability of sodium carriers with aging. Furthermore,
since membrane responsiveness is voltage-dependent, it would be
determined in part by the duration of repolarization. Since the
repolarization phase is increased to the same extent by quinidine
at all ages studied, the effect on membrane responsiveness is
most likely due to its greater effect on sodium reactivation
with increasing age.

Quinidine has been shown to decrease both atrial and ventricular pacemaker rates, with its effect occurring to a greater extent at the ventricular site (Methods and Results, B, 3, a). This was somewhat surprising in view of previous reports that the intensity of quinidine action in rabbit and cat hearts is rate-dependent; that is, the faster the rate, the greater the effect (31,32). According to this, the effect of quinidine would have been expected to be greater on the faster atrial pacemakers. The deviant effect may be due to species variation. An alternate explanation may be that the distribution of quinidine in the heart is not uniform, with more of the drug concentrating in the ventricle. We have evidence that there is an increase in collagen in the ventricle and an increased incidence in myocarditis and fibrosis as rats age. Such changes may account for increased quinidine concentration in the extracellular space of ventricle, and may indeed contribute to the increased incidence of arrhythmia as aging proceeds. With respect to the slowing effect on pacemakers within the same tissue, the action of quinidine was as expected, i.e., decreased effectiveness with increasing age. In atrial and ventricular pacemakers, the degree of depression brought about by quinidine decreased with increasing age (Figure 10), paralleling the decreasing intrinsic rate of the pacemaker with increasing age (Figures 8 and 9).

Another point of interest regarding the decreased sensitivity of the ventricular pacemaker to quinidine as the animal ages refers to its clinical implications. If this occurs in man, the administration of quinidine in the geriatric patient to depress ventricular arrhythmia might not be too successful since it may require doses of drug which will at the same time depress the normal pacemaker. Under these circumstances, restoration of normal sinus rhythm would be difficult to achieve.

The action of propranolol in producing its antiarrhythmic effects have been reported to be similar to that of quinidine (33,34). Yet in the rat atrium, its effects on the membrane action potential was found to be equivalent at all ages (Table III). Although comparable concentrations to those producing the effects in other species were used, it may be that the rat atrium is particularly resistant to propranolol. A more likely alternative, however, is that aging affects drugs of a given type differently. Again, this may be due to differences in drug distribution or may reflect age related differences on the cardiac membrane.

In conclusion, the use of basic physiologic techniques coupled with the use of pharmacologic agents have revealed striking changes in the electro-physiological behavior of cardiac muscle as the animal ages. Several suggestions for future experimentation are now apparent and with these experiments more definite characterization of the status of cardiac membranes in animals as a func-

tion of age whose hearts are free of atherosclerosis will be revealed. These studies should provide further insight into the
nature of the aging process in general.

SUMMARY

    The effects of aging on myocardial membranes were investi-
gated in CD Fisher strain rats by several in vivo and in vitro
techniques. In the intact non-anesthetized animals, heart rate
did not appear to change dramatically with increasing age. In
isolated heart preparations, intrinsic pacemaker rates decreased
with increasing age, regardless of whether rate was monitored
in the whole isolated preparation or in preparations with surgical-
ly-induced heart block. Furthermore, chemical sympathectomy with
6-OHDA unmasked an age related decreasing heart rate in the in
vivo situation but failed to alter the age versus rate relationship in the isolated heart situation. These data indicate that
age associated changes in heart rate are due to basic alterations
in the membrane of the pacemaker itself and that in vivo, neuro-
endocrine influences may mask the expression of such changes.

    Additional evidence for age related changes occurring in
cardiac membranes is presented from microelectrode recordings of
atrial action potentials. Changes observed to occur by this
technique with increasing age are: decreased maximum rate of rise
of phase 0 of the action potential; increased duration of plateau
and repolarization phases.

    Changes in sensitivity to drugs with increasing age were
studied. The depressing effect of quinidine was found to be more
pronounced on ventricular pacemakers than on atrial pacemakers.
In atrial single cell recordings of action potential, quinidine
depressed membrane responsiveness. Quinidine's effect was greatest in heart from young animals and decreased with increasing age.
In contrast, the effect of lidocaine on the action potential of
atrial cells generally increased with increasing age. Propranolol,
whose mechanism of action is thought to be similar to that of
quinidine, produced equivalent effects at all ages studied.

    The consequences of the observed functional changes in the
heart as well as of the alterations in the sensitivity of the
heart to drugs as the animal ages were discussed with reference
to the possible mechanisms underlying membrane changes and the
clinical implications of using antiarrhythmic drugs in geriatric
patients.

ACKNOWLEDGEMENTS

This work was supported by Program Project Grant # HD 06267.

The authors gratefully acknowledge the technical assistance of Sylvan Hemingway and Sallie Stoner.

REFERENCES

1. Shah, G. B., S. R. Shah, and H. C. Merchant. Indian Heart J. 20:278 (1968).
2. Cheraskin, E. and W. M. Ringsdorf. J. Amer. Geriatric Soc. 19:271 (1971).
3. Willems, J. H., J. Roelandt, H. DeGeest, H. Kesteloot, and J. V. Joossens. Circulation 42:37 (1970).
4. Rothbaum, D. A., D. J. Shaw, C. S. Angell, and N. W. Shock. J. Gerontol. 28:287 (1973).
5. Berg, B. N. J. Gerontol. 10:420 (1955).
6. Everitt, A. V. Gerontologia 2:204 (1958).
7. Jones, D. C., G. K. Osborn, and D. J. Kimeldorf. Gerontologia 13:211 (1967).
8. Bender, A. D. J. Amer. Geriatric Soc. 12:114 (1964).
9. Raisbeck, M. J. Geriatrics 7:12 (1952).
10. Wilson, G. M. In: Modern Trends in Geriatrics. (Ed.) W. Hobson, Harper and Bros., New York (1957) p. 272.
11. Fine, W. Med. Press (London) 242:4 (1959).
12. Sprague, H. B. In: Geriatric Medicine. (Ed.) E. J. Streglitz, Lippincott, Philadelphia (1954) p. 359.
13. Frolkis, V. V. Farmakol. i. Toksikol. 28:612 (1965).
14. Kostrzewa, R. M. and D. M. Jacobowitz. Pharmacol. Rev. 26:199 (1974).
15. Hollander, P. B. and J. L. Webb. Circ. Res. 3:604 (1955).
16. Blinks, J. R. J. Pharmacol. Exp. Ther. 151:221 (1966).
17. Brown, H. F. and S. J. Noble. J. Physiol. 204:717 (1969).
18. Muller, P. Helv. Physiol. Acta 23:C38 (1965).
19. Trautwein, W. Pharmacol. Rev. 15:277 (1963).
20. Beeler, G. W. and H. Reuter. J. Physiol. 207:165 (1970).
21. Tarr, M. J. Gen. Physiol. 58:523 (1971).
22. Beeler, G. W. and H. Reuter. J. Physiol. 207:191 (1970).
23. deHemptinne, A. Pflugers Arch. 329:321 (1971).
24. Cranefield, P. F., A. L. Wit, and B. F. Hoffman. J. Gen. Physiol. 59:227 (1972).
25. Wit, A. L., P. F. Cranefield, and B. F. Hoffman. Circ. Res. 30:11 (1972).
26. Wit, A. L., B. F. Hoffman, and P. F. Cranefield. Circ. Res. 30:1 (1972).
27. Arnsdorf, M. F. and J. T. Bigger, Jr. J. Clin. Invest. 51:2252 (1972).
28. Davis, L. D. and J. V. Temte. Circ. Res. 24:639 (1969).
29. Johnson, E. A. J. Pharmacol. Exp. Ther. 117:237 (1956).
30. Vaughan Williams, E. M. Brit. J. Pharmacol. 13:276 (1958).
31. West, T. C. and D. W. Amory. J. Pharmacol. Exp. Ther. 130:183 (1960).

32. Nye, C. E. and J. Roberts. J. Pharmacol. Exp. Ther. 152:67 (1966).
33. Davis, L. D. and J. V. Temte. Circ. Res. 22:661 (1968).
34. Pitt, W. A. and A. R. Cox. Amer. Heart J. 76:242 (1968).

CHANGES IN PROTEIN SYNTHESIS IN HEART

J.R. Florini, S. Geary, Y. Saito, E.J. Manowitz, and
R.S. Sorrentino
Biology Department, Syracuse University

Syracuse, N.Y. 13210

Our initial decision to undertake an investigation of protein
synthesis in cardiac muscle as a function of age was prompted by
the conviction that the general question of age related changes in
protein synthesis might usefully be studied in a tissue obviously
essential to the survival of the animal. Heart certainly meets
that criterion, and it offers some other advantages, too. The perfused heart system we selected occupies what is (to us at least) a
satisfying intermediate position between whole-animal studies and
their problems in controlling conditions, and cell-free preparations
with their argueable physiological significance. There was one
small problem at the start of this research; no one had reported
procedures for the perfusion of isolated mouse hearts, but we were
reasonably confident that it would be possible to adapt the standard
rat system we had been using for some time (Florini and Dankberg,
1970) to studies on the mouse heart. Surprisingly, this turned out
to be true.

The central position of protein synthesis in gene expression
has prompted a number of theories regarding the role of this process in senile deterioration. From the error theory of Orgel (1963)
to the codon-restriction theory of Strehler (1971), investigators
have suggested that changes in rates or kinds of protein synthesized
might play major roles in the aging processes. However, when we
first looked into it, a question as simple as the direction of age
related changes in rate of protein synthesis had not reached any
generally-accepted answer; reports that protein synthesis decreased
(Von Hahn, 1966; Short, 1969), remain unchanged (Barrows, 1969;
Lang et al., 1966), or increased (Perry, 1966) were found. Obviously, much of this disagreement could be attributed to differences
in the kinds of measurements made. Furthermore, it is reasonable

149

to assume that not all tissues change in parallel throughout the lifespan of the animal. Finally, there was some suspicion that some of the disagreement resulted from questionable choices of experimental systems, especially the failure to consider possible variations in intracellular amino acid pools and consequent variations in specific activity of the precursors incorporated into proteins. This can be a problem in any rate study when radioisotope tracers are used, but in spite of its widespread discussion, it remains an infrequent part of experimental designs in studies on aging. We resolved that our determinations would include measurements of intracellular specific activities of the labeled precursors, and that the determinations would be done individually for each heart studied. We felt rather virtuous about this, and considered ourselves properly rewarded when variations in leucine pools caused important differences in interpretation of our data in which hearts from young or sexually mature mice were compared with those from retired breeders or mice which had reached the mean lifespan of their strain. However, as you will see, some of that reward has now been withdrawn.

In our experiments, hearts from male C57B1/6J mice were perfused by a variation of the technique of Morgan et al. (1961). The perfusion medium was Krebs-Henseleit bicarbonate buffer equilibrated with O_2 and CO_2 (95:5) and containing unlabeled amino acids at the concentrations found in rat plasma by Scharff and Wool (1965). ^{3}H-leucine (48 Ci/mmole) was added to give a final concentration of 1 μCi/ml; dilution by unlabeled leucine in the medium reduced the final specific activity to 4.33 mCi/mmole, but this was adequate to give count rates of 1000 or more cpm range for all protein samples. Details of sample preparations and counting techniques are presented by Geary and Florini (1972).

As there had been no previous reports on perfusion of mouse hearts, we did some characterization of the system before proceeding to measure changes in incorporation rates with age. Not surprisingly, flow rate through the heart varied with perfusion pressure, and there was some effect of these variations on rate of amino acid incorporation into protein. However, in the approximately physiological range used in our perfusions (60 mm Hg, 8 ml/min), incorporation did not vary with pressure over a range of $\pm$ 10 mm Hg, and hearts continued to beat at the normal rate of about 600 beats/min. Uptake of radioactive amino acid occurred rapidly under these conditions, and incorporation into protein was linear with time for at least one hr; routine perfusions were done for 30 min. In all age groups studied, the labeled precursor was present in large excess (compared to that incorporated into protein) within 5 min and remained so throughout the perfusion period so it seems unlikely that precursor uptake was rate-limiting for protein labeling in any of the perfusions.

As expected ^{3}H-leucine incorporation was quite sensitive to cycloheximide (70% inhibition by 0.25 μg/ml) and insensitive to Actinomycin D (no detectable inhibition at 3 μg/ml). Acid hydrolysis and chromatography of the acid-insoluble fraction indicated that all radioactivity was associated with leucine. We concluded that the mouse heart perfusion system would provide a useful assay for rates of protein synthesis in hearts of animals of various ages.

It is apparent that isotope incorporation data must be corrected for variations in dilution of the labeled precursor upon mixing with unlabeled endogenous precursor; otherwise the radioactivity data do not provide any real information about actual reaction rates. In these studies, we measured specific activity of acid-soluble leucine in samples from each heart individually, so that appropriate corrections could be made. In the first experiments (Geary and Florini, 1972), this was done using an amino acid analyzer to measure amounts of leucine. Subsequently, we used the ^{14}C-fluorodinitrobenzene method of Regier and Kafatos (1971) as modified for one-dimensional thin layer chromatography by Saito and Florini (1973); this facilitated determination of the specific activities of rather large numbers of small samples of acid-soluble fractions containing ^{3}H-leucine. We found that there were substantial changes in amounts of intracellular leucine in mouse hearts with age, and correction for variations in dilution made significant differences in the apparent effects of age (Table 1). However, as will be seen later, it appears that even this laborious and time-consuming determination of precursor specific activity may not give unambiguous measurement of rates of protein synthesis in intact tissues.

Table I summarizes our results in a series of determinations of rates of protein synthesis in normal mice of various ages. It is clear that consideration of the free unlabeled leucine pool in the hearts has a substantial effect on interpretation of the results. If only raw counting data (dpm/mg protein) is considered, it appears that there is a progressive decrease in rate of protein synthesis throughout the lifespan of the animal. However, the free leucine pool is substantially larger in hearts of adult animals; the lower values for specific activity at 8 and 25 months result from changes in the denominator, not the numerator, of the radioactivity/mole leucine ratio at the end of the perfusion. When these changes are considered, protein synthesis does not increase progressively; the levels in young animals are as low as, or slightly lower than in the senile group. In fact, this pattern illustrates the crucial importance of selecting an appropriate group for comparison to old animals. If comparison is made to young mice, it could be concluded that protein synthesis is unchanged or increases, whereas comparison to adult animals (3 months) indicates a substantial decrease in protein synthesis in hearts

TABLE I

EFFECT OF AGE ON ^{3}H-LEUCINE INCORPORATION, INTRACELLULAR SPECIFIC
ACTIVITY, AND PROTEIN SYNTHESIS IN MOUSE HEARTS.*

Mouse Age (Months)	^{3}H-Leu Incorporation (dpm/mg protein)	Average Intracellular Specific Activity (Ci/mole)	Calculated Protein Synthetic Rate (pmoles leu/mg prot.)
	$(\times 10^{-3})$		$(\times 10^{-2})$
1	4.63 ± 0.072	4.74 ± 0.146	4.03 ± 0.098
2.8	3.71 ± 0.063	5.18 ± 0.109	3.20 ± 0.011
8	$2.98 \pm 0/048$	1.15 ± 0.066	13.1 ± 0.25
25	2.22 ± 0.036	1.16 ± 0.073	5.91 ± 0.28

* Hearts were perfused in triplicate for 30 minutes; uptake, incorporation, and
specific activity of ^{3}H-leucine were determined as described by Geary and Florini
(1972). Average intracellular specific activity of ^{3}H-leucine during the perfusion time was calculated from the measured final value and the time course of
^{3}H-leucine uptake into the hearts; it averaged 70% of the final value. Means
are presented here to allow comparisons; however, specific activities of intracellular leucine determined separately for each heart were used to convert incorporation rates into calculated rates of protein synthesis.

of the old animals. The latter seems to us to be more reasonable
choice in gerontological studies. However, these results do not
provide a simple explanation for increased cardiac diseases in old
animals, as the rate of protein synthesis in old animals is at
least as great as that in rapidly-growing young mice. Of course,
the possibility remains that older animals might be less able to
respond to stress which could require elevated rates of protein
synthesis.

To test this hypothesis, we investigated the induction of cardiac hypertrophy in adult and old mice (Florini et al., 1973).
Initially, we hoped to use the aortic constriction techniques we
had used in earlier studies on rats (Florini and Dankberg, 1971),
but we found the surgical problems insuperable in mice. Consequently, we then turned to induction of cardiac hypertrophy by
repeated injections of thyroxine. In a series of range-finding
experiments, we found that adult (8 month) and old (26 month)
mice responded essentially identically when treated with thyroxine
in the range 50 to 200 µg/mouse (30-40 g body wt.) on alternative
days for two weeks. Administration of the hormone each day, or

extension of the treatment period to four weeks, had no effect
on the final heart/body wt. ratio. A maximal response was obtained with doses of 100 μg thyroxine/mouse. Thus the lower
"basal" level of protein synthesis in hearts of older animals had
no apparent effect on ability of these organs to respond to thyroxine stress over a two-week period.

Adelman (1972) has shown that hormonal induction of a number
of liver enzymes exhibits a longer lag period in old rats than in
young rats, although in many cases the same levels are eventually
attained. It occurred to us that this might also be true of cardiac hypertrophy, so we compared the time-course of hypertrophy in
adult and old mice given 100 μg thyroxine on alternate days; the
results are summarized in Figure 1. It is apparent that the adult
animals responded more rapidly than the older mice, although the
latter group achieved equal hypertrophy after 9 days.

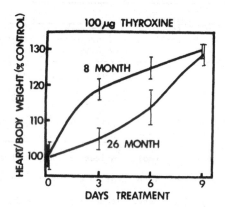

Figure 1. Time course of thyroxine-induced cardiac hypertrophy.
Mice received intraperitoneal injections of 100 μg thyroxine in
0.2 ml 0.9% (w/v) saline - 0.01 M NaOH during the specified number
of days. All mice received either saline-NaOH of thyroxine on days
1, 3, 5, 7, and 9; animals were sacrificed and heart/body wt. ratios
determined as described by Florini et al. (1973). Points are means
of 8 animals in each group and vertical bars are standard errors
of the mean. Heart/body wt. ratios (i.e., 100% values) in control
8-month-old mice were 4.04 ± 0.12, and in 26-month-old mice they
were 4.45 ± 0.16 mg/g. (Reproduced by permission from the Journal
of Gerontology.)

In an attempt to localize the effects of thyroxine on protein
synthesis (as distinguished from changes in breakdown, accumulation
of fat or water, or some other process possibly unrelated to the
differences in protein synthesis we had observed previously), we
measured rates of ^{3}H-leucine incorporation into protein of isolated perfused hearts from mice treated with thyroxine for various
times. The results are summarized in Table II; large changes in
rates of protein synthesis preceded the increase in heart/body wt.
ratios illustrated in Figure 1. This was true of both the adult
and the old groups, and the latter lagged in absolute rate of protein synthesis only because they started at a lower point. Indeed,
within five days they were approaching the same absolute rate of

TABLE II

TIME COURSE OF THE THYROXINE-INDUCED INCREASE IN PROTEIN SYNTHESIS
IN HEARTS FROM ADULT AND OLD MICE*

Days Treat-ment	Adult (8 month)		Old (26 month)		
	Protein Synthesis Rate	% Adult Control	Protein Synthesis Rate	% Old Control	% Adult Control
0	3.23 ± 0.12	100	2.33 ± 0.20	100	72
3	5.29 ± 0.38**	164	3.92 ± 0.19**	168	121
5	6.07 ± 0.46**	188	5.34 ± 0.33**	229	165

*Protein synthesis is expressed as pmoles ^{3}H-leucine incorporated per µg

protein in a 30-minute perfusion. Incorporation data (dpm ^{3}H-leucine per

µg protein) were divided by measure specific activity of the intracellular

leucine as described in the text. Values reported are means ± S.E.M., with

five animals per group in the controls and three per group in the treated

sets. Double asterisks denote means significantly different from same-age

controls with p values of 0.005 or less. Control animals received 0.2 ml

saline-NaOH on days 1,3, and 5; 3-day mice received vehicle on day 1 and

100 µg thyroxine on days 3 and 5, and the 5-day group received 100 µg

thyroxine on days 1, 3, and 5. All animals were sacrificed and hearts per-

fused on day 6. (Reproduced with permission from the Journal of Gerontology.)

protein synthesis as the hearts from adult animals. These observations are quite similar to those obtained in studies of enzyme induction in liver and adipose tissue (Adelman, 1972); regeneration
of liver after partial hepatectomy has also been reported to occur
more slowly in older animals (Bucher and Glinos, 1950).

It is possible that decreased cardiac protein synthesis in old
mice results simply from a decrease in thyroxine secretion with age
and we happened to treat the mice with a hormone they were lacking.
For example, Mainwaring (1968) demonstrated a somewhat similar restoration of function in prostate glands of old mice following
androgen administration. However, reported changes in circulating
levels of thyroid hormones with age are matters of controversy
(McGavack, 1967; Gregerman, 1967). Interpretation of the significance of our data is complicated by uncertainties concerning the
variations in serum protein-binding of thyroid hormones, and the
role of thyroxine as a precursor of triiodothyronine. Moreover,
Grad (1969) suggests that any decrease in thyroid hormone secretion with age in rats is offset by increased responsiveness
or decreased inactivation or excretion of the hormone.

Considering these uncertainties, we have recently begun to
explore other models for age related changes in cardiac tissue.
In our view, the most interesting of these is the hypertensive
and hypotensive lines of mice by Schlager (1972) and recently
established in Syracuse by M.F. Elias of our Psychology Department.
In cooperation with Elias, we have begun to study protein synthesis
in hearts of mouse strains with chronic hyper- and hypo-tension.
As illustrated in Table III, our initial results indicate that
there are substantial differences in cardiac protein synthesis
in these animals. Thus it seems reasonable to suspect that there
will be changes with age in cardiac function or response to stress
in the hypotensive and hypertensive mice as they reach senility,
and the parallels with human cardiac diseases make this line of
approach particularly attractive.

On the basis of these results, we feel we now have an interesting and useful system for the study of biologically significant
age related changes in protein synthesis in heart muscle, a tissue
obviously crucial for survival of the animal. Initially, we were
rather complacent about our techniques which permitted determination
of specific activity of intracellular leucine on individual hearts,
so we could avoid the ambiguities which are an inevitable part
of studies in which only gross isotope incorporation is measured.
However, it has now become apparent that some ambiguities still
remain, and I will spend the rest of the talk describing our recent
struggles with them.

While our studies on protein synthesis in isolated perfused
hearts were in progress, a controversy regarding the role of extra-

TABLE III

EFFECTS OF CHRONIC HYPERTENSION AND HYPOTENSION IN MOUSE HEARTS*

Measurement	Hypotensive	Hypertensive
Blood Pressure (Systolic) (mm Hg)	79.2 ± 3.8	137 ± 2.4**
Heart Weight (mg)	123.1 ± 5.2	144 ± 8.3
Heart/Body Weight Ratio (x 10^3)	4.85 ± 0.25	5.33 ± 0.34
Heart Protein Content	108.8 ± 2.9	120.9 ± 5.0
^{3}H-Leucine Incorporation	10.3 ± 0.76	14.1 ± 0.52**
Intracellular Leucine Sp. Act. (µCi/mmole)	123.1 ± 5.2	144.1 ± 8.3
Protein Synthetic Rate (pmoles leu/µg protein)	6.00 ± 0.45	10.05 ± 0.68**

*Hearts from untreated male mice of the Schlager strains were studied; in this preliminary experiment ages ranged from 14 to 23 months. Blood pressure was determined by the tail cuff procedure of Schlager (1972). Hearts were perfused as described by Geary and Florini (1972), and specific activity of intracellular leucine determined separately for each heart by the method of Florini et al. (1973). Mean specific activities are listed for informational purposes, but protein synthesis was calculated separately for each heart using the specific activity measured for that heart. All data are presented as means ± S.E.M. for groups of six mice; double asterisks denote differences between hypotensive and hypertensive groups which were significant at the 0.005 level.

cellular and intracellular amino acids as direct precursors of proteins was developing. Hider, Fern, and London (1969, 1971) reported studies on isolated muscles which indicated that extracellular amino acids were incorporated into protein without dilution by intracellular pools, and Venrooij et al. (1972) made similar observations in studies of leucine and lysine incorporation into protein by pancreas fragments. On the other hand, Morgan et al., (1971) concluded that the intracellular free amino acid pool was an intermediate in protein synthesis in perfused hearts, and Mortimore et al., (1972) agreed that this was also true in perfused livers. Even Fern (Fern and Garlick, 1973) reached the conclusion that the extracellular pool is not the direct precursor of amino acids in protein in vivo, no matter what the situation in isolated muscle.

Indeed, it struck us as noteworthy that systems in which amino acids
enter cells through the circulatory system (as in intact animals
and perfused tissues) lead to the conclusion that intracellular amino
acids are intermediates, whereas systems in which entry is by diffusion through tissue membranes indicate that extracellular amino
acids are not diluted before incorporation. Although the latter
results may be considered artifactual, if they do in fact result
from "unnatural" supply of amino acids through non-capillary
channels, they are nevertheless important to note because a good
many biochemical experiments are done on isolated tissues and tissue minces.

Most of the experiments described above involve somewhat indirect kinetic estimates of relative contributions of the amino
acid pools or comparisons of ratios of two amino acids in various
compartments; the direct comparisons of free amino acid pool and
aminoacyl-tRNA specific activities by Schrieber et al. (1973) provide more direct information. They found that "the quantities of
lysine released by protein degradation may be large enough to dilute the intracellular pool and are available for new protein synthesis." In other words, the specific activity of lysine in tRNA
was lower than that of the free intracellular amino acid. This
surprising result suggests that neither extracellular or intracellular amino acids serve simply as direct precursors of amino
acids in protein.

We felt that our adaptation of the Regier-Kafatos procedure
offered special advantages for investigation of this question, as
it allows relatively convenient analyses of a rather large number
of samples. Furthermore, resolution of this question was essential
to understanding of the significance of some of our results (Table
I), although fortunately the senile decrease in protein synthesis
from 8 to 25 months of age was not substantially affected by corrections for variation in intracellular precursors. To facilitate
isolation and characterization of tRNA, initial experiments were
done on isolated perfused rat hearts, from which larger quantities
of tRNA could be obtained. Following perfusion of the hearts for
the indicated periods, the tissue was homogenized in isotonic su-
crose-phosphate, pH 6.8 (low pH was essential to avoid hydrolysis
of leucyl-tRNA and phosphate buffer was used to avoid reaction
between tris and DNFB). A portion of the homogenate was used to
determine incorporation into protein and specific activity of
leucine in the acid-insoluble fraction by our usual techniques
(Florini et al., 1973); the remainder was centrifuged at 147,000 g
for one hour to isolate the soluble fraction. The pH 5 precipitate
was prepared from this, and RNA isolated by standard phenol extraction techniques at pH 6.8. Following dialysis and reprecipi-
tation from ethanol, the RNA preparation was further purified by
gel electrophoresis at pH 5.8 in 7.5% acrylamide-0.5% agarose.
Gels were scanned using a Gilford spectrophotometer; the UV ab-

sorbing peak coincided with the radioactivity peak observed by slicing and counting the gels, and both were eliminated by prior incubation of the RNA fraction with RNase. Thus it seemed that we had a reasonably clean preparation of soluble RNA with no apparent contamination by free leucine.

To determine specific activity of ^{3}H-leucine in leu-tRNA, the preparation of the gel containing the UV-absorbing peak was incubated in dilute NH_4OH (pH 8.0) at 37° for one hour and the solution collected by filtration. This extract was dried under vacuum and used to determine the specific radioactivity of the solubilized leucine by the FDNB procedure (Regier and Kafatos, 1971; Saito and Florini, 1973). Figure 2 presents the results of four experiments which were normalized by setting initial specific activity of leucine in the perfusion medium to 100%.

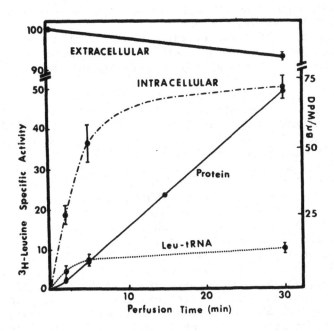

Figure 2. Specific radioactivity of leucine in fractions from isolated perfused hearts. Hearts from normal rats were perfused with Krebs-Ringer buffer (containing glucose) in a recirculating system similar to that described by Morgan et al. (1961); amino acid concentrations were those determined by Scharff and Wool (1965) as corresponding to blood levels of amino acids. At the indicated times, perfusions were terminated; the hearts were rinsed, homogenized in dilute buffer, and the homogenates divided into two

equal portions. Proteins were precipitated with trichloroacetic acid and the acid-soluble fraction collected from one portion. The 147,000 g supernate of the other portion was isolated by ultra-centrifugation and soluble RNA prepared by phenol extraction. The RNA was precipitated twice with ethanol, dialyzed, and purified by preparative electrophoresis on polyacrylamide gels. Amino acids were released from tRNA by incubation at pH 8.5. Specific activity of leucine in all fractions was determined in triplicate by the ^{14}C-DNFB procedure of Regier and Kafatos (1971) as modified by Saito and Florini (1973). Results of four experiments were combined, normalized by setting initial specific activity of the perfusion medium to 100%, and plotted as means with vertical bars indicating standard errors of the mean for the four experiments.

These determinations were designed to determine whether the specific activity of leucine in tRNA was equal to that in the intracellular pool or in the extracellular fluid (which is generally assumed to equilibrate rapidly with the perfusion medium). It appears that the answer to this "either-or" question is "none of the above", and the experiments do not allow a simple choice between intracellular leucine and extracellular leucine as direct precursors of amino acids in proteins. Thus, of the reports described above, our results agree most closely with those of Schrieber et al. (1973), who found the specific activity of lysine in tRNA to be lower than that in the intracellular fluid, and still lower than that of the perfusion medium.

Obviously, we were surprised to find that the specific activity of leucine in tRNA was barely 1/5 that of that in the intracellular space, long after the former had apparently reached equilibrium. Although we have been puzzling over these results for some time, we do not yet have a solid explanation for them, but we do have some possibilities to consider and are investigating one approach that may allow us to avoid the problem.

It seems clear that the results in Figure 2 do not allow simple distinction between possible roles of intracellular and extracellular amino acids as protein precursors. Our results could be explained if protein breakdown involved direct incorporation of the freed amino acids into tRNA without equilibration with the total intracellular amino pool, or some other form of compartmentation which maintained separation of these freed amino acids from the general cytoplasm. These are not, in our opinion, very attractive suggestions. There is no direct evidence to support them, and they require the postulation of compartments or reactions which are very difficult to examine experimentally.

An alternative explanation can be devised by a slight extension of the codon modulation theory of aging and development

of Strehler et al. (1971). If certain messenger RNA's cannot be
translated because the aminoacyl-tRNA synthetase charging the tRNA
bearing a crucial anticodon is inactive at that stage of development, then it follows that subsequent codons on that mRNA will
not be expressed. Although it seems likely that these codons
may occur on other mRNA's which can be expressed, it is possible
that some tRNA's for a particular amino acid may not be used at
a particular stage of development, even though they are saturated
with amino acid. (Of course, any other mechanism which restricted
translation of a set of messenger RNA's bearing certain specific
codons could have the same effect.) This could then mean that
some populations of leucine-tRNA's might be relatively stable,
neither transferring their amino acids into protein nor exchanging
with free leucine molecules in the cytoplasm. Thus these leucyl-
tRNA's would be effectively separated from the general pathway of
protein synthesis, and any unlabeled leucine attached to them would
simply dilute the radioactivity concentration of leucine on the
several leucyl-tRNA's present in the cell. If something like this
is happening, then leucine is a particularly unsatisfactory choice
as labeled precursor for measurement of protein synthesis because
it has more codons than any other amino acid, and thus seems particularly likely to have some variant tRNA's which do not participate in the protein synthetic pathway at any given time in the
animal's development. This is a great disappointment; a good many
investigators have used leucine as the labeled precursor for several
good reasons: it is one of the most abundant amino acids in proteins, it is generally considered to be rather slowly metabolized,
and (in our case, at least) it could be obtained at high specific
activity at very low cost by a simple do-it-yourself radiochemical
synthesis (Florini, 1964). It now appears that the first point
may be a disadvantage (if it really is associated with the presence of non-participating species of leu-tRNA), and the second is
not true in muscle, especially during starvation (Goldberg and
Odessey, 1972), so it turns out that the low cost really represents
a very poor bargain.

This suggestion that some species of leucyl-tRNA do not participate in protein synthesis at all stages of development is
obviously open to experimental testing, although the experiments
are not easy; such work is now in progress. But resolution of
this question is, in our opinion, much less important than investigation of the phenomena it is obscuring; what happens to protein synthesis and degradation in hearts as a function of age and
stress? Thus it would be more interesting to find a way around
the problem, so we could go ahead and find unambiguous answers
to the questions that are our principal concerns. It is possible
that the more judicious choice of a labeled amino acid may allow
us to avoid - or at least delay facing - the leucine problem.
At present, phenylalanine seems the best choice for this purpose.

Intracellular pools of phenylalanine are very small in muscle, so the intracellular and extracellular specific activities are nearly identical in perfused hearts (Morgan et al., 1971; Schreiber et al., 1973). In addition, there are only two codons reported for phenylalanine, and only one phenylalanine-accepting tRNA peak was found in muscle in Ortwerth's (1971) extensive survey of iso-accepting tRNA's in bovine tissues. Furthermore, Goldberg and Odessey (1972) found that phenylalanine was not metabolized by muscle under conditions in which extensive leucine metabolism occurred. Accordingly, we are currently repeating the perfusion experiments with phenylalanine with some hope that it will be possible to calculate protein synthetic rates directly from specific activity of the amino acid in the perfusion medium; in other words, that extracellular, intracellular, and aminoacyl-tRNA phenylalanine will all exhibit the same specific radioactivity. If this happy result occurs, we can continue our studies of cardiac protein synthesis without first finding some resolution of the awkward questions about the role of various subcellular pools of leucine as precursors of this amino acid in proteins.

ACKNOWLEDGEMENTS

Thiw work was supported by grants from the National Heart and Lung Institute, USPHS (HL11551), the Heart Association of Upstate New York, and the Muscular Dystrophy Association of America. We are grateful to Drs. Howard Morgan, L.S. Jefferson, and Ira Wool for stimulating discussions, to Dr. Samuel Mallov for initial instruction in the heart perfusion technique, to Dr. Thomas P. Fondy for use of his amino acid analyzer, and to Dr. Frederick G. Sherman for providing the old mice used in this study.

REFERENCES

1. Adelman, R. C. Advances in Gerontological Research 4:1 (1972).
2. Barrows, C. H. Proc. 8th International Congress of Gerontology 1:179 (1969).
3. Bucher, N. L. R. and A. D. Glinos. Cancer Res. 10:324 (1950).
4. Fern, E. B. and P. J. Garlick. Biochem. J. 134:1127 (1973).
5. Florini, J. R. Biochemistry 3:209 (1964).
6. Florini, J. R. and F. L. Dankberg. Biochemistry 10:530 (1971).
7. Florini, J. R., Y. Saito, and E. J. Manowitz. J. Gerontology 28:293 (1973).
8. Geary, S. and J. R. Florini. J. Gerontology 27:325 (1972).
9. Goldberg, A. L. and R. Odessey. Am. J. Physiol. 233:1384 (1972).
10. Grad, B. J. Gerontology 24:5 (1969).
11. Gregerman, R. I. In "Endocrines and Aging" (L. Gitman, Ed.) C.C. Thomas, Springfield, Ill., pp. 161-173 (1967).
12. Hider, R. C., E. B. Fern, and D. R. London. Biochem. J. 114:171 (1969).

13. Hider, R. C., E. B. Fern, and D. R. London. Biochem. J. 121:817 (1971).

14. Lang, C. A., H. Y. Law, and D. J. Jefferson. Biochem. J. 95:372 (1966).

15. Mainwaring, W. I. P. Biochem. J. 110:79 (1968).

16. McGavack, T. H. In "Endocrines and Aging" (L. Gitman, Ed.) C.C. Thomas, Springfield, Ill., pp. 36-50 (1967).

17. Morgan, H. F., D. C. N. Earl, A. Broadus, E. B. Wolpert, K. E. Giger, and L. S. Jefferson. J. Biol. Chem. 246:2152 (1971).

18. Morgan, H. E., J. J. Henderson, D. M. Regan, and C. R. Park. J. Biol. Chem. 236:253 (1961).

19. Mortimore, G. E., K. H. Woodside, and J. E. Henry. J. Biol. Chem. 247:2776 (1972).

20. Ortwerth, B. J. Biochemistry 10:4190 (1971).

21. Perry, K. W. Ph.D. Dissertation, Syracuse University, Syracuse, N.Y. (1966).

22. Regier, J. C., and F. C. Kafatos. Chem. 246:6480 (1971).

23. Saito, Y. and J. R. Florini. Analyt. Biochem. 54:266 (1973).

24. Scharff, R. and I. G. Wool. Biochem. J. 97:257 (1965).

25. Schlager, G. J. Heredity 63:35 (1972).

26. Schreiber, S. S., M. Oratz, C. Evans, F. Reff, I. Klain, and M. Rothschild. Am. J. Physiol. 217:307 (1973).

27. Strehler, B., G. Hirsch, D. Gusseck, R. Johnson, and M. Bick. J. Theor. Biol. 33:429 (1971).

28. Van Venrooij, V. J., C. Poort, M. F. Kramer, and M. T. Jansen. Eur. J. Biochem. 30:427 (1972).

29. von Hahn, H. P. J. Gerontology 21:291 (1966).

SENESCENCE AND VASCULAR DISEASE

George Martin, Charles Ogburn, and Curtis Sprague

Department of Pathology, University of Washington

Seattle, Washington 98195

SENESCENCE AND VASCULAR DISEASE

It is with considerable humility that I approach my task of discussing some aspects of cell senescence as it pertains to vascular disease. First of all, the literature of arteriosclerosis and related subjects, if comprehensively and critically analyzed, would surely saturate my aging nervous system. I therefore apologize to all those scholars -- living or dead -- whom I offend by my restricted knowledge and special viewpoints. Secondly, I must emphasize that our own experimental work in this area is still quite preliminary. Our message is primarily to indicate some relatively simple approaches to the assessment of the replicative potentials of various cell types within and around blood vessels, how these may change as a function of age and what significance such changes may have for the pathogenesis of certain types of vascular disease.

Our interest in these questions evolved from experiments with human skin fibroblast cultures, in which we confirmed and extended the pioneering work of Hayflick and Moorhead on the limited replicative life spans of diploid human fibroblast culture (Martin et al., 1970). Three types of experiments supported the view that this in vitro phenomenon had biological significance and was not an artefact of tissue culture. Firstly, there was an inverse correlation of replicative life-span with donor age. Secondly, cultures from patients with Werner's syndrome, an autosomally inherited progeroid syndrome, had sharply limited growth potentials in comparison with age-matched controls. Thirdly, the replicative potentials of "fibroblasts" varied with the tissue

of origin, being greatest with explants from upper arm skin, least
with explants from lumbar vertebral bone marrow and of intermediate life span with explants of psoas muscle.

As a pathologist, I am acutely aware of the probability that,
in vivo, a limited replicative life span of subepidermal fibroblasts or of sweat gland myoepithelial cells (it is conceivable
that such cells also participate in the establishment of mass
cultures) are not life-threatening phenomena. Perhaps they contribute to the pathogenesis of senile elastosis or to the progressive age dependent atrophy of skin appendages. It is of
course also possible that the depletion or functional decline
of such cohorts of cells contribute to host susceptibility to
epidermal carcinogenesis, or to tumor progression, once such neoplasms have arisen; that would be life-threatening and is probably a subject worthy of investigation.

In our opinion, however, a more urgent question is whether
or not the cells which make up blood vessels have limited growth
potentials and, if so, how such clonal senescence might play a
role in the development of important vascular pathology, especially in atherogenesis.

Let us first briefly review the major age related vascular
diseases in humans; they are tabulated in Table I.

TABLE I

MAJOR AGE RELATED VASCULAR DISEASES IN HUMANS

A.   ARTERIOSCLEROSIS

  1.   Atherosclerosis

  2.   Medial Calcinosis

  3.   Arteriolosclerosis

B.   VARICOSE VEINS

C.   MICROANGIOPATHY

We see immediately that arteriosclerosis is a generic term for
at least three different disease entities: atherosclerosis,
medial calcinosis (or Monckeberg's sclerosis) and arteriolosclerosis (Robbins, 1974). Arteriolosclerosis is frequently sub-
divided (Robbins, 1974) into two entities: hyaline arteriolosclerosis and hyperplastic arteriolosclerosis. The latter is a

proliferative lesion associated with fibrinoid necrosis and occurring in patients with malignant hypertension, not infrequently
in a young adult. Hyaline arteriolosclerosis is characterized
by lumenal narrowing attributable to a thickening of the arteriolar
wall by eosinophilic, homogeneous material which, under the
electron microscope, includes what appears to be thickened base-
ment membrane material and trapped smooth muscle cells. Although,
to the best of my knowledge, well controlled quantitative studies
of the rate of progression of this lesion in specific subsets of
arterioles have not yet been carried out, these lesions are very
common in the aged, especially in those with benign essential
hypertension and/or diabetes mellitus. Hyaline change of
arterioles may be associated with a degree of proliferation and
hyaline change may affect small arteries, as in nephrosclerosis
(Figure 1f).

Although the replacement of medial smooth muscle by dense
deposits of calcium (and sometimes bone) in Monckeberg's sclerosis
is a very striking lesion (Figure 1d), the disease is of less
clinical significance than other forms of arteriosclerosis. Age
dependency is commonly acknowledged, but once again, we lack
quantitative data.

Atherosclerosis is, of course, the most important class of
arteriosclerosis, being in fact the leading underlying cause of
morbidity and mortality in the so-called "developed" societies.
Thanks to the work of the International Project on Atherosclerosis
(McGill, 1968), a great deal of interesting quantitative data is
available (much of it still to be digested) as to its extent in
various human population subgroups. The term "class" of arteriosclerosis is here used deliberately, since atherosclerosis, even
on morphological grounds, may yet prove to be a heterogeneous
group of diseases. Certainly, in terms of the complex interactions of genetic and environmental factors which produce the
phenotype(s) (Martin and Hoehn, 1974), it is heterogeneous --
witness, for example, the different mendelian genes which strongly
determine the rates of progression of the lesions (Goldstein,
1973). One pathogenic factor, however, seems to be at the top
of everyone's list, and that is age.

Figure 2 illustrates the striking increase in the extent of
coronary artery atherosclerosis in human males as a function of
age, beginning at about age 20. This curve was drawn from pooled
data from various population groups of individuals who died of
causes other than those associated with atherosclerosis. Different slopes and different kinetics were observed with specimens
from specific ethnic, geographical and sex subgroups, including
some with clearly exponential rises in the extent of the disease
with age (Eggen and Solberg, 1968). Figure 2 shows essentially

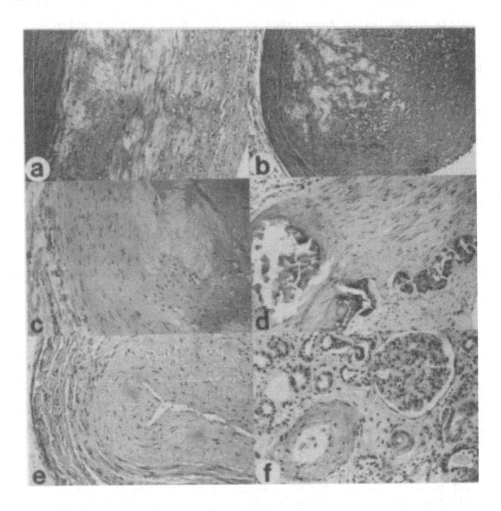

Figure 1.   Some examples of major age related vascular
diseases in humans.   a.   atherosclerotic plaque of abdominal
aorta.   The intima is markedly thickened as a result of both intimal cellular proliferation and, in this instance, especially
extracellular materials.   Histochemical and fine structure studies
generally reveal atypical smooth muscle cells with both intracellular and extracellular lipid, collagen, elastin and muco-
polysaccharides.   Note also the light infiltration of lymphocytes.   (X 100)   b.   atherosclerotic plaque of coronary artery.
This illustrates a very discrete, focal nodular lesion producing
tremendous fibrous and lipid-rich intimal thickening with destruc-
tion of adjacent media.   There are scattered lymphocytes.   The
adventitial connective tissue is normal.   (X 100)   c.   atherosclerosis of coronary artery.   This illustrates the classical
picture of "cholesterol clefts" (aggregates of cholesterol were

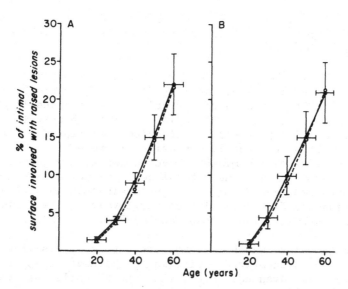

Figure 2. Extent of gross lesions of coronary artery atherosclerosis in human males as a function of age by decades. Solid
circles are unweighted means of the means (+ 95% confidence limits)
for 19 different location-race groups involving 9031 subjects
dying from causes other than coronary heart diseases, diabetes or
hypertension. Open circles are weighted means, obtained by nor-
malizing the sample sizes of the various location-race groups.
Panel A: data from the three major coronary arteries. Panel B:
data from the anterior descending branch of the left coronary
artery. (after Eggin and Solberg, 1968.)

dissolved by solvents employed in the tissue preparation).
(X 100) d. medial calcinosis or Monckeberg's sclerosis of a
medium-sized artery of the lower extremity. Nodular, multifocal
deposits of calcium in the media and, in this instance, the internal elastica. As is commonly the case, internal thickening
and fibrosis may occur concommitantly. Fibrosis also was found
in the media and adventitia. (X 100) 3. varicose veins from
the lower extremity. Marked thickening of the intima (proliferation & fibrosis); replacement of medial smooth muscle by fibrous
connective tissue. (X 100) f. benign nephrosclerosis. There
is arteriolosclerosis and a hyaline arteriosclerosis of a small
artery. Note also interstitial fibrosis and focal lymphocytic
infiltrate. (X 140) All specimens were formalin fixed, paraffin
embedded and stained with H&E. (Magnifications are before reduction.)

linear kinetics, at least after the age of 30 -- i.e., it does
not show a Gompertz function. Of interest is the increase in
variance as a function of age.

The histopathology has been exhaustively reviewed. With the
exception of the newer electron microscopic observations indicating that cells with characteristics of smooth muscle pre-
dominate in the intimal proliferation (Geer and Haust, 1972), not
much has been added to the older classical descriptions. While
lipid depositions are usually emphasized (Figure 1a, b, c), in
some lesions they may be minimal. For example, the spontaneous
disease in the elephant, whose total serum cholesterol concentration averages about 85 mgm %, is predominantly one of intimal
proliferation and fibrosis, with comparatively little lipid
(McCullagh and Lewis, 1967; McCullage, 1972).

Varicose veins, another common age dependent vascular disease, is also characterized by intimal proliferation and fibrosis
(Figure 1e). In advanced stages, the smooth muscle coat is
typically partially replaced by fibrous connective tissue. It is
of interest that a time-dependent intimal proliferative lesion is
also noted in veins (saphenous) grafted to coronary arteries
(Kern et al., 1972).

Finally, we should mention microangiopathy -- a thickening
of the walls of precapillaries, capillaries, and venules. While
such lesions are characteristic of diabetes mellitus (Vracko,
1970), they may also be found in individuals without overt evidence of the disease and are probably age dependent (Ashworth
et al., 1960; Bloodworth et al., 1969), although here we are
on shaky grounds, since age regression studies are needed,
especially in humans. Electron micrographs of such lesions have
revealed concentrically arranged lamellae of basal lamina with
intervening cell debris, and with the interesting interpretation
of a centripetal quantum synthesis of basal lamina by endothelial
cells; like rings of a tree trunk the layers of basal lamina are
thought to give an index of the number of cell generations which
transpired in the life history of the capillary (Vracko and
Benditt, 1970).

In what ways could the aging of cells of vascular walls
contribute to the pathogenesis of these various vascular diseases?
One generic proposition might be that, as post-replicative,
mature, differentiated cells become senescent (metabolically insufficient), and are no longer replaced at suitable rates from
progenitor cells, various secondary effects ensue. Paramount
among these is the seemingly paradoxical effect of cellular proliferation. Even in the case of medial calcinosis, we are im-
pressed with how difficult it is to find an example in which

there is no associated intimal proliferative thickening. But
it is dangerous to make sweeping generalizations about such a
heterogeneous group of disorders, so we will consider one of them,
atherosclerosis, in greater detail. This task is difficult enough
since, as we have indicated, it is already clear that the pathogenesis of atherosclerosis is itself heterogeneous.

Atherosclerosis is a multi-focal disease which preferentially
involves certain segments of the arterial tree, such as the distal
abdominal aorta (Roberts et al., 1959), certain segments of the
coronary arteries (Vlodaver et al., 1972) and, as a generalization,
bifurcations; this is probably true even in the case of predis-
posing inborn errors of metabolism, such as familial hypercho-
lesterolemia. In a series of transplantation studies, Haimovici
and his colleagues (1958, 1964) have shown that there are factors
intrinsic to a particular vascular segment which determine its
relative susceptibility to atherogenesis. Could one such factor
be the replicative potential of the component cells of the particular segment? A complex of variables may determine the sizes and
distribution of regional stem cell pools and the rates at which
such stem cells and their differentiating and mature progeny are
depleted: 1) Programmed genetic information, a factor which could
result in substantial differences in stem cell compartments and
kinetics among the species and therefore could be of prime importance in determining differences in general and regional suscep-
tibilities to the disease (Lindsey and Nichols, 1971). These could
include point mutations, such as the autosomal recessively inherited progeroid syndromes (Epstein et al., 1966). Such genes
could limit the initial sizes or distributions of stem cell pools.
Recently, we have also suggested that such genes may result in
increased rates, premature onsets or defective types of differentiation within the proliferative pools of certain cell types during
growth and cell turnover (Martin et al., 1974). 2) Differential
morphogenetic growth and necrosis (Glucksmann, 1951; Gillman, 1959;
Saunders et al., 1962), as in bifurcations, elongations and various
remodelings. 3) A great variety of cell injuries, such as those
caused by infections, heavy metals, cytotoxic compounds, and immune reactions (Poston and Davies, 1974). 4) A variety of mitogens.
In this connection, it is of interest that two classical athero-
genetic factors, cholesterol and hypertension, have been shown to
be mitogenic for vascular smooth muscle (Daoud et al., 1970;
Schmitt et al., 1970) (Table II).

TABLE II

SOME VASCULAR SMOOTH MUSCLE MITOGENS

A.   CHOLESTEROL (Daoud et al., 1970)
B.   HYPERTENSION (Schmitt et al., 1970)
C.   PLATELET FACTOR (Ross et al., 1974)

It is also of interest that the effects of hypertension are thought
to be especially pronounced in the abdominal aorta (Wolinsky and
Glagov, 1969). If depletion of regional stem cells (clonal
senescence) (Martin et al., 1974) is in fact an important event
in determining the increase in the frequency of atherosclerotic
lesions as a function of age, how then does one explain the widespread observation that the first observable histopathologic
lesion is a proliferation of atypical myointimal cells (Geer
and Haust, 1972)? We have speculated (Martin and Sprague, 1972
and 1973) that such proliferation may result from a release from
feed-back inhibition by regulatory macromolecules operating within
a family of related differentiated cell types, such as was originally postulated by Weiss and Kavanau (1957). Figure 3

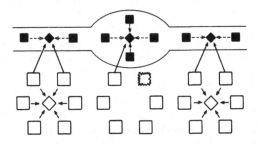

Figure 3. A schematic drawing of the hypothetical cell interactions transpiring in senescing aortas which might lead to a
proliferation of myointimal cells, a lesion which many pathologists
now believe to be of paramount importance in the genesis of progressive atherosclerosis. ◇ = smooth muslce stem cell of media;
□ = differentiated smooth muscle cell of media; ◆ = myointimal
stem cell; ■ = differentiated myointimal cell. Under equilibrium
conditions (groups of cells in the left and right portions of the
diagram), there is normal feed-back inhibition of stem cells;
a loss of differentiated cells in such regions would presumably
be exactly compensated by derepression and replication of medial
stem cells. In specific vascular segments in which there is a
partial depletion or functional failure of medial stem cells
(groups of cells in the central portion of the diagram), effete
differentiated smooth muscle cells (▢) are no longer replaced at
suitable rates, so that the regional concentration of molecules
which inhibit replication of myointimal stem cells falls below a
critical threshold; this leads to focal proliferation until a new
equilibrium can be established. It is presumed that the major
regulation (solid arrows) is via the quantitatively larger mass
of differentiated smooth muscle cells of the media; the total
contribution from differentiated myointimal cells (broken arrows)
would be less significant. A qualitatively distinctive and less
effective regulation via differentiated myointimal cells would
have to be considered, however (after Martin and Sprague, 1972).

gives a diagrammatic outline of this admittedly speculative proposition. It is of considerable interest, however, that recent
studies by the Albany group (Florentine et al., 1973) have provided evidence for the existence, in crude extracts of pig aorta,
of a substance which inhibits the mitosis of carotid artery smooth
muscle, but not of isologous epidermis (Table III).

TABLE III

MEAN RATIOS (+ S.E.) OF MITOTIC COUNTS IN PIG CAROTID ARTERIES AS
   BIOASSAYS FOR CRUDE EXTRACTS OF ENDOGENOUS TISSUE-SPECIFIC
   INHIBITOR(S) OF AORTIC SMOOTH MUSCLE CELL PROLIFERATION

[Ratios < 2.0 are indicative of inhibition (after Florentine et
                  al., 1973)]

	S.M.C.	EPIDERMIS
Saline Control	1.95 ± 0.18	1.38 ± 0.15
Aortic Extract	1.08 ± 0.06	1.59 ± 0.15
	$p < 0.001$	$p > 0.05$

This result is compatible with a specific "chalone" as postulated
by our theory.

    There are of course other explanations for why myointimal
cells begin to proliferate (Table IV). A particularly imaginative
idea is that the focal lesions are neoplastic proliferations
resulting from mutation or transformation (Benditt and Benditt,
1973). The evidence for this was derived from electrophoretic
studies of glucose-6-phosphate dehydrogenase (G6PD) derived from
early lesions in female subjects heterozygotic for A and B alleles
of G6PD; the results suggested a monoclonal or oligoclonal origin
of the lesions. However, cell culture studies have raised the
question that small healing wounds or hyperplastic foci could
be monoclonal or oligoclonal in derivation (Martin et al., 1974).

TABLE IV

ATHEROSCLEROSIS: SELECTED PATHOGENETIC THEORIES BASED UPON A
PRIMACY OF MYOINTIMAL CELL PROLIFERATION

A. ENDOTHELIAL INJURY + PLATELET FACTOR

    (Ross et al., 1973, 1974; Harker et al., 1974)

B. NEOPLASIA (Benditt, 1973)

C. CLONAL SENESCENCE -- with release from feed-back

    inhibition (Martin and Sprague, 1972, 1973)

This could occur by clonal selection or genetic drift. Certainly,
evidence for monoclonicity cannot be regarded as synonymous with
evidence for mutation or transformation; the clonal senescence
theory outlined above would also predict oligoclonicity or
monoclonicity. Many neoplasms are of course strongly age dependent, so that it would not be difficult to reconcile a cell aging
theory with the theory of Benditt and Benditt.

    A leading contemporary conception of atherogenesis has been
summarized by Ross and Glomset (1973). Exciting new studies by
Ross et al. (1974) and Harker et al. (1974a and b) have once again
focused upon the platelets (Mustard, 1967) as an important component of atherogenesis (Table IV). These workers have emphasized
that the premature intimal proliferation and fibrosis which occurs
in connection with homocystinuria may serve as an important model for
the study of the pathogenesis of atherosclerosis. It is thought
that a platelet-dependent proliferation of arterial smooth muscle
cells follows chronic endothelial injury; pharmacologic inter-
ruption of the associated platelet consumption prevents the intimal lesions.

    A disturbing aspect of the homocystinuria model is that the
distribution of lesions and some aspects of the histopathology
are quite unlike what is observed in the naturally occurring
disease. For example, the aorta may be spared, while unusual
sites are affected (McCully, 1969). Peri-vascular proliferation
of connective tissue is a very conspicuous component (McCully,
1969) and this is not usual for the spontaneous disease. If loss
of the integrity of endothelium should prove to be a vital event
in the natural history of atherosclerosis, however, this too could
be reconciled with a theory implicating clonal senescence (of endothelial cells).

    By now, one would naturally wish to know if tissue culture

studies have lent any credibility to the proposition of a limited
replicative life span of vascular cells or have provided evidence
of differential growth as a function of site of biopsy or age of
donor. Of four published studies (Table V),

TABLE V

GROWTH OF THORACIC (T) VS. ABDOMINAL (A) AORTIC
EXPLANTS IN CULTURE

SPECIES	INVESTIGATORS	RESULTS
Dogs	Parshley et al., 1953	T > A
Rabbits	Kokubu and Pollak, 1961	T > A
Rats	Wexler and Thomas, 1967	A > T
Monkeys	Martin and Sprague, 1973	T > A

three gave evidence that explants from the thoracic aorta (a
region relatively resistant to atherosclerosis) grew better than
explants from the abdominal aorta (a region relatively susceptible to atherosclerosis). Ours was the only study which addressed
itself primarily to this question, but it certainly could not be
regarded as definitive.

TABLE VI

COMPARATIVE CELL GROWTH FROM EXPLANTS OF MONKEY THORACIC (N = 12)
AND ABDOMINAL (N = 11) AORTAS

	EXP	TID	TIY
Thoracic	5.8	29.8	10.6
Abdominal	3.1	55.3	2.4

EXP = mean number of explants (of total of eight per animal) producing growth. TID = mean time (days) before first passage or to
termination for lack of growth. TIY = mean yield of cells ($X10^3$)
per set of explants at first passage or at termination (after
Martin and Sprague, 1973).

In Table VI, we summarize data from that study indicative of superior cell growth from monkey distal thoracic aortic explants, in comparison with explants from the distal abdominal aorta. Individual clones of cells of various types underwent clonal senescence, with cumulative population doublings (CPD) ranging from 7.5 to 20.5 (n = 7). Interpretation of the longevities of long-term established mass cultures was complicated by the almost routine emergence of cytopathogenic effects (CPE), presumably related to latent viruses. However, the two best-growing abdominal aortic cultures without CPE yielded only 8.3 to 8.6 CPD whereas the two best-growing thoracic cultures yielded 20.0 to 27.9 CPD.

The widespread problem of virus contamination in subhuman primate cell cultures (Rogers et al., 1967), particularly the potential biohazard (Hull, 1973), prompted us to investigate other experimental models. We also turned our attention to enzyme dissociation methods of obtaining cell cultures, since they have several potential advantages over explant techniques, such as the opportunity for improved quantitation and the possibility of primary cloning. While we have not yet explored a range of combination of different enzymes, elastase, at suitable concentrations and for suitable time periods proved most useful. In the experiments to be reported, a Worthington Co. (Freehold, N.J.) preparation of elastase, 120 units/mgm (ESFF 53 J 422) was used at a final concentration of 120 units/ml of phosphate buffered saline (PBS) [0.145 M, pH 7.5 (adjusted to this final pH after addition of elastase)]. Two ml were used to dissociate 0.1 to 0.5 mgm of minced (0.5 mm^3), washed (PBS) tissue in a 40 ml round-bottom pyrex centrifuge tube with magnetic stirring at 37°C. After various time intervals (usually 15 min) elastase action was slowed by dilution with 10 ml complete medium (including a 5 ml wash for transfer to a 15 ml pyrex conical centrifuge tybe) followed by centrifugation (1000 rev/min X 5 min in a clinical centrifuge) and resuspension of the cells in complete media, which was a fortified (Martin, 1974) Dulbecco-Vogt medium with 16% heat-inactivated fetal calf serum, 9 mM bicarbonate and 33 mM Hepes buffer (pH 7.4); this medium was used in an atmosphere of 1% CO_2 in air. In the experiments to be described with mouse tissues, penicillin (100 units/ml), streptomycin (50 µg/ml), aureomycin (50 µg/ml) and nystatin (50 units/ml) were added.

In Figure 4, the effects of time of elastase treatment upon cell yield and viability are given for a group of rodents (Buffalo rats). Such treatments have yielded primary clones of presumptive smooth muscle cells (Ross, 1971; Martin and Sprague, 1973) from the aortic medias of rabbits (sexually mature New Zealand white), pigs (9- to 12-month-old random bred Poland China and Hampshire), rats (sexually mature Buffalo and Sprague-Dawley) and humans (neonatal to adult). While quantitative comparative studies have not been done, human cells, or at least post-mortem human cells

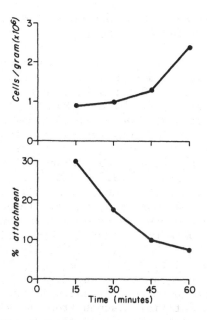

Figure 4. Effect of duration of treatment with elastase upon cell yield and cell viability. Six three-month-old male Buffalo rats were killed by cervical fracture, their aortas removed aseptically, washed with complete medium and stripped of their adventitial tissues. The pooled weighed aortas were diced into ∿ 16 hr incubation (see text).

(< 8 hr) appear to be more sensitive to such treatments. It is also possible that there are fewer clonable stem cells in the human aorta; only rare primary clones have been observed with human material. This important point awaits future investigations.

Because of the availability of an aging colony of outbred white mice, provided through the courtesy of Dr. Donald Gibson (Adult Aging Branch, National Institute of Child Health and Human Development), the first experiments we carried out on the replicative potential of aortic cells as a function of age were done with this strain (designated ICR, after the Institute of Cancer Research, Philadelphia, but originally developed from the Swiss Webster strain of Rockefeller University). These animals were randomly bred and maintained by the Charles River Breeding Laboratories under an NICHD contract. Details of maintenance and longevity are available from Dr. George J. Pucak of Charles River. Approximately 50% of males survived to age 24 months and approximately 2% survived to age 30 months. Detailed reports of

the pathology are not available, but there are apparently no unusual or specific patterns of mortality.

The animals were equilibrated to new quarters for five days
after shipment to Seattle, during which time they were housed
in groups as shipped (9 to 10 per age group per cage) and given
Purina Chow and tap water ad libitum. Non-filter-topped cages
were provided with white pine bedding. Beginning on the sixth
day, one group of animals per day were sacrificed by cervical
translocation, in the following sequence of ages (months): 25, 18,
6, 24, 12. Means (with standard deviations) of body wt. at times
of sacrifice were as follows: 33.7 $\pm$ 3.5, 49.1 $\pm$ 3.5, 52.9 $\pm$ 6.1,
28.4 $\pm$ 4.0 and 44.4 $\pm$ 5.6 (6 through 25 months, respectively).
Because of fighting behaviour, many animals (especially those
18 months and older) had crusted excoriations over the dorsum;
in no case, however, were these lesions suppurative. At autopsy,
one 12-month animal had a small ($\sim$ 1 cm^3), discrete, well differentiated hepatoma. Intact aortas were dissected out aseptically
from the arch to the common iliacs and divided approximately into
thoracic and abdominal portions. Because it was not possible to
cleanly strip the adventitial tissues from the small mouse aortas
(especially from abdominal segments), elastase treatments were
carried out on pooled segments (9 to 10 thoracic or 9 to 10 abdominal) of aortas together with their surrounding areolar connective tissues. Figure 5 shows the pre-elastase histology, illustrating the variability of the amounts and types of adventitial
tissues in thoracic segments. Note the ganglion in section d.
A larger extent and more variable degree of adventitial contamination was observed in abdominal segments, in which, for example,
lymphoid tissue was frequently detected. There is no evidence of
aortic histopathology as a function of age. Figure 6 illustrates
the range of histology after a 15 min period of elastase digestion of the minced fragments of aortas. Some fragments were
extensively depleted of medial wall cells, while others, including
those in identical incubations (a) retained large numbers of cells;
these residual cells often showed bizarre morphologies (b, c).
Ganglia and, at least in some segments, areolar connective tissues, were more resistant to digestion (d).

Because of the large amounts of adventitial tissues (especially the fatty tissues) with their associated cell fragmentation and
debris, it proved quite difficult to derive reliable hemocyto-
meter cell counts of suspensions of elastase-treated cells and
therefore quantitative assessments of primary cloning efficiencies
were not possible. However, it was possible to determine the
proportion, among all morphologic types of primary clones, of
presumptive "smooth muscle" clones, a typical example of which is
illustrated in Figure 7. It must be emphasized that the evidence
that such clones may be derived predominantly from the media of

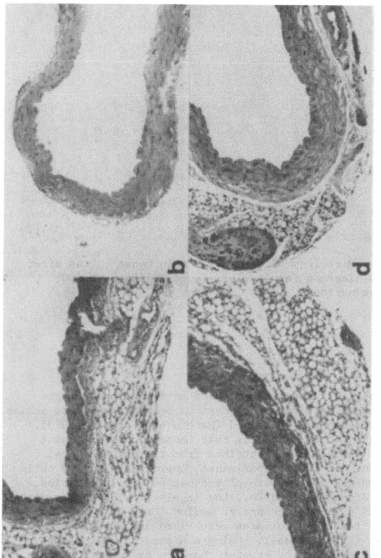

Figure 5. Histology of segments of strain ICR male mouse thoracic aortas before elastase treatments, illustrating the variety and variability of adventitial tissue and the absence of histopathology in the older specimens. a. age 6 months. b. age 18 months. c. age 12 months. d. age 25 months. Fixed in 10% neutral phosphate buffered formalin, embedded in paraffin and stained with H&E. (X 150 before reduction)

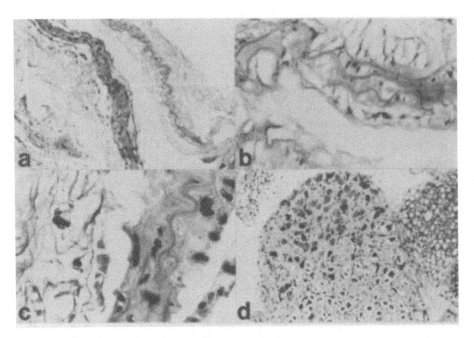

Figure 6. Histology of strain ICR male mouse aortas after treatment with elastase for 15 min. (a, d X 150; b, X 600; c, X 900 before reduction)

the aorta is quite tenuous, being based solely upon the light microscopic resemblance to clones derived from monkey aorta medias which we have previously described (Martin and Sprague, 1973). All one can say with certainty is that these clones are quite different from those usually obtained from the skin of mice, monkeys and men. In these experiments, approximately 1000 cells in 4 ml of complete medium were plated per 60 mm plastic tissue culture petri dishes (Falcon Co., Los Angeles). The dishes were incubated at 37°C without change of medium for 9 days, after which time the resulting colonies were fixed and stained with 1% crystal violet in 20% ethanol. Using a dissecting microscope, all clonal foci equal to or greater than six cells were counted. The numbers of colonies per dish ranged from 20 to 158. There was also a substantial range of colony sizes (6 to $\sim$ 900 cells per colony), but only a small proportion (< 10%) were "mini clones" in the range of six to ten cells. We do not believe that these small clones derived via seeding from more vigorously growing parental clones, since 1) the total growth period was comparatively

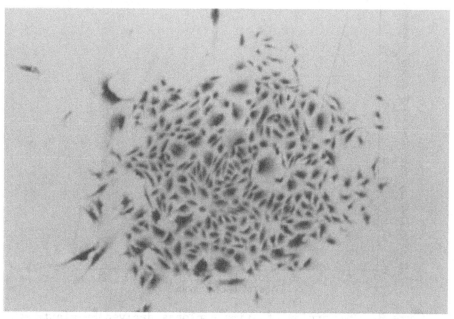

Figure 7. Typical morphology of a primary clone of presumptive "smooth muscle" cells derived by elastase treatment of
aortas of strain ICR male mice. The morphology is strikingly
similar to that derived from medias of monkey aortas (Martin and
Sprague, 1973) and is distinctly different from skin fibroblast
clones derived from mice, monkeys and men. (X 10 before reduction)

short (nine days), 2) the cultures were left undisturbed and unfed,
3) the small groups of cells were often quite large, reminiscent
of slowly growing senescent cultures (Martin et al., 1974) and
4) such clonal heterogeneity of growth potential is well established with diploid cultures (Martin et al., 1974). A graph of
the proportion of these primary clones which were of the presumptive "smooth muscle" type, plotted as a function of donor
age, is given in Figure 8. More specifically, what was scored
for were clones large enough to be reliably classified as "smooth
muscle"; most of the very large clones were of this type. The
data could therefore reflect the numbers of surviving stem cells
of this character. There is a quite convincing decline in the
proportion of such clones with advancing donor age. One cannot
conclude from the lower figures for the abdominal aortas that
these contained fewer such clonable cells, since there was quite
clearly a larger amount of contaminating adventitial tissues in
those samples.

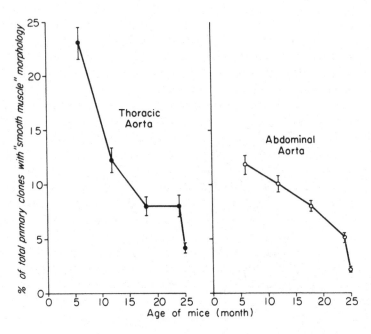

Figure 8. Proportion of primary clones derived by elastase treatments of strain ICR male mouse aortas which were of the presumptive "smooth muscle" type, plotted as a function of age of donor. Means ± standard errors (see text).

A second series of 60 mm petri dishes, inoculated with approximately 2000 cells from the initial elastase digests of pooled aortic segments from each of the age groups, was harvested with trypsin-versene (Martin, 1964) after 10 days of growth in a single feeding of complete medium (4 ml per dish). A series of "secondary" cloning dishes were initiated simultaneously with cells pooled from these harvested. Four-hundred cells per 60 mm dish, each with 4 ml complete media, were grown for 14 days at 37°C with a single change of medium, then fixed and stained with 1% crystal violet in 20% ethanol. Unlike the cell suspensions obtained by primary elastase digestions, accurate cell counts now permitted a determination of "secondary" cloning efficiencies as a function of donor age; these are plotted in Figure 9.

There is a clear decline with age of this parameter also. Again, one has to be cautious in concluding that cells from the abdominal aortic segments grew less well, in view of the possibility that a larger proportion of input cells from the abdominal segments were those exogenous to the aortic wall of a type with lesser in vitro growth potential (like fat cells, perhaps).

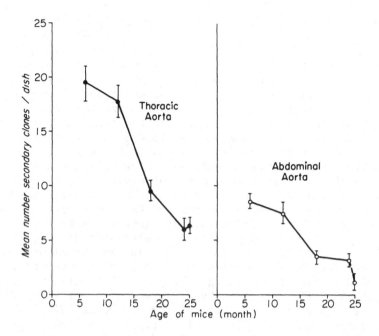

Figure 9.   Mean (± S.E.) numbers of "secondary" clones from strain ICR male mouse aortas plotted as a function of age of donor.   (see text)

In a separate set of experiments, performed with a second group of comparably aged male ICR mice from the identical stock and initiated within one week of the elastase experiments, an evaluation of the replicative potential of aortic cells was carried out with an entirely independent method and, moreover, one which permitted an unambiguous diagnosis of the cell type being evaluated.

Age-matched pairs of mice were chosen at random from among the five age groups for sacrifice by cervical translocation. One 24-month-old mouse was found to have a hepatoma involving 20% of the liver and a 25-month-old mouse had a presumptive renal carcinoma (not studied histologically), as well as a necrotic abscess of one testis.   Crusted excoriations of skin of the back were again observed and were especially marked in the 18 month age group.   Representative animals were weighed from each group and these showed no unusual group-specific deviations.   Aorta specimens from all of these animals were utilized in the experiments to be described.

Thoracic aortas were removed as previously described. From each pair of mice, one organoid culture was set up in a 60 mm plastic tissue culture petri dish with 2.5 ml of complete media, containing two intact thoracic aortic segments. The amounts and varieties of adventitial tissue were as previously described. Special "organ culture dishes" were not used; the tissues were simply totally immersed in the media and maintained under conditions identical to those employed for the cell culture studies (i.e., at pH 7.4 in an atmosphere of 1% CO_2 in air, bicarbonate being the minor buffer and Hepes the major buffer). The rationale was to induce the tissues to undergo a controlled reaction to injury (hopefully to include a phase of preparation for cell division) in a nonphysiologic environment, but one which was known to be compatible with semi-conservative DNA synthesis. The latter was evaluated by ^{3}H-thymidine autoradiography. A basically similar approach had been previously employed by Sade et al. (1972) and in fact had given evidence of a decline in the mitotic index of rat aortic endothelial cells as a function of donor age. A series of cultures from each age group were subjected to sequential 24 hr pulses of thymidine (methyl-^{3}H), specific activity 6.7 Ci/mmole (New England Nuclear, Boston, Mass., lot no. 744-289), at a final concentration of 2.0 µc/ml of complete medium. The medium of all cultures was completely replaced with fresh medium (with or without the radioisotope) at the end of each 24 hr period. At the completion of each pulse period, the specimens were washed with three changes of PBS, fixed in Bouin's for four hours, and transferred to 35% alcohol, in which they were stored until further dehydration and embedding in paraffin. Two micron thick step sections (10 µ intervals) were prepared from paraffin blocks, each of which consisted of trisected cross sections of the pair of aortic segments, giving sets of six cross sections per culture dish; usually three step sections were mounted on a standard 3 X 1 inch microscope slide, giving 18 cross sections of thoracic aorta per slide. These slides were dipped (Kopriwa, 1967) in NTB-2

Figure 10. Autoradiographic sections of segments of strain ICR male mouse thoracic aortas after variable periods of time in organoid culture, including differential 24-hr pulses with tritiated thymidine. There was multifocal and variable degeneration, especially of adventitial tissues, but the integrity of the aortic wall was relatively preserved. a. in culture one day with 24-hr. pulse of ^{3}H-thymidine (age 6 months). b. in culture four days with 24-hr. pulse of ^{3}H-thymidine between days three to four (age 12 months); note the conspicuous labeling by silver grains of mesothelium and of aortic endothelium. c. in culture for five days with 24-hr. pulse of ^{3}H-thymidine between days four to five (age 25 months). Fixed in Bouins and stained with H&E after autoradiographic development. (see text) (X 150 before reduction)

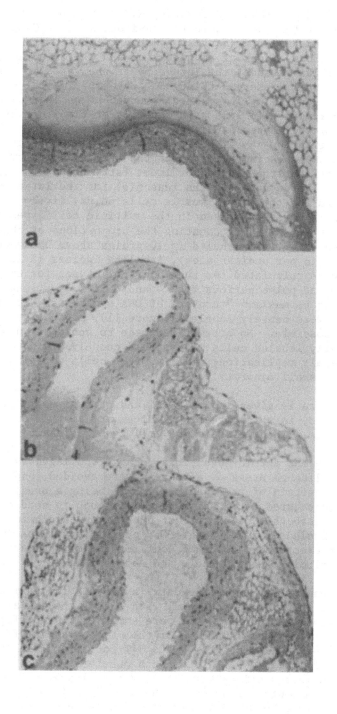

emulsion (Eastman Kodak, Rochester, N.Y.), incubated for four
days in a light-proof, dessicated environment at 4°C and processed
with D-19 and Rapidfix (Eastman Kodak). Although there were
small multifocal areas of degeneration and necrosis, especially
of adventitial tissues, the integrity of the vascular wall was
remarkably well preserved throughout the experimental period
(Figures 10 and 11). This was documented by nuclear counts, which
failed to reveal cell loss as a function of time in culture for
the several cell types studied (Figure 12). In fact, there was
an increase in the number of mesothelial cells. We attribute
the large variance in the data for the areolar connective tissue
to the fact that the amounts of input fatty tissue varied considerably. We do not know the reason(s) for the large variance
in the data for the smooth muscle cells on day five. DNA synthesis was clearly expressed in the multiple cell types examined
(Figures 10 and 11). By counting the proportions of these various
cell types which were labeled ($\geq$ 10 grains above background, which
was < 1 grain per nuclear area), labeling indices (% labeled
nuclei) were calculated for the major cell types for the various
age groups at pulse periods 3 to 4 and 4 to 5 days, when there
appeared to be maximun "turn on" of DNA synthesis. The bulk of
the cells were densely labeled (Figure 11), so that grain counts
were not possible. No attempt was made to score for a subset of
less heavily labeled cells which could conceivably have represented repair replication; clearly, such cells would have con-
stituted a small minority.

The data is given in Table VII and summarized in graphic form
in Figure 13, in which labeling indices are plotted as a function
of donor age. Identification of cell type was unambiguous except
in the case of the areolar connective tissue (adipose tissue)
surrounding the aortic adventitial coat of collagenous connective
tissue. Although areas of autolysis were avoided, one could not
always be certain of the exact cell type being scored; the majority were considered to be adipocytes, although in some cases, endothelial, histocytic or fibroblast nuclei may have been labeled
and were included in the data. Obviously, it will be important
to obtain electron microscopic confirmation of the various cell
types, including smooth muscle and endothelium.

The general trend of the data is clearly indicative of a
decline in replicative potential with age of the animal for both
pulse periods. Moreover, there are some striking differences in
labeling indices as a function of cell type, varying from a high,
in 6-month-old animals, of ∿ 40 to 54% for adventitial mesothelium
to a low of ∿ 0.3 to 0.7% for smooth muscle of media. Three obviously anomalous points (graphs A, B and E) are each derived from
a pair of 12 month aortas pulsed between days 4 to 5; the results
could therefore be attributable to a single animal with an

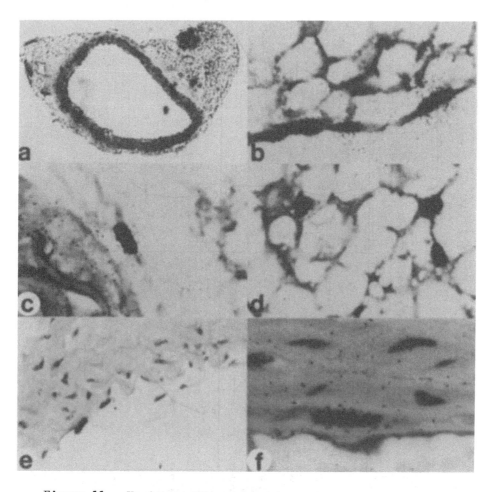

Figure 11. Various cell types which incorporated tritiated
thymidine during days three to four or four to five of organoid
culture of strain ICR male mouse aortas. A. ring of aorta illustrating extent of adventitial tissues and degree of preserva-
tion of the tissue after four days of culture. b. silver grains
over mesothelial cells. c. labeled adventitial fibroblast. d.
labeled areolar connective tissue cells. e. labeled aortic endothelium. f. labeled subintimal smooth muscle cell. (see text)
a X 30; b-d, f X 960; e X 480 (before reduction)

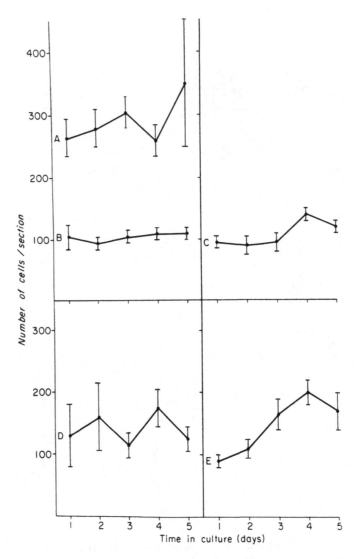

Figure 12.   Total number of cells per 2 μ thick histologic
cross section of Bouin's fixed paraffin embedded aortas as a
function of time in culture and cell type.   Strain ICR male mouse
thoracic aortas in organoid culture.   Means and 95% confidence
limits are calculated from pooled data from all age groups (five
sections per age group).   A.   smooth muscle of media.   B.   endothelial lining of intima.   C.   adventitial fibroblasts.   D.
areolar connective tissue (predominantly adipocytes).   E.   mesothelium.

TABLE VII

TOTAL CELLS COUNTED AND PERCENT LABELED WITH ^{3}H-THYMIDINE (SEE TEXT) OF VARIOUS CELL TYPES IN ORGANOID CULTURES OF THORACIC AORTAS AND ADVENTITIAL TISSUES DERIVED FROM STRAIN ICR MALE MICE OF DIFFERENT AGES

	6 Months		12 Months		18 Months		24 Months		25 Months	
	Total Cells	Percent Labeled	Total Cells	Percent Labeled	Total Cells	Percent Labeled	Total Cells	Percent Labeled	Total Cells	Percent Labeled
Endothelium	881	4.1	1,208	2.6	1,030	< 0.1	1,329	< 0.1	1,401	0.4
(Intimal)	883	3.6	1,301	11.5	969	2.2	1,169	< 0.1	1,219	0.2
Smooth Muscle	2,056	0.7	2,279	0.4	3,291	0.2	3,277	0.03	3,634	< 0.03
(Medial)	1,244	0.3	3,198	0.6	2,331	0.1	2,875	0.1	3,705	< 0.03
Fibroblasts	1,089	6.2	1,428	7.2	1,235	4.3	1,056	4.0	1,611	1.4
(Adventitial)	1,169	10.4	1,200	8.3	947	3.9	1,409	1.5	1,241	1.2
Adipose	1,443	9.2	1,097	8.1	1,287	6.4	1,349	5.3	1,472	7.7
Tissue	1,400	12.5	1,395	11.3	1,049	2.6	997	0.7	1,116	2.3
Endothelium	340	1.8	413	< 0.25	544	< 0.2	505	< 0.2	509	< 0.2
(Adventitial)	324	.3	932	3.9	304	0.3	88	< 1.0	416	< 0.25
Mesothelium	1,440	39.7	1,077	32.0	1,702	17.0	1,423	20.7	2,545	16.3
	1,342	54.0	1,099	27.6	1,421	24.0	1,528	8.9	1,394	11.2

For each cell type, the upper row of data is for specimens pulsed with thymidine during days 3-4 of culture, and the lower row, for specimens pulsed between days 4-5.

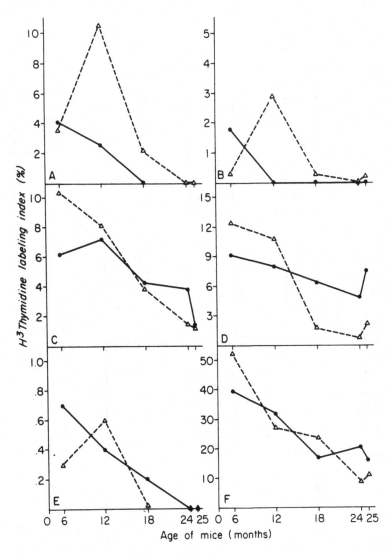

Figure 13. Tritiated thymidine labeling indices (percent labeled cells) plotted as a function of donor age for various cell types within thoracic aortas and adventitial tissues of strain ICR male mouse. o——o pulsed during days three to four of culture; △——△ pulsed during days four to five of culture. (see text; data derived from Table VII) A. endothelial lining of intima. B. endothelium of adventitial blood vessels. C. adventitial fibroblasts (collagenous connective tissue layer contiguous to the media). D. adventitial areolar connective tissue (predominantly adipocytes). E. smooth muscle of media. F. adventitial mesothelium.

unusually large number of endothelial and smooth muscle cells
capable of undergoing DNA synthesis. Since these were outbred
animals, it is interesting to speculate that there could have been
genetic factors responsible for this result. One means to investigate this hypothesis, and to evaluate the alternative explanation of environmental factors (including those related to the
methodology) is to compare the results of replicate experiments
with those obtained using various inbred strains of mice. This
is a general principle of experimental pathology which I would
urge my colleagues in aging research to consider in the design of
their experiments. It is unfortunate that, because of an almost
total lack of interest on the part of investigators, the N.I.H.
no longer subsidizes the production of any outbred line of mice
for aging research.

We conclude from both types of experiments that the replicative potential of vascular wall cells does in fact decline as a
function of age, at least in this particular outbred strain of
mice. Moreover, at least in the first type of experiment, involving cloning, there was evidence for a _differentially_ rapid
rate of decline of a particular cell type (presumptive medial
smooth muscle stem cell); such a differential loss is consistent
with the clonal senescence theory of atherogenesis. In the case
of the autoradiographic experiments, the data (Figure 13) is not
sufficient to confirm or deny such a differential rate of decline.
Although a statistical analysis of data from additional experiments could clarify this point, the interpretation would still be
subject to the uncertainty that the _in vitro_ assay may not reflect,
in a proportional way, the _in vivo_ behaviour. On the other hand,
in vitro assays have the great merit of minimizing many of the
variables which confuse the interpretation of _in vivo_ experiments
(for example, the effects of neurological, endocrinological,
circulatory and nutritional parameters as a function of age).

Finally, we should like to mention the results of some preliminary experimens, performed with the assistance of W.R.
Pendergrass and P. Bornstein, on an evaluation of one potential
mechanism which could explain the decline of replicative potential
of various cell types (including vascular cells) as a function of
age. The protein synthesis error catastrophe theory of Orgel
(1963, 1970, 1973) predicts an increasing proportion of abnormal
proteins in aging cells. Support for (Holliday and Tarrant, 1972;
Lewis and Tarrang, 1972; Holliday _et al._, 1974) and against
(Holland _et al._, 1973; Pendergrass _et al._, 1974) this theory has
been obtained with diploid human fibroblasts aged _in vitro_.
Using a slight modification of methods employed by Pendergrass
_et al._ for fibroblast cultures (details to be published), we have
so far been unable to detect any differences in the amounts of
heat-labile glucose-6-phosphate dehydrogenase in extracts of old
(24 months) and mature (8 months) C57B16J male mice (Charles

River, Boston). It seems quite possible that what we suppose takes place in senescencing "fibroblast" cultures, may also explain clonal senescence of vascular cells -- namely that stem cells, or cells of varying degrees of "stemness," eventually "differentiate themselves to death." It is reasonable to expect that the initial pools of such stem cells and/or their rates of depletion would vary as a function of cell type and genotype (both interspecifically and intraspecifically). Thus, qualitative and quantitative aspects of stem cell depletion of the vascular walls of mice and men may be quite different, and this could be one of the reasons men are more subject to degenerative vascular diseases as they age.

SUMMARY

After briefly reviewing the pathology of the major age related vascular diseases, we discussed some recent theories on the pathogenesis of the most important of these, atherosclerosis, and considered how, within the framework of any of these theories, aging could predispose to atherogenesis. The authors believe that clonal senescence (i.e., an intrinsically limited replicative life span) of cells of the aortic wall may be an important factor in determining the initiation and rate of progression of atheromas.

Published evidence was then reviewed suggestive of an inverse correlation between the susceptibility of a given arterial segment to atherosclerosis and the growth potential of cells of that particular segment (at least in the case of thoracic versus abdominal aorta).

New results from the authors' laboratory were then reported indicative of a decline in the replicative potential of various cell types from the aorta and its adventitial tissues. This conclusion was derived with two independent in vitro methods, both employing aortas from an outbred male mouse (strain ICR), ages 6, 12, 18, 24 and 25 months. In one series of experiments, clones of cells were derived from primary elastase digests and from the first subsequent passage by trypsinization. In the latter situation, reliable determinations of cloning efficiencies were possible, and these showed a negative regression as a function of age for both thoracic and abdominal segments. In the primary cloning experiments, the proportion of total clones which were of presumptive "smooth muscle" origin could be determined and these were also shown to decline as a function of age for both aortic segments.

In a second series of experiments, autoradiographic assays of DNA synthesis were carried out with organoid cultures of thoracic aorta subjected to pulses of ^{3}H-thymidine. For all cell types examined there was a fall-off of the labeling index (% thymidine labeled nuclei) as a function of donor age. For specimens labeled during days 3 to 4 in culture, for example, values for 6 months → 25-month-old animals were as follows: endothelium of aortic intima, 4.1 → 0.4; endothelium of adventitial vessels, 1.8 → 0.2; adventitial fibroblasts, 6.2 → 1.4; areolar connective tissue (predominantly adipocytes), 9.2 → 7.7 (5.3 for 24 month specimens); smooth muscle of media, 0.7 → < 0.03; adventitial mesothelium, 39.7 → 16.3.

Finally, mention was made of preliminary experiments which failed to support a protein synthesis error catastrophe theory as an explanation for the clonal senescence of these vascular and peri-vascular cells.

ACKNOWLEDGEMENTS

This work was supported by N.I.H. research grants AM4826 and GM13543.

REFERENCES

1. Ashworth, C. T., R. R. Erdmann, and N. J. Arnold. Amer. J. Path. 36:165 (1959).
2. Benditt, E. P. and J. M. Benditt. Proc. Nat. Acad. Sci. 70:1753 (1973).
3. Bloodworth, J. M. B., Jr., R. L. Engerman, and K. L. Powers. Diabetes 18:455 (1969).
4. Daoud, A. S., K. E. Fritz, and J. Jarmolych. Exp. Mol. Path. 13:377 (1970).
5. Eggen, D. A. and L. A. Solberg. Lab. Invest. 18:571 (1968).
6. Epstein, C. J., G. M. Martin, A. L. Schultz, and A. G. Motulsky. Medicine 45:177 (1966).
7. Florentine, R. A., S. C. Nam, K. Janakidevi, K. T. Lee, J. M. Reiner, and W. A. Thomas. Arch. Path. 95:317 (1973).
8. Geer, J. C. and M. D. Haust. In: Monographs in Athero-sclerosis. (Eds.) O. J. Pollak, H. S. Simms, and J. E. Kirk, Vol. 2, Smooth Muscle Cells in Atherosclerosis, S. Karger, Basel, Switzerland.
9. Gillman, T. A.M.A. Arch. Path. 67:48/624 (1959).
10. Glucksmann, A. Biol Rev. 26:59 (1951).
11. Goldstein, J. L. Hosp. Practice 8:53 (1973).
12. Haimovici, H. and N. Maier. Arch. Surg. 89:961 (1964).
13. Haimovici, H., N. Maier, and L. Strauss. Arch. Surg. 76:282 (1958).
14. Harker, L. A., S. J. Slichter, C. R. Scott, and R. Ross. New Eng. J. Med. 291:537 (1974a).
15. Harker, L. A., R. Ross, S. J. Slichter, and R. C. Scott. J. Clin. Invest. 25:31a (1974b).

16. Holland, J. J., D. Kohne, and M. V. Doyle. Nature 245:316 (1973).
17. Holliday, R. and G. M. Tarrant. Nature (London) 238:26 (1972).
18. Holliday, R., J. S. Porterfield, and D. D. Gibbs. Nature 248:762 (1974).
19. Hull, R. N. "Biohazards associated with simian viruses", In: Biohazards in Biological Research. (Eds.) A. Hellman, M. N. Oxman, and R. Pollack, Cold Spring Harbor Laboratory, New York (1973) pp. 3-40.
20. Kern, W. H., G. B. Dermer, and G. G. Lindesmith. Amer. Heart J. 84:771 (1972).
21. Kokubu, T. and O. J. Pollak. J. Atherosclerosis Res. 1:229 (1961).
22. Kopriwa, B. M. J. Histochem. & Cytochem. 14:932 (1967).
23. Lewis, C. M. and G. M. Tarrang. Nature (London) 239:316 (1972).
24. Lindsay, S. and C. W. Nichols. Exp. Med. Surg. 29:42 (1971).
25. Martin, G. M. "Dilution plating on coverslip fragments", In Tissue Culture Methods and Applications. (Eds.) P. F. Kruse, Jr. and M. K. Patterson, Jr.) (1973) pp. 264-266.
26. Martin, G. M. Proc. Soc. Exp. Biol. Med. 116:167 (1964).
27. Martin, G. M. and H. Hoehn. Human Path. 5:387 (1974).
28. Martin, G. M. and C. A. Sprague. Lancet 2:1370 (1972).
29. Martin, G. M. and C. A. Sprague. Exp. Molec. Path. 18:125 (1973).
30. Martin, G. M., C. A. Sprague, and C. J. Epstein. Lab. Invest. 23:86 (1970).
31. Martin, G. M., C. A. Sprague, T. H. Norwood, and W. R. Pendergrass. Amer. J. Path. 74:137 (1974).
32. McCullagh, K. G. Atherosclerosis 16:307 (1972).
33. McCullagh, K and M. G. Lewis. Lancet 2:492 (1967).
34. McCully, K. S. Amer. J. Path. 56:111 (1969).
35. McGill, H. C., Jr. Lab. Invest. 18:465 (1968).
36. Mustard, J. F. Molec. Path. 7:366 (1967).
37. Orgel, L. E. Proc. Nat. Acad. Sci. 49:517 (1963).
38. Orgel, L. E. Proc. Nat. Acad. Sci. 67:1476 (1970).
39. Orgel, L. E. Nature 243:441 (1973).
40. Parshley, M. S., R. A. Deterling, Jr., and C. C. Coleman, Jr. Amer. J. Anat. 93:221 (1953).
41. Pendergrass, W. R., G. M. Martin, and P. Bornstein. Gerontologist 14(2):34 (1974).
42. Poston, R. N. and D. F. Davies. Atherosclerosis 19:353 (1974).
43. Robbins, S. L. In: Pathologic Basis of Diseases. W. B. Saunders, Philadelphia (1974).
44. Roberts, J., Jr., C. Moses, and R. H. Wilkins. Circulation 20:511 (1959).
45. Rogers, N., M. Basnight, C. Biggs and D. Gajdusek. Nature (London) 216:446 (1967).

46. Ross, R. J. Cell Biol. 50:172 (1971).
47. Ross, R. and J. A. Glomset. Science 180:1332 (1973).
48. Ross, R., J. Glomset, B. Kariya, and L. Harker. Proc. Nat. Acad. Sci. 71:1207 (1974).
49. Sade, R. M., J. Folkman, and R. S. Cotran. Exp. Cell Res. 74:297 (1972).
50. Saunders, J. W., Jr., M. T. Gasseling, and L. C. Saunders. Devel. Biol. 5:147 (1962).
51. Schmitt, G., H. Knoche, G. Junge-Hulsing, R. Koch, and W. H. Hauss. Z. Krieslaufforsch. 59:481 (1970).
52. Vlodaver, Z., H. N. Neufeld, and J. E. Edwards. Seminars in Roentgenology 7:376 (1972).
53. Vracko, R. Circulation 41:271 (1970).
54. Vracko, R. and E. P. Benditt. J. Cell Biol. 47:281 (1970).
55. Weiss, P. and J. Kavanau. J. Gen. Physiol. 41:1 (1957).
56. Wexler, B. C. and L. L. Thomas. Nature 214:243 (1967).
57. Wolinsky, H. and S. Glagov. Circ. Res. 25:677 (1969).

CHANGES IN HORMONE BINDING AND RESPONSIVENESS IN TARGET CELLS

AND TISSUES DURING AGING

George S. Roth

Endocrinology Section, Clinical Physiology Branch
Gerontology Research Center, National Institute of Aging
NIH, Baltimore City Hospitals, Baltimore, MD 21224

INTRODUCTION

One very obvious manifestation of aging is a generalized decrease in vitality. This change can be quantitated, at least in
part, in the form of ability to respond biochemically to various
stimuli (for reviews see Adelman, 1972; Roth and Adelman, 1974;
Gusseck, 1972). Many responses of this type directly involve or
are mediated by hormones (Roth and Adelman, 1974; Gusseck, 1972).

Table 1 is a partial list of some representative post maturational changes in responsiveness to hormonal stimuli. Several
points regarding this table should be emphasized. 1) Most of the
responses are decreased during senescence but a few actually
exhibit increases. 2) Such differences may be related to the fact
that the responses in Table 1 are measured at a hierarchy of regulatory levels; from the individual cell to the entire organism.
The more complex the system, the greater the chance of multiple
responses regulating one another. Hence, an increased sensitivity
for one response may be due to decreased sensitivity at a related
regulatory response. 3) Great diversity is also evident with
respect to types of hormones as well as target cells and tissues.

Obviously it is important to understand how such generalized
age related changes in biochemical vitality occur. First, however,
the mechanisms of hormone action at the cellular and molecular
levels must be elucidated. Fortunately, such investigations have
been reasonably productive to date. We now know that binding of
hormones to target cell receptors is the initial requirement for
most of their documented actions (for reviews see Roth and Adelman,
1975; King and Mainwaring, 1974). Moreover, although control may

195

TABLE I

POST MATURATIONAL CHANGES IN RESPONSIVENESS TO HORMONES AND SIMILAR STIMULI

STIMULUS	RESPONSE	TARGET CELL OR TISSUE	ANIMAL	CHANGE	REFERENCE
Isoproterenol	Muscle relaxation	Aorta	Rabbit	→	Fleisch et al., 1970.
"	Stimulation of DNA syn.	Salivary gland	Rodent	→	Roth and Adelman, 1973.
Cortisol	TAT induction	Liver	Rat	→ at high dosages	Frolkis, 1970.
"	"	"	"	← at low dosages	" "
Insulin	Glucose oxidation and lipid synthesis	Adipocyte	Human	→	Gries and Steinke, 1967.
Epinephrine	Neurosecretion	Hypothalamus	Rat	←	Frolkis et al., 1972.
Acetylcholine	"	"	"	←	" "
Thyroxin	BMR, O_2 consumption		Thyroidectomized rat	←	Grad, 1969.
"	Induction of hypertrophy	Heart	Mouse	→	Florini et al., 1973.
Estradiol	Acetylcholinesterase induction	Brain	Rat	→	Moudgil and Kanungo, 1973.
ACTH	Androgen excretion	Adrenal	Human	→	Moncloa et al., 1963.
Norepinephrine	Lipolysis	Non-obese adipocytes	Human	→	Berger et al., 1971.

be exerted at various levels, the degree of response in many of
these cases is dependent upon the amount of hormone binding to
receptor. It is thus possible, at least in theory, that some age
related changes in responsiveness may be due to alterations in hormone binding by target cells and tissues. Since binding is the
initial step, probably the best understood step, and common to
most hormonal responses, it seems a logical starting place to
examine aging effects on hormonal responsiveness.

POST MATURATIONAL CHANGES IN HORMONE BINDING BY TARGET CELLS AND
TISSUES

If a case is to be made for possible changes in hormone binding being responsible for generalized post maturational changes in
responsiveness, two phenomena must obviously be demonstrated. 1)
Post maturational changes in the binding of a variety of hormones
to a variety of target cells and tissues must occur. 2) Such
binding changes must be proven at least partially responsible for
post maturational changes in responsiveness to the same hormones
in the same target cells and tissues.

As a first step, it was decided to examine steroid hormone
binding in liver, adipose, prostate, skeletal muscle and brain.
These tissues are responsive to steroids and exhibit a spectrum
of morphological and physiological changes during aging. Steroid
hormones were chosen for several reasons. Among them 1) their
mechanism of action has been extensively studied. In most instances
steroids enter target cells by passive diffusion and bind to cytoplasmic receptor proteins. The steroid receptor complex is then
translocated into the nucleus, where it interacts with the chromatin
to allow synthesis of RNA and translation into enzyme proteins for
a recent review see King and Mainwaring, 1974). 2) Steroid binding
is easily and rapidly assessed using activated charcoal to adsorb
unbound hormone (Rousseau et al., 1972). 3) Many tissues are responsive to steroids (King and Mainwaring, 1974).

Figure 1 shows that specific binding of nanomolar concentrations of cortisol in vitro by cytoplasmic macromolecules of all
tissues examined except liver decreases during the senescence phase
of the rat lifespan. Such determinations at low hormone concentrations generally reflect high affinity binding sites, but are complicated by possible low affinity cortisol binding to contaminating
plasma proteins and "non-receptor" tissue proteins (Roth, 1974a).
In addition, these values are functions of both numbers and affinities of such binding sites. In order to determine whether the
age alterations shown in Fig. 1 reflect qualitative and/or quantitative changes in specific high affinity glucocorticoid binders,
analyses by the method of Scatchard were performed. Such analyses
measure both numbers and affinities of binding sites (Scatchard,

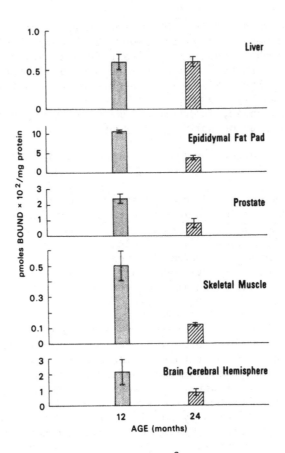

Figure 1. In vitro binding of ^{3}H-cortisol to tissue
cytosols of 12- and 24-month-old adrenalectomized, male, retired
breeder Sprague Dawley (C-D strain of Charles River Laboratories)
rats. Tissue cytosols were prepared and incubated with 10^{-9} M
[3]H-cortisol for 60-90 min at 0°C. Specifically bound steroid
was determined by the charcoal adsorption technique previously
described (Roth, 1974a). Values represent the means ± standard
errors for 6 individual rats.

1949). ^{3}H-dexamethasone which binds to high affinity tissue receptors but not plasma proteins was employed instead of ^{3}H-cortisol
(Beato et al., 1972; Rousseau et al., 1972; Roth, 1974a). Changes
in binding affinity were found to be negligible, but Fig. 2 shows
that actual concentrations of specific binding sites decrease
during senescence (Roth, 1974a).

   Around the time of this preliminary survey, other reports of
post maturational changes in hormone uptake and binding began to
appear (Table II). Singer <u>et al</u>. (1973) demonstrated decreased
concentrations of corticoid binding proteins in livers of 70–80–
year–old humans relative to 30–40–year–old subjects. Such a
change was not found in the study on rats cited above (Fig. 2)
(Roth, 1974a) nor in an <u>in vivo</u> study of corticosterone binding in
rat liver performed by Britton <u>et al</u>. (1975). It is possible
that species differences or difficulties associated with the use

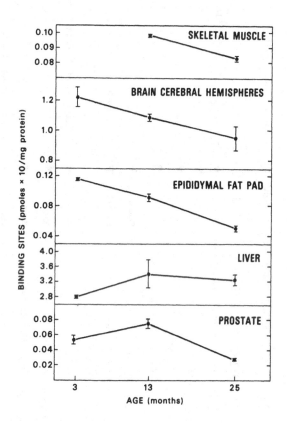

   Figure 2. <u>In vitro</u> ^{3}H–dexamethasone binding to tissue
cytosols of 3–, 13–, and 25–month–old adrenalectomized male,
virgin Wistar rats. Numbers of specific ^{3}H–dexamethasone binding sites in these tissue cytosols were determined by Scatchard
analyses as previously described (Roth, 1974a). Values represent
means ± standard errors for 2–4 individual rats. Reprinted from
Roth, G. S., 1974, <u>Endocrinology</u> 94:82.

TABLE II

POST MATURATIONAL CHANGES IN HORMONE UPTAKE AND BINDING

HORMONE	TARGET CELL OR TISSUE	ANIMAL	CHANGE	REFERENCE
Glucocorticoids	Brain Cerebral Hemispheres	Rat	↓ Concentration of Binding Sites	Roth, 1974a.
"	Prostate	"	↓ "	" "
"	Adipose	"	↓ "	" "
"	Skeletal Muscle	"	↓ "	" "
"	Liver	Human	↓ "	Singer et al., 1973.
Estradiol and Progesterone	Uterus and Skeletal Muscle	Rabbit	↓ Uptake	Larson et al., 1972.
Progesterone	Oviduct	Chicken	↓ Concentration of Binding Sites	O'Malley, 1974.
5α Dihydrotestosterone	Prostate	Rat	↓ "	Shain and Axelrod, 1973.
Corticosterone	Brain Hippocampus	Mouse	↓ "	Finch and Latham, 1974.
Acetylcholine	Brain	Rat	↑ Apparent Binding of Low Concentrations	Rogova and Khilko, 1973.

of post mortem human livers (such as proteolysis or pathologic change) may account for this discrepancy.

Finch and Latham (1974) have recently reported reduced concentrations of a specific dexamethasone binding protein in brain hippocampi of aged mice. Although brain regions differ markedly in structure and function, such observations may be related to reduced concentrations of glucocorticoid binders reported in brain cerebral hemispheres of senescent rats (Fig. 2) (Roth, 1974a). These findings may reflect a trend of neural tissue toward loss of steroid receptors with aging (see also next section).

A trend toward loss of steroid binders with increased aging may also occur in prostrate gland. Shain and Axelrod (1973) have reported that cytoplasmic extracts of ventral prostrates from castrated rats aged 10-14 months contain substantially less high affinity macromolecular binder for 5α-dihydrotestosterone than those of 2-3-month-old animals. Dramatic loss was observed after 10 months of age, with little change between 2 and 10 months. Since prostate is currently reported to have little or no true glucorticoid receptor (Ballard et al., 1974), the physiological significance of decreased concentrations of prostate glucorticoid binding sites in aged rats (Fig. 2) (Roth, 1974a) is not known. Nevertheless, these androgen binding observations are strikingly similar to the above mentioned glucocorticoid binding changes (Fig. 2) (Roth, 1974a) which occur between 13 and 25 months of age, with little change occuring between 3 and 13 months.

Decreased uptake and binding of female sex steroids with increasing age is also evident. Progesterone receptors of chicken oviduct appear to be decreased in concentration during senescence (O'Malley, 1974). This reduction may be due to lower levels of estrogen secreted by aged ovaries. Toft and O'Malley (1972) have demonstrated that oviduct progesterone receptor concentration is estrogen dependent. Meanwhile, Larson et al. (1972) showed that slices of uterus and skeletal muscle from 49-72-month-old rabbits take up estradiol and progesterone less than half as rapidly in vitro as the same tissues from 6-13-month-old animals. It would be very interesting to know whether specific estradiol and progesterone binding is altered to the same extent.

Finally, Rogova and Khilko (1973) reported that a brain cholinoreceptor protein changes sulfhydryl groups in response to smaller concentrations of acetylcholine in 24-month-old rats than in 10-month-old animals. This suggests that binding affinity for acetylcholine is actually increased in the older rats. Such post maturational increases in binding seem to be the exception rather than the rule, however.

Although most of these reports deal with alterations in steroid

hormone uptake and binding, the binding of other type hormones also
seems to change with age. However, most of the changes seem to
occur prior to the senescence phase of the lifespan. It should also
be pointed out that the present methods for determining the binding
of at least one group of membrane associating hormones, the catecholamines, have recently been questioned (Tell and Cuatracanas, 1974;
Cuatracasas et al., 1974). Much of this type binding may be to
sites which are not true receptors, since stereoisomer specificity
is lacking and bound hormone can be displaced by analogs without
inhibition of response. Whether or not these same criticisms can
be leveled at binding assays for other membrane associating hormones
remains to be determined. Freeman et al. (1973) have observed a
progressive decrease in specific binding of insulin to purified
hepatic plasma membranes as rats aged from 2 to 24 months. About
80% of the loss occurs between 2 and 12 months. Along the same
lines, Manganiello and Vaughn (1972) showed that rat adipocyte
adenyl cyclase responsiveness to glucagon decreases progressively
during early life and has been essentially lost by 4-6 months of
age. Unfortunately, exact age was not reported and must be estimated from rat wt. No direct hormone binding studies were performed. However these investigators felt that the change was due
to selective loss of glucagon receptors since epinephrine and
ACTH stimulation of adenyl cyclase remain relatively constant
over this period. Such reasoning is dependent upon the assumption
that fat cells possess only one adenyl cyclase with multiple hormone receptors. Livingston et al. (1974) later did perform the
crucial binding studies. Although part of the reduction in activity was due to increased phosphodiesterase levels, glucagon binding was indeed decreased in the cells of the larger (older) rats.
Despite the fact that these binding changes occur relatively early
in the lifespan and may be growth phenomena, their contributions
to generalized alterations in responsiveness during senescence
should not be overlooked.

RELATIONSHIP BETWEEN AGE CHANGES IN HORMONE BINDING AND RESPONSIVENESS

Having thus presented a variety of evidence for post maturational changes in hormone binding, it must next be determined
whether such alterations are responsible for changes in responsiveness to the same hormones in the same target cells and tissues. Efforts in this regard have been relatively limited to date.

One of the earliest attempts was a developmental study by
Singer and Litwack (1974). These investigators fractionated the
corticoid binding proteins of rat liver from animals aged up to
40 days. The ability to induce tyrosine aminotransferase is first
apparent at 11 days and increases up to at least 40 days, paral-

leling the increasing amount of cortisol association with one of
these binders. More recently, Van Der Meulen and Sekeris (1973)
have correlated an increase in chromatin RNA synthetic capacity
in vitro with the concentration of a specific glucocorticoid receptor of rat liver over the same age range.

King and Mainwaring (1974) have correlated the concentration
of rat uterine estradiol receptors determined by Clark and Gorski
(1970) with the estradiol stimulation of uterine wt. increase between birth and 25 days of age (Price and Oritz, 1944). Another
developmental study by Livingston et al. (1974) suggested that
loss of glucagon receptors from adipocytes during growth is partially responsible for reduction of lipolytic response to this
hormone.

Work by Roth and Adelman (1973) suggested that a post maturational age related reduction and delay in stimulated salivary gland
DNA synthesis in vivo is due at least partially to a reduced rate
of isoproterenol entry into the glands of aging rats. In another
investigation during later life Moudgil and Kanungo (1973)
suggested that age related decreases in brain estradiol receptors
may be one possible cause of decreased sensitivity for acetylcholinesterase induction with increased age in rats. Unfortunately
binding studies were not performed by these investigators. Such
steroid binding changes would be consistent, however, with the
previously mentioned findings of decreased brain glucocorticoid
receptors (Roth, 1974a, Finch and Latham, 1974).

Unfortunately, in one way or another all these investigations
lack definite proof of a causal relationship between post maturational binding and responsiveness changes. In an effort to obtain such proof glucocorticoid binding and responsiveness were
examined in splenic leukocytes from mature and senescent rats.
The mechanism by which glucocorticoids inhibit transport of
nutrients into lymphoid cells has been extensively documented
(Makman et al., 1971; Hallahan et al., 1973; Turnell et al., 1974).
Specific binding of glucorticoids to cytoplasmic receptors is the
initial required step for this effect, since prevention of binding
with certain other steroids prevents inhibition of substrate transport (Turnell et al., 1974; Roth, 1974b and c). Binding is followed by translocation to the nucleus and subsequent synthesis
of RNA and a postulated "transport inhibitory protein" (Makman
et al., 1971; Hallahan et al., 1973). Another advantage of the
splenic leukocyte system is the opportunity to immunologically
and physically isolate functionally defined cell populations.
Hopefully, this will allow distinction between age changes intrinsic to the target cell population and changes in the concentration
of target cells relative to the rest of the cell population.

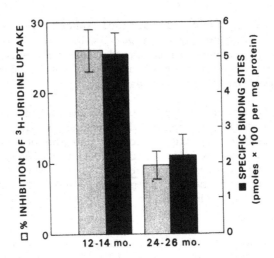

Figure 3. Glucocorticoid binding and inhibition of ^{3}H-uridine uptake in splenic leukocytes of mature and senescent rats. Splenic leukocytes were prepared from 12-14- and 24-26-month-old male, virgin Wistar rats as previously described (Roth, 1974b and c). Numbers of specific ^{3}H-dexamethasone binding sites and glucocorticoid induced inhibition of ^{3}H-uridine uptake were also determined as previously described (Roth, 1974b and c). Histograms represent means ± standard errors for 3 separate ^{3}H-uridine uptake experiments, each using pooled spleens from 5 rats of each age, and binding experiments using 6 individual spleens from rats of each age. Under the cell preparation and assay conditions employed adrenalectomy did not alter the values reported here.

Figure 3 shows that the degree of cortisol inhibition of uridine uptake in cells from senescent (24-26-month-old) rats is 63% less than that in cells from mature (12-14-month-old) counterparts (Roth, 1974b and c). When cells are cultured in the presence of tracer concentrations of ^{3}H-cortisol, a 40% reduction in specific binding of the hormone by cytoplasmic macromolecules is observed in the senescent group (Roth, 1974b and c). Scatchard Analyses (Scatchard, 1949) were performed on cytosols in vitro at 0°C to determine the actual numbers of binding sites at saturating concentrations of glucocorticoids and conditions of minimal metabolism. Fig. 3 shows that a 57% reduction in binding site concentration occurs. This corresponds almost exactly to the reduction in inhibition of uridine uptake. Since specific binding is required for inhibition of uridine uptake (Turnell et al., 1974;

TABLE III

REGULATION OF HORMONE BINDING

BINDER FOR	CELL OR TISSUE	REGULATOR	EFFECT	REFERENCE
Corticosterone	Hippocampus	Adrenalectomy	↑ Binding	McEwen et al., 1974.
Androgen	Testis	FSH	↑ Conc. of binding sites	Sanborn et al., 1974.
Estradiol	Anterior Pituitary	Estradiol	↑ Receptor conc. per cell	Wise et al., 1974.
Progesterone	Uterus	Estradiol	↑ Concentration of receptor	Milgrom et al., 1974.
"	"	Progesterone	↓ "	" " " "
Insulin	Lymphocytes	Insulin	↓ "	Gavin et al., 1974.
"	Hepatocytes	Dexamethasone	↑ Concentration of receptor per cell	Olefsky et al., 1974.
Growth hormone	Lymphocytes	Estradiol	↑ Binding affinity	Ranke et al., 1974.
CAMP	Mammary gland	Prolactin	↑ Concentration	Majumder and Turkington, 1971.
"	Ovary	LH	↑ "	DeAngelo et al., 1974.

Roth, 1974b) the decreased responsiveness of splenic leukocytes
of senescent rats appears largely due to decreased concentrations
of glucocorticoid receptors.

FUTURE WORK ON AGE CHANGES IN HORMONE BINDING AND RESPONSIVENESS

It must now be determined whether loss of glucocorticoid
binding and responsiveness during senescence is due to decreased
receptor concentration within a given population of target cells
or decreased numbers of target cells in the total splenic leukocyte population. Localization and purification of the glucocorticoid target cells is currently being pursued using antisera to
specific lymphocyte types as well as physical separation on density
gradients.

It must also be determined whether correlations between age
changes in hormone binding and responsiveness can be made in other
systems; particularly cell types that do not undergo appreciable
proliferation or turnover during the adult lifespan (e.g. neurons,
adipocytes, muscle cells, etc.). Neuronal cell bodies have been
purified from cerebral hemispheres by the density gradient methods
of Sellinger et al. (1971). These perikaryons specifically take
up and bind glucocorticoids in short term culture. Concentrations
of glucocorticoid receptors in the cells are presently being assessed. If decreased concentrations of receptors are evident in
these aged neurons, as was shown in whole cerebral hemispheres
(Roth, 1974a) and in hippocampi (Finch and Latham, 1974), it will
be most interesting to determine whether neuronal responsiveness
to glucocorticoids is concommitantly reduced.

Should linked age changes in target cell hormone binding and
responsiveness be shown to be a generalized manifestation of
senescence it will be necessary to examine the mechanisms by which
they occur. Those factors which control the quality and quantity
of hormone receptors in target cells and tissues must be elucidated
in order to localize the effects of aging on these processes.
At present the regulation of hormone sensitivity and receptor
concentration is fast becoming a subject of major interest. Table
III shows some representative examples of such regulation. Considerable diversity is apparent with respect to both binders and
regulatory agents. Although most of these manipulations alter the
concentration of receptors, binding affinity may also be controlled.
Already, the molecular mechanisms responsible for estrogen and progesterone control of uterine progesterone receptor levels have
been partially worked out by Milgrom et al. (1973). Doubtlessly,
other laboratories will follow with the biochemical regulatory
schemes for other receptors.

Information as to the control of hormone binding can be of

great value to aging research. Such findings may ultimately allow cellular and molecular localization of changes responsible for alterations in hormone binding and responsiveness. It may even be possible to restore lost responsiveness in aged target cells by reconstitution of altered hormone receptor systems through appropriate biochemical manipulations.

REFERENCES

1.   Adelman, R. C. In "Advances in Gerontological Research," (B. Strehler, ed.), Academic Press, New York, pp. 1-24 (1972).
2.   Ballard, P., J. Baxter, S. Higgins, G. Rousseau, and G. Tomkins. Endocrinology 94:998 (1974).
3.   Beato, M., M. Kalimi, and P. Feigelson. Biochem. Biophys. Res. Commun. 47:1464 (1972).
4.   Berger, M., H. Preiss, C. Hesse-Wortmann, and F. A. Gries. Gerontologia 17:312 (1971).
5.   Cristofalo, V. J. In "Perspectives in Aging Research," (V. J. Cristofalo, J. Roberts, and R. C. Adelman, eds.), Plenum Publishing Inc., New York, pp. 57-79 (1975).
6.   Clark, J. H., and J. Gorski. Science 169:76 (1970).
7.   Cuatrecasas, P., G. Tell, V. Sica, I. Parikh, and K. Chang. Nature 247:92 (1974).
8.   DeAngelo, A. B., L. M. Skrypack, and R. A. Jungman. Program of the Fifty-sixth Annual Meeting of the Endocrine Society A-236 (1974).
9.   Finch, C. E., and K. R. Latham. Program of the Fifty-Sixth Annual Meeting of the Endocrine Society A-236 (1974).
10. Fleisch, J. H., H. M. Maling, and B. B. Brodie. Circulation Res. 26:151 (1970).
11. Florini, J. R., Y. Saito, and E. J. Manowitz. J. Gerontology 28:293 (1973).
12. Freeman, C., K. Karoly, and R. C. Adelman. Biochem. Biophys. Res. Commun. 4:1573 (1973).
13. Frolkis, V. V. Exp. Gerontology 5:37 (1970).
14. Frolkis, V. V., V. V. Berzukov, Y. K. Duplenko, and E. D. Genis. Exp. Gerontology 7:169 (1972).
15. Gavin, J., J. Roth, D. Neville, P. DeMeyts, and D. Buell. Proc. Nat. Acad. Sci. 71:84 (1974).
16. Grad, B. J. Gerontology 24:5 (1969).
17. Gries, F. A., and J. Steinke. J. Clin. Invest. 46:1413 (1967).
18. Gusseck, D. In "Advances in Gerontological Research," (B. Strehler, ed.), Academic Press, New York, pp. 105-166 (1972).
19. Hallahan, C., D. Young, and A. Munck. J. Biol. Chem. 248: 2922 (1973).
20. King, R. J. B., and W. I. P. Mainwaring. "Steroid-Cell Interactions," University Park Press, Maryland (1974).
21. Larson, L. L., C. H. Spilman, and R. H. Foote. Proc. Soc. Exp. Biol. Med. 141:463 (1972).
22. Livingston, J. N., P. Cuatracasas, and D. H. Lockwood. J. Lipid Res. 15:26 (1974).

23. Majunder, G. C., and R. W. Turkington. J. Biol. Chem. 246:
     5545 (1971).
24. Makman, M. H., B. Dvorkin, and A. White. Proc. Nat. Acad.
     Sci. 68:1269 (1971).
25. Manganiello, V., and M. Vaughan. J. Lipid Res. 13:12 (1972).
26. McEwen, B. W., G. Wallach, and C. Magnus. Brain Res. 70:
     321 (1974).
27. Milgrom, E., L. Thi, M. Atger, and E. Bauleiu. J. Biol.
     Chem. 248:6366 (1973).
28. Moncloa, R., R. Gomez, and E. Pretell. Steroids 1:437 (1973).
29. Moudgil, V. K., and M. S. Kanungo. Biochem. Biophys. Res.
     Commun. 52:725 (1973).
30. Olefsky, J., J. Johnson, F. Liu, P. Jen, and G. Reaven.
     Program of the Fifty-sixth Annual Meeting of the Endocrine
     Society A-282 (1974).
31. O'Malley, V. W. Personal communication (1974).
32. Price, D., and E. Oritz. Endocrinology 34:215 (1944).
33. Ranke, M. B., J. S. Parks, and A. M. Bongiovanni. Program
     of the Fifty-sixth Annual Meeting of the Endocrine Society
     A-73 (1974).
34. Rogova, A. N., and O. R. Khilko. "Starenie kleli," Kiev
     (1973).
35. Roth, G. S. Endocrinology 94:82 (1974a).
36. Roth, G. S. Manuscript submitted (1974b).
37. Roth, G. S. Fed. Proc. (in press) (1974c).
38. Roth, G. S., and R. C. Adelman. J. Gerontology 28:298 (1973).
39. Roth, G. S., and R. C. Adelman. Exp. Gerontology (in press)
     (1975).
40. Rousseau, G. C., J. D. Baxter, and G. M. Tomkins. J. Mol.
     Biol. 67:99 (1972).
41. Sanborn, B. M., J. S. H. Elkington, and E. Steinberger.
     Program of the Fifty-sixth Annual Meeting of the Endocrine
     Society A-199 (1974).
42. Sellinger, O. Z., J. M. Azcurra, D. E. Johnson, W. G. Ohlsson,
     and Z. Lodin. Nature N. Biol. 230:253 (1971).
43. Scatchard, G. Ann. N. Y. Acad. Sci. 51:660 (1949).
44. Shain, S. A., and L. R. Axelrod. Steroids 21:801 (1973).
45. Singer, S., H. Ito, and G. Litwack. Int. J. Biochem. 4:
     569 (1973).
46. Singer, S., and G. Litwack. Endocrinology 88:1488 (1971).
47. Tell, G., and P. Cuatrecasas. Biochem. Biophys. Res. Commun.
     57:793 (1974).
48. Toft, D. O., and B. W. O'Malley. Endocrinology 90:1041 (1972).
49. Turnell, R., N. Kaiser, R. Millholland, and F. Rosen. J.
     Biol. Chem. 249:1133 (1974).
50. Van Der Meulen, N., and C. E. Sekeris. F.E.B.S. Letters
     33:184 (1973).
51. Wise, P. M., A. H. Payne, F. J. Karsch, and R. B. Jaffe.
     Program of the Fifty-sixth Annual Meeting of the Endocrine
     Society A-316 (1974).

REGULATION OF CORTICOSTERONE LEVELS AND LIVER ENZYME ACTIVITY IN AGING RATS

Gary W. Britton[1,2], Samuel Rotenberg[1,3], Colette Freeman[4], Venera J. Britton[1,5], Karen Karoly, Louis Ceci, Thomas L. Klug[1], Andras G. Lacko and Richard C. Adelman[6]

Fels Research Institute and Departments of Biochemistry and Medicine, Temple University School of Medicine

INTRODUCTION

The ability to regulate the activities of a large number of enzymes in response to a broad spectrum of environmental stimuli is altered during aging (1-4). For example, following administration of glucose to three-day fasted, male, Sprague-Dawley rats, more time is required to increase the activity of hepatic glucokinase to the same degree in older rats (5). The duration of the adaptive latent period increases progressively and is directly proportional to chronological age between two and at least 24 months (1-3). Many other enzyme adaptations in a variety of tissues from several different species also are altered in time course and/or magnitude of response during aging (4).

The mechanisms responsible for these biochemical manifestations of senescence are not yet understood. The complexity of the problem relates to the multiple levels of regulation to which

[1] Postdoctoral Trainee, Training Grant CA-05280 from the NCI.
[2] Recipient of Postdoctoral Fellowship, HD-00412 from the NICHD.
[3] Current address: Department of Biological Sciences, Drexel Univ., Phila., PA.
[4] Portions of these data are included in the Ph.D. thesis by C.F. approved by the Department of Biochem. Current address: Section of Intermediary Metabolism, NIAMDD, Bethesda, MD.
[5] Current address: School of Allied Health, Temple Univ., Phila., PA.
[6] To whom all inquiries should be directed at the Fels Research Institute, Temple Univ., School of Medicine, 3420 N. Broad St., Phila., PA 19140.

enzyme activity is susceptible in vivo. The biological reactivity
of any population of enzyme molecules is determined by the catalytic behavior of individual molecules, their synthesis de novo,
and their post-synthetic fate. These expressions of cellular
regulation can be influenced by the functional integrity of various
subcellular organelles, the availability of effector molecules
and amino acid precursors, the performance of hormonal and neural
receptor systems, etc. In turn, capacity for performance of a
target cell population in vivo can be influenced by the availability of extracellular hormonal and neural signals, metabolic
nutrients such as blood glucose and amino acids, etc. Furthermore,
the number of responsive cells which comprise a whole tissue at
different ages may contribute to the pattern of enzyme adaptation.

The importance of circulating hormones to the adaptive regulation in vivo of certain enzyme activities is well recognized.
For example, the availability of at least corticosterone and
insulin probably is crucial to the adaptive responsiveness both
of hepatic tyrosine aminotransferase activity following injection
of ACTH into intact fed rats and of hepatic glucokinase activity
following intragastric administration of glucose to fasted rats
(6,7). It was suggested previously that impaired control of
hepatic glucokinase and tyrosine aminotransferase activities during
aging may reflect alterations in the availability of key hormonal
factors (5,6,8). Therefore, the purpose of the present work is
to examine effects of aging on adaptation in corticosterone levels
under experimental conditions that lead to altered responses of
hepatic glucokinase and tyrosine aminotransferase activities during
aging (1,5,6).

EXPERIMENTAL PROCEDURES

A. Animals

Intact, male rats of the Sprague-Dawley strain were obtained
at 2, 12 and 24 months of age from a special aging rat colony
maintained for R. C. Adelman at The Charles River Breeding Laboratories. Intact, male Fisher 344 rats and C57B1/6 mice of the
indicated ages were obtained from the NICHD contract colonies
of Dr. Donald Gibson, and also were maintained at Charles River.
All of these animals are caesarean-derived and barrier-maintained
under rigorously controlled environmental and genetic conditions,
as will be described in separate publications. Prior to experimentation these animals were maintained in our own facility under
the following conditions: in air-conditioned rooms at approximately 72°F; alternating 12-hr periods of light (six a.m. to
six p.m.) and dark; fed a pasteurized, sterilized Charles River
diet reported to be of constant composition and component source;
and additional factors required for individual protocols, as
described below.

B.   Treatments

ACTH and corticosterone were administered in the forms and
amounts, and at the constant times of day, as described below.
All periods of fasting were initiated at approximately 10:00 a.m.,
after which time animals were allowed free access to tap water.
Bilateral adrenalectomies were performed following anesthetization
with ether in our laboratory, after which surgically treated rats
were allowed free access to an aqueous solution of one percent
NaCl in place of tap water, and killed at the times indicated
below.

C.   Materials

Porcine ACTH (20 U/ml in 0.5% phenol) was purchased from
National Drug; unlabeled corticosterone from Schwarz-Mann; ^{3}H-
corticosterone (84.6 c/mM) from New England Nuclear; and radioactive human serum albumin, either ^{131}I (11.1 µc/mg)- or ^{125}I
(one µc/mg)-labeled, from Abbott Laboratories.

D.   Assay Methods

In all experiments reported below, exposure to stress was
minimized by employment of the following precautions: animals
were maintained under the criteria of nutrition, lighting, temperature and humidity mentioned above; all treatments were initiated and biological samples collected at approximately 10:00
a.m., except where noted otherwise; all animals were housed singly
at least 24 hr prior to experimentation; and animal rooms were
frequented by caretaker personnel only following appropriate experimentation.

Blood samples were collected by inserting a needle directly
into the aorta or portal vein approximately three min following
initial exposure to ether anesthesia. Blood was collected in
disposable polystyrene tubes, chilled on ice, and centrifuged
at 2200 x g for 10 min in an I.E.C. PR-6000 refrigerated centrifuge
at 4° in a type 259 rotor. The fibrin clot was removed by use
of wooden applicator sticks, and the entrapped serum transferred
into another set of polystyrene tubes. The serum above the pelleted blood cells was combined with the originally fibrin-entrapped
serum and recentrifuged as above. The supernatant solution was
collected and used as the serum source for the appropriate measurements described below.

Serum concentrations of corticosterone were measured fluoro-
metrically with a Turner fluorometer equipped with a blue lamp,
according to the method of Kitabchi and Kitchell (9), using corticosterone as a standard. Identity and quantitation of corticosterone were confirmed, and possible interference of the assay
procedure by fluorescing metabolites was ruled out by means of

thin layer chromatographic analysis of serum samples of blood collected 30 min following intraperitoneal injection of 7.5 mg of corticosterone per 100 g of body wt. Quanta/Gram* thin layer plates (Quantrum Industries, Fairfield, N.J.) were used following pretreatment with solvent: 95% chloroform, five percent ethanol. Microliter quantities of serum and corticosterone standard in methanol were applied to each slot and chromatographed. Dried plates were sprayed with a reagent (10) containing 25 g of ammonium molybdate per 450 ml of water, 21 ml of concentrated sulfuric acid, and three g of $Na_2HAsO_7 \cdot H_2O$, and heated in an oven at 140° for 15 min.

Macromolecular binding of corticosterone in serum was determined by a modification of the procedure of Beato and Feigelson (11). Intact 2-, 12- and 24-month-old Sprague-Dawley rats were injected under ether anesthesia into the inferior vena cava with ^{3}H-corticosterone. Two-month-old rats received 20 μc and the larger 12- and 24-month-old rats 40 μc of ^{3}H-corticosterone. Blood was collected and serum treated as follows at 4°. To 0.5 ml of serum was added 0.05 ml of Norit A suspension (2.5 mg/ml in 0.01 M Tris-HCl, pH 7.4). This amount of charcoal removes all unbound radioactivity and precipitates no protein. The samples were thoroughly mixed on a Vortex Genie mixer, and centrifuged as above. The radioactivity in 0.1-ml samples of the charcoal-treated and untreated supernatant solution, solubilized by addition of 0.5 ml of NCS solubilizer, was measured with an Intertechnique model SL-40 liquid scintillation spectrometer in a toluene scintillation cocktail described previously (12). The amount of bound steroid was calculated from the radioactivity ratio of the treated to untreated serum samples after appropriate correction for dilution by the added charcoal suspension.

Tyrosine aminotransferase activity was assayed in 105,000 x g supernatant solutions from liver according to the discontinuous procedure of Rosenberg and Litwack (13), which measures the rate of formation of p-hydroxyphenylpyruvate (PHPP).

Volumes of circulating blood in 2-, 12- and 24-month-old Sprague-Dawley rats were determined by isotopic dilution of ^{131}I- or ^{125}I-labeled human serum albumin, following injection into the tail vein as specified in the Abbott Laboratories manual.

Serum concentration of glucose was determined by the methods of Somogyi (14) and Nelson (10); and free fatty acids by the method of Trout et al. (15).

In order to assess the rate of utilization of corticosterone from aortal blood in vivo, Sprague-Dawley rats of the indicated ages were fasted for 24 hr, anesthetized with ether for 40 (2 month) or 50 (12 month) min in order to raise corticosterone levels, subjected to bilateral adrenalectomy, and then maintained on one percent NaCl without food for the duration of the experiment.

RESULTS

A. Availability of Corticosterone in Fed Rats

Observing the precautions and methodology described above, the basal concentration of corticosterone in blood collected from the aorta of Sprague-Dawley rats at 9:00 a.m. to 11:30 a.m. is approximately 10 μg per 100 ml of serum at all ages examined, as shown in Table 1.

TABLE I

CIRCULATING CORTICOSTERONE LEVELS AT DIFFERENT AGES

Age (months)	BW[a] (g)	Circulating[b] corticosterone level (μg/100 ml serum)	Blood[b] volume (ml)	Total[c] circulating corticosterone (μg/animal)	^{3}H-corticosterone[b] bound to serum proteins (%)
2	175	8.0 ± 0.9	10.9 ± 0.2	0.5	95.9 ± 0.9
12	500	12.5 ± 1.8	18.3 ± 0.6	1.3	98.1 ± 1.6
24	700	10.3 ± 1.0	22.8 ± 1.2	1.3	98.7 ± 1.0

[a]Body weights represent approximate values determined during the 3-year history of our Sprague-Dawley rat colony.

[b]The concentration of serum corticosterone in aortal blood at 9–11:30 a.m., total blood volume, and percentage of ^{3}H-corticosterone bound to serum proteins, were determined as described in the METHODS section for rats of the indicated ages.

[c]Total circulating corticosterone was calculated from the determined serum hormone concentrations and blood volumes corrected for hematocrit (Freeman, 1974).

Experimental values represent the mean ± standard error for 6 to 9 rats. Environmental conditions are described in the text.

Values obtained at 12 and 24 months may be slightly greater than that seen in 2-month-old rats. In these experiments blood was collected at approximately three min subsequent to anesthetization with ether. Thus, it is conceivable that small differences in the concentration of this hormone are masked by rapid response to the stresses of ether treatment and animal handling. Although the observed concentrations of corticosterone are nearly the same at all three ages, the total amount of circulating hormone increases more than two-fold between 2 and 12 months of age, accompanying considerable increases both in body wt. and in blood volume. The relative amount of corticosterone associated with serum proteins remains the same, only slightly less than 100%, as rats age from 2 to 24 months.

The increase in concentration of corticosterone in blood collected from the aorta following injection of ACTH into intact 2-, 12- and 24-month-old Sprague-Dawley rats is shown in Figure 1.

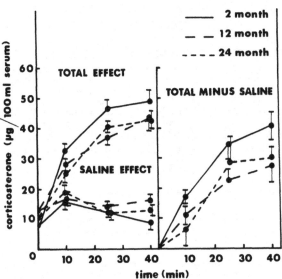

Figure 1. ACTH-stimulated corticosterone levels in aortal blood. Sprague-Dawley rats of the indicated ages were injected subcutaneously at 10:00 a.m. either with 5.0 units of ACTH or an equivalent volume of 0.9% saline per 100 g of body wt., and serum corticosterone levels determined as described in the text. Data in the panel labeled TOTAL MINUS SALINE were obtained by subtraction of appropriate mean measurements of the response to saline from the response to ACTH injection. Values labeled TOTAL EFFECT and SALINE EFFECT were determined in different groups of rats, and the standard errors indicated under TOTAL MINUS SALINE are additive. Each experimental value represents the mean ± standard error of three to eight rats. Environmental conditions are described in the text.

Five units of ACTH per 100 g of body wt. were injected subcutaneously at the lower abdomen, as described in the methods section.
Rats were anesthetized with ether approximately three min prior
to collection of blood at the indicated time points, as described
immediately above. It is essential to avoid anesthetization at
the time of injection of ACTH or saline, because in a sufficient
period of time ether treatment alone evokes a corticosterone
response similar to that of ACTH.

The data indicate at most only a small decrease in responsiveness of 12- and 24-month-old rats relative to 2-month-old
rats. The degree to which these increases in the concentration
of corticosterone reflect the stresses of handling and injection
probably is small at all three ages examined, as shown by the
responses to injections of 0.9% saline. Injection of 0.5% phenol,
which is present as a preservative in our commercial preparations
of ACTH, evokes only a minimal response identical at least at
12 months to that of saline, as shown in Table II. As also shown
in Table II, the increases in concentration of corticosterone
collected from aortal blood 30 min following injection of dosages
of ACTH ranging from 0.025 to 5.0 units per 100 g of body wt.
are very similar at 2, 12 and 24 months of age.

The ability of corticosterone, once delivered to the liver
of Sprague-Dawley rats, to stimulate an adaptive increase in
hepatic tyrosine aminotransferase activity is identical at 2,
12 and 24 months of age, as shown in Figure 2. This observation
is consistent throughout the range of intraperitoneally injected
dosages of corticosterone that evoke a detectable increase in
enzyme activity, 0.5 to 7.5 mg per 100 g of body wt., although
results of only the highest dosage are indicated. These dosages
of corticosterone, which are required for detection of the liver
enzyme adaptation, generate serum concentrations of hormone which
are far greater than those detected in vivo either in unstimulated
rats (Table I) or following treatment with ACTH (Figure 1), as
shown in Table III. The absence of an increase in enzyme activity
following injection of identical volumes of water containing no
corticosterone was shown previously (6,7).

B. Availability of Corticosterone during Fasting

The concentrations of corticosterone collected from aortal
blood of fed and one- to six-day fasted Sprague-Dawley rats aged
2, 12 and 24 months are shown in Figure 3. At 2 months of
age, the concentration of corticosterone increases more than
four-fold following four days of starvation, and is maintained
at approximately these high levels for at least two additional
days. At 12 months of age, only a 50-to-100% increase is evident
during days one and two of the fast. At 24 months of age, the

TABLE II

STIMULATION OF CORTICOSTERONE LEVELS AT DIFFERENT AGES

Stimulus	Dosage[a] (amt/100 g body wt)	Corticosterone level[b] (µg/100 ml serum)		
		2-mo	12-mo	24-mo
0.5% phenol	0.3 ml	-----	10.7 ± 0.6(6)	-----
0.9% saline	0.3 ml	8.5 ± 2.1(4)	10.3 ± 1.3(5)	12.7 ± 1.5(3)
ACTH	5.0 units	49.9 ± 2.4(4)	43.2 ± 2.8(6)	41.8 ± 2.6(7)
	0.5 units	45.2 ± 4.2(4)	45.1 ± 2.3(6)	35.3 ± 3.7(4)
	0.05 units	38.5 ± 1.0(6)	37.5 ± 4.1(6)	35.8 ± 4.4(3)
	0.025 units	26.0 ± 1.0(5)	31.8 ± 3.6(6)	27.1 ± 2.9(4)

[a]All injections were administered subcutaneously to Sprague-Dawley rats, as described in the text, in volumes of 0.3 ml per 100 g of body weight.

[b]The concentration of serum corticosterone in aorta blood was determined as described in the text.

Experimental values represent the mean ± standard error for the number of rats indicated in parentheses. Environmental conditions are described in the text.

increase observed in younger rats within the first few days of starvation may be effectively abolished. However, a delayed response similar in magnitude to that observed at day one in 12-month-old rats occurs at day four of the fast. Furthermore, as indicated previously in Table I, Sprague-Dawley rats undergo a large increase in body wt. as they age from 2 to 24 months. Therefore, it is difficult to distinguish between relative contributions by growth and aging to the absence of an increase in corticosterone levels in older fasted rats. However, as shown

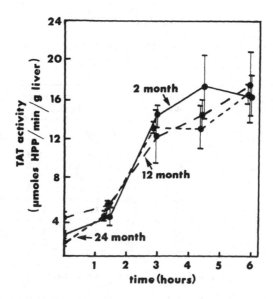

Figure 2. Corticosterone-induced hepatic tyrosine aminotransferase activity. Sprague-Dawley rats of the indicated ages
were injected intraperitoneally at nine a.m. with 7.5 mg of corticosterone in 0.75 ml of 20% DMSO per 100 g of body wt. Liver
cytosol extracts were prepared at the indicated times following
injection of corticosterone, and assayed for enzyme activity, as
described in the text. Each value represents the mean ± standard
error for four to six rats.

in Figure 3, the diminished increase in corticosterone levels
is evident also in male Fisher 344 rats whose body wt. increases
to a lesser extent than that of the Sprague-Dawley by 12 months,
and also in male C57Bl/6 mice whose body wt. is constant beyond
sexual maturity. As demonstrated in Table IV, a two-fold increase
in hormone concentration is expressed at a time of day other than
10:00 a.m. in 24-month-old Sprague-Dawley rats that are fasted
for three days.

As indicated by the data in Table V, it is apparent that
the older rats recognize and respond to the absence of food when
alternative physiological manifestations of starvation are assessed. Liver wt., body wt. and the serum concentration of glucose
decrease significantly at all three ages studied, although more
notably at two months. Serum levels of free fatty acids increase
similarly at all three ages.

TABLE III

LEVELS OF CORTICOSTERONE IN THE PORTAL VEIN FOLLOWING ITS
INTRAPERITONEAL INJECTION

Dosage (mg/100g body weight)	Age (months)	Corticosterone (μg/ml serum) time after injection	
		(10 min)	(45 min)
1	2	4.4 ± 1.2(5)	1.8 ± 0.1(5)
	12	9.2 ± 2.6(4)	2.4 ± 0.4(4)
	24	7.7 ± 2.8(4)	2.7 ± 0.2(5)
5	2	16.9 ± 3.9(5)	5.9 ± 0.9(5)
	12	20.8 ± 6.8(4)	15.3 ± 1.6(5)
	24	24.7 ± 8.1(5)	12.8 ± 1.5(4)
7.5	2	15.5 ± 5.2(5)	9.8 ± 2.6(4)
	12	30.5 ± 7.2(4)	14.5 ± 1.1(5)
	24	48.6 ± 7.3(5)	15.2 ± 4.1(4)

Experimental conditions are identical to those described in the

legend to Figure 2. The concentration of corticosterone was

determined in serum from portal vein blood, as described in the

text, at the indicated times, ages and intraperitoneal dosages.

Each experimental value represents the mean ± standard error for

the number of rats indicated in parentheses.

    Although fasting may increase the rate of hormone utilization
to a greater extent in older rats, the differences are small.
As illustrated in Figure 4, the rate of disappearance of corticosterone from aortal blood of bilaterally adrenalectomized Sprague-
Dawley rats may be slightly greater at 2 than it is at 12 months
of age following approximately one day of starvation. In contrast,
by the third day of starvation, the rate of disappearance of
corticosterone appears slightly greater in the 12-month-old rats.

    As shown in Table VI, the increase in concentration of cor-
ticosterone in blood collected from the aorta following injection
of ACTH to three-day fasted, 12-month-old Sprague-Dawley rats
is even greater than the maximal increase detected in 2-month-old
rats in response to starvation (Figure 3). The small decrement
in magnitude of response to ACTH between 2 and 12 months of
age is similar to that detected previously in fed rats (Figure
1). It also is noteworthy that responsiveness of the adrenal
cortex to exogenous ACTH in vivo apparently increases during
fasting.

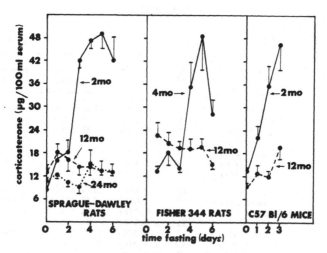

Figure 3.   Corticosterone levels during fasting. Rats
and mice of the indicated strains and ages were fasted from three
to six days beginning at 10:00 a.m. The concentration of corticosterone was determined in serum from aortal blood collected at
24-hr intervals, as described in the text. Each experimental
value represents the mean ± standard error of three to eight
rats. Environmental conditions are described in the text.

TABLE IV

CORTICOSTERONE LEVELS IN THREE-DAY FASTED 24-MONTH-OLD RATS
AT DIFFERENT TIMES OF DAY

Time of Day	Corticosterone (μg/100 ml serum)
10 p.m.	12.9 ± 1.6(3)
2 a.m.	18.7 ± 2.5(3)
6 a.m.	14.4 ± 1.5(3)
10 a.m.	9.4 ± 1.0(13)
2 p.m.	23.4 ± 2.7(4)
6 p.m.	24.4 ± 3.4(4)
10 p.m.	22.7 ± 1.1(3)

Experimental conditions are identical to those described

in the legend to Figure 3 for Sprague-Dawley rats, except

that values were obtained at 4-hr intervals beginning 12

hr before and terminating 12 hr after the 72nd hr of

starvation (10:00 a.m.) at 24-months of age. Each value

represents the mean ± standard error for the number of

rats indicated in parentheses.

TABLE V

EFFECT OF AGING ON VARIOUS CRITERIA OF SHORT-TERM STARVATION

Age (mo)	Time fasting (days)	Body weight[a] (g)	Liver weight (g)	Glucose[b] (mg/100ml)	Free fatty acids[b] (μ equiv/1)
2	0	200	9.8 ± 0.4(6)	140 ± 3(6)	344 ± 21(5)
	1	176 ± 1(6)	5.8 ± 0.1(6)	83 ± 5(6)	790 ± 62(4)
	2	161 ± 3(6)	5.5 ± 0.1(6)	93 ± 8(6)	–
	3	145 ± 2(6)	4.6 ± 0.1(6)		–
	4	142 ± 4(6)	4.2 ± 0.2(6)		776 ± 85(3)
	5	126 ± 3(6)	3.4 ± 0.3(8)		
	6	124 ± 2(6)	2.7 ± 0.2(9)		
12	0	500	17.0 ± 0.5(6)	151 ± 5(6)	378 ± 22(6)
	1	466 ± 2(6)	13.5 ± 1.0(6)	127 ± 5(6)	565 ± 44(5)
	2	450 ± 1(6)	12.3 ± 0.7(6)	111 ± 4(6)	–
	3	450 ± 2(6)	11.4 ± 0.5(6)	97 ± 10(6)	–
	4	440 ± 3(6)	9.7 ± 0.3(6)		665 ± 70 (6)
	5	431 ± 3(6)	10.6 ± 0.9(6)		
	6	422 ± 4(6)	10.4 ± 0.7(6)		
24	0	700	20.1 ± 1.4(6)	120 ± 6(6)	277 ± 67(6)
	1	657 ± 4(6)	14.6 ± 0.7(6)	107 ± 7(5)	457 ± 57(4)
	2	642 ± 6(6)	14.8 ± 1.1(6)	96 ± 9(6)	–
	3	638 ± 4(6)	14.1 ± 1.5(6)	88 ± 7(6)	–
	4	628 ± 4(6)	13.8 ± 0.4(6)		527 ± 36(4)
	5	612 ± 2(6)	13.5 ± 0.5(6)		
	6	592 ± 13(6)	13.2 ± 0.8(6)		

[a]Body weights of the same six Sprague-Dawley rats of each age were determined each day. Values were normalized to fed values of 200 g at 2-months of age, 500 g at 12-months and 700 g at 24-months.

[b]Concentrations of glucose and free fatty acids in serum obtained from aortal blood were determined as described in the METHODS section.

All data were obtained at constant time of day, as described in the METHODS section. Except where noted otherwise, each experimental value represents the mean ± standard error for the number of rats indicated in parentheses.

The inability to increase the circulating concentration of corticosterone during short-term starvation of aging rats is accompanied by an alteration in the pattern of liver enzyme adaptation. As shown in Figure 5, an increase in hepatic tyrosine aminotransferase activity in response to short-term starvation of 4-month-old rats progressively deteriorates as they age to 24 months. Although data obtained only with Fisher 344 rats are presented, similar results were obtained in Sprague-Dawley rats and C57Bl/6 mice.

DISCUSSION

A. Regulation of Corticosterone Concentration

Unstimulated levels of corticosterone in aortal blood, described above for our male Sprague-Dawley rats aged 2 to 24

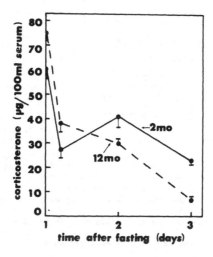

Figure 4. Turnover of circulating corticosterone during
fasting. Sprague-Dawley rats of the indicated ages were fasted
for 24 hr beginning at 10:00 a.m. and then treated with ether,
as described in the text, in order to elevate levels of corticosterone. At the indicated times following adrenalectomy, hormone levels were measured in serum of blood collected from the
aorta, as described in the text. Days one, two and three after
fasting correspond to days zero, one and two after adrenalectomy.
Each value represents the mean ± standard error for five to six
rats.

months, are approximately 10 μg per 100 ml of serum at 9:00 a.m.
to 11:30 a.m. This value is comparable to, although slightly
higher than, previously reported values for 5- and 12-month-old
male Long-Evans rats (16). The amount of corticosterone associated
with serum proteins remains the same as rats age from 2 to 24
months, only slightly less than 100%. Of course, this type of
measurement does not preclude the possibility that the concentration and/or affinity of one or more of the steroid-binding proteins
in serum, e.g., transcortin, may be altered during aging.

TABLE VI

REGULATION OF CORTICOSTERONE LEVELS IN
FASTED RATS OF DIFFERENT AGES

Age (mo)	Treatment[a] of 3-day fasted rats	Corticosterone[b] (µg/100 ml)
2	-------	41.4 ± 3.4(23)
	ACTH	81.1 ± 2.3(6)
12	-------	14.0 ± 1.6(23)
	ACTH	66.6 ± 2.8(6)

[a]Fasted Sprague-Dawley rats either were injected

subcutaneously with 5 units of ACTH per 100 g of

body weight and sacrificed after 40 min., or were

not treated further.

[b]Corticosterone concentration was determined in serum

prepared from aortal blood, as described in the METHODS

section. Each value represents the mean ± standard

error for the number of rats indicated in parentheses.

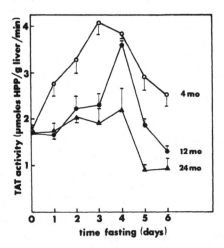

Figure 5. Hepatic tyrosine aminotransferase (TAT) activity
during fasting. Experimental conditions are identical to those
reported for Fisher 344 rats in the legend to Figure 3. Enzyme
activity was assayed as described in the text. Each value represents the mean ± standard error for six rats.

Although the serum concentration of corticosterone is approximately the same at all three ages examined, the total amount
of circulating hormone increases more than two-fold between 2
and 12 months. That the increased total amount is a consequence
of growth and/or maturation, rather than senescence, is indicated
by three factors: 1) the large increase in body mass during this
period of the lifespan; 2) a concomitant increase in blood volume
at this time; and 3) the maintenance of constant total amounts
between 12 and 24 months. Relative contributions to the increased
amount of hormone by altered feedback control of steroidogenesis,
increased steroidogenic capacity of adrenocortical cells, diminished rates of steroid turnover, etc., are unknown.

Responsiveness of the adrenal cortex in vivo to administration
of ACTH (Figure 1 and Table II) does not decline during aging.
Earlier claims of impaired steroidogenic capacity in vivo in aged
experimental animals compared rodents at approximately six months
of age to those of approximately two years of age; neglecting
intermediate ages (16-18). We apparently confirm a small reduction
in ACTH-stimulated levels of circulating corticosterone in our
rats between 2 and 12 months of age, but not later. The possibility that adrenocortical responsiveness to more physiological
conditions may decline during aging will be addressed in more
detail below. However, it is clear that the delayed increase
in hepatic tyrosine aminotransferase activity of aging rats following treatment with ACTH (1,6) is not the consequence of delayed
steroidogenesis.

The apparently impaired ability to increase circulating levels
of corticosterone when rats of increasing age are subjected to
the stress of starvation may reflect either of two distinct general
mechanisms. On the one hand, this may represent yet another
example of regulatory capacity which deteriorates during aging.
On the other hand, since our Sprague-Dawley rats continue to grow
as they age beyond puberty (Table I), starvation simply may not
represent a significant stress to the older and larger rats.
However, it was shown (Table V) that the older rats recognize
and respond to the absence of food when alternative manifestations
of starvation are examined; e.g., changes in liver and body wt.
and in serum levels of glucose and free fatty acids. It also
was shown previously that levels of immunoreactive insulin in
portal vein blood decrease precipitously during starvation of
2-, 12- and 24-month-old Sprague-Dawley rats (19). Furthermore,
the diminished increase in circulating levels of corticosterone
during starvation also was demonstrated in animals which exhibit
completely different patterns of growth as they age beyond sexual
maturity (Figure 3). Thus, the diminished ability to increase
the circulating level of this hormone in response to starvation

probably represents a specific lesion of aging, that is not related
to growth. This may be of extreme importance to age associated
impairments in the regulation of glucocorticoid-sensitive enzymes
in fasted rats. For example, the age dependent adaptation of
hepatic glucokinase following administration of glucose was observed in three-day fasted rats (5). The progressively increasing
delay in the time required to initiate this enzyme adaptation
in rats aged 2, 12 and 24 months is accompanied by the apparent
progressively reduced ability of the three-day fasted rat to
stimulate the circulating concentration of corticosterone (Figure 3); i.e., 400% at 2 months, 50% at 12 months, and not at
all at 24 months.

The age dependent impairment in regulation of corticosterone
levels probably cannot be ascribed to an enhanced rate of hormone
utilization in older fasted rats (Figure 4). Therefore, the
inability to increase corticosterone levels probably is the consequence of an alteration in the control of hormone production.
The steroidogenic capacity of the adrenal cortex in vivo in response to exogenous ACTH is not impaired during short-term starvation in aging rats (Table VI). Therefore, the aging lesion
may relate to regulation of the availability and/or effectiveness
of endogenous ACTH. One previous report of hypoadrenalism in
vivo accompanied by adequate adrenal responsiveness to exogenous
ACTH was the apparent consequence of a circulating pool of inactive
endogenous ACTH (20). Furthermore, a previously reported increase
in corticosterone levels during fasting of young adult rats is
nearly abolished by thyroidectomy (21). The conceivable importance
of age dependent changes either in the availability or action
of thyroid hormone (22) or in the accumulation of an inhibitor
of throxine action (23) remains to be determined.

It was suggested recently that modification of circadian
activity rhythms may be of importance to aging (24). Starvation
of fed humans of various ages probably is not associated with
changes in the circadian periodicity of circulating levels of
cortisol (25). However, a 12-hr shift in the time of the circadian
peak of corticosterone concentration in approximately one-year-old
Sprague-Dawley rats may be induced by restriction of the feeding
schedule (26). Thus, it is conceivable that short-term starvation
modulates this circadian rhythm differently at different ages.
Circulating levels of corticosterone increase in three-day fasted
24-month-old rats, although only at a later time of day than that
observed at younger ages (Figure 3, Table IV). Ascertainment
of relative contributions by a delayed response to the stress
of short-term starvation and by alterations in circadian activity
awaits further experimentation.

B. On the Nature of Lesions in Liver Enzyme Regulation during

Aging

One or more of at least three general mechanisms may account
for the occurrence of impaired enzyme adaptation in liver during
aging. 1) The deficiency may be intrinsic to the liver. Adaptive
increases in the activities of hepatic tyrosine aminotransferase
following injection of glucocorticoids (Figure 2), insulin or
glucagon (6-8), and of hepatic glucokinase following administration
of insulin (5,7) do not deteriorate during aging. However, for
example, as demonstrated for the corticosterone-mediated increase
in tyrosine aminotransferase activity, the amount of injected
hormone required for detection of the liver enzyme adaptation
results in blood levels of the hormone which are considerably
greater than physiological (Table III) (27). Thus, age dependent
deficiencies in the adaptation of tyrosine aminotransferase may
be detectable only in the face of more physiological conditions,
such as any of the large number of phenomena resulting from
administration of ACTH (6,7). Clearly, any such deficiency may
be related to any of a large number of factors, including: status
of the hormone receptor system (19,28-30); regulation of enzyme
synthesis, degradation and catalytic behavior; the number of cells,
which comprise the whole tissue, that respond to hormonal stimulation; etc.

2) The observations described above also represent the first
data that are consistent with earlier suggestions that specific
neuroendocrinological deficiencies during aging may be amplified
via subsequent cascading events in endocrine and peripheral tissues, such as liver enzyme adaptation (5-8). For example, age
dependent deterioration of the adaptive increase in hepatic
tyrosine aminotransferase activity during short-term starvation
(Figure 5) may reflect the inability to increase the circulating
concentration of corticosterone observed under identical experimental conditions (Figure 3). As discussed above, this impaired
regulation of corticosterone levels may reflect age dependent
alterations in the availability and/or effectiveness of endogenous
ACTH.

3) The modified ability to express at least certain enzyme
adaptations during aging may be the consequence of alterations
in specific relevant rhythms of circadian activity. However,
the impaired regulation of hepatic tyrosine aminotransferase
activity in fasted aging rats (Figure 5) probably is consistent
with such a possibility only to the extent that the enzyme adaptation may reflect the effects of starvation on circulating
levels of corticosterone. The daily rhythm in hepatic tyrosine
aminotransferase activity of fed two-month-old rats, which persists

in the absence of pituitary or adrenal glands (31-33), is not
evident during the first 24 hr of starvation of intact rats (34).
After this time, enzyme activity increases sharply and is maintained at these high levels for at least several hr (34).   Thus,
the increase in enzyme activity during fasting probably reflects
a stress response which presumably is mediated, at least in part,
by the ACTH-adrenal axis.

SUMMARY

The ability to increase circulating levels of corticosterone
and the activity of hepatic tyrosine aminotransferase in response
to the stress of starvation is progressively diminished as male
Sprague-Dawley rats age from 2 to 24 months.   This phenomenon
also is demonstrable in Fisher 344 rats and C57Bl/6 mice up to
at least 12 months of age, each of which exhibits markedly different patterns of growth as they age beyond sexual maturity.
Alternative physiological expressions of starvation, such as the
appropriate fluctuations in body and liver wt. and in serum concentrations of glucose, free fatty acids and immunoreactive insulin, are evident throughout this period of the life span in
the Sprague-Dawley rat.   The inability to increase corticosterone
levels probably is not the consequence of an enhanced rate of
utilization of the hormone from blood or reduced capacity of the
adrenal cortex to secrete corticosterone in response to exogenous
ACTH.   The most likely cause is a deficiency in the regulation
of ACTH levels or potency.

The ability to increase hepatic tyrosine aminotransferase
activity following injection of corticosterone to fed, intact,
male Sprague-Dawley rats does not deteriorate during aging.   In
contrast, initiation of this enzyme adaptation following injection
of ACTH is progressively delayed as the rats age from two to 24
months.   Basal levels of corticosterone are approximately 10 µg
per 100 ml of serum between 9:00 a.m. and 11:30 a.m. in aortal
blood of these rats as they age from 2 to 24 months.   Nearly
100% of the hormone is associated with serum proteins during this
period of the life span.   The total amount of circulating hormone
increases more than two-fold between 2 and 12 months of age.
accompanying similar increases in both body wt. and blood volume.
The capacity to increase circulating levels of corticosterone
following injection of ACTH does not deteriorate during aging.

REFERENCES

1.   Adelman, R. C.   Nature 228:1095 (1970).
2.   Adelman, R. C.   Exper. Geront. 6:75 (1971).
3.   Adelman, R. C.   In: Advances in Gerontological Research.
     (Ed.) B. L. Strehler, Academic Press, New York (1972) p. 1.

4. Adelman, R. C. In: Enzyme Induction. (Ed.) D. V. Parke,
    Plenum Press Ltd., London. In press.
5. Adelman, R. C. J. Biol. Chem. 245:1032 (1970).
6. Adelman, R. C. and C. Freeman. Endocrinol. 90:1551 (1972).
7. Adelman, R. C., C. Freeman, and B. S. Cohen. In: Advances
    in Enzyme Regulation. (Ed.) G. Weber, Pergamon Press, New
    York (1972) Vol. 10, p. 365.
8. Finch, C. E., J. R. Foster, and J. E. Mirsky. J. Gen. Physiol.
    54:690 (1969).
9. Kitabchi, A. E. and L. C. Kitchell. Anal. Biochem. 34:529
    (1970).
10. Nelson, N. J. Biol. Chem. 153:375 (1944).
11. Beato, M. and P. Feigelson. J. Biol. Chem. 247:7890 (1972).
12. Florini, J. R. Biochemistry 9:909 (1970).
13. Rosenberg, J. S. and G. Litwack. J. Biol. Chem. 245:5677
    (1970).
14. Somogyi, M. J. Biol. Chem. 160:61 (1945).
15. Trout, D. L., E. H. Estes, Jr., and S. J. Friedberg. J.
    Lipid Res. 1:199 (1960).
16. Hess, G. C. and G. D. Riegle. J. Gerontol. 25:354 (1970).
17. Rapaport, A., Y. Allaire, F. Bourliere, and F. Gerard.
    Gerontologia 10:20 (1964).
18. Grad, B., V. A. Kral, R. C. Payne, and J. Berenson. J.
    Gerontol. 22:66 (1967).
19. Freeman, C., K. Karoly, and R. C. Adelman. Biochem. Biophys.
    Res. Commun. 54:1573 (1973).
20. Krieger, D. T. J. Clin. Endocrinol. Metab. 38:964 (1974).
21. Hainer, V., V. Kubik, and S. Stoilov. Hormone and Metab.
    Res. 4:314 (1972).
22. Frolkis, V. V., N. V. Verzhikovskaya, and G. V. Valueva.
    Exper. Geront. 8:285 (1973).
23. Denckla, W. D. J. Clin. Invest. 53:572 (1974).
24. Pittendrigh, C. S. and S. Daan. Science 186:548 (1974).
25. Marti, H., H. Studer, W. Dettwiler, and R. Rohner. Experientia
    25:320 (1969).
26. Krieger, D. T. Endocrinol. 95:1195 (1974).
27. Finch, C. E. In: Cellular Activities during Aging in Mammals
    MSS Information Corp., New York (1969) p. 141.
28. Roth, G. S. Endocrinol. 94:82 (1974).
29. Singer, S., H. Ito, and G. Litwack. Internat. J. Biochem.
    4:569 (1973).
30. Roth, G. S. and R. C. Adelman. Exper. Geront. 10:1 (1975).
31. Wurtman, R. J. and J. Axelrod. Proc. Nat. Acad. Sci. USA
    57:1594 (1967).
32. Civen, M., R. Ulrich, B. R. Trimmer, and C. B. Brown. Science
    157:1563 (1967).
33. Shambaugh, G. E., III, D. A. Warner, and W. R. Beisel.
    Endocrinol. 81:811 (1967).

34. Wurtman, R. J., W. J. Shoemaker, and F. Larin. Proc. Nat. Acad. Sci. USA 59:800 (1968).
35. Freeman, C. Ph.D. Dissertation, p. 39.

AGING AND THE REGULATION OF HORMONES: A VIEW IN OCTOBER 1974

C. E. Finch, Ph.D.

Chief, Laboratory of Neurobiology, Andrus Gerontology
Center, University of Southern California, Los Angeles,
California

The last ten years of research have shown a number of significant changes in hormonal regulation during aging. For example,
there is virtually complete halt of estrogen production by the
ovary after menopause (1); in contrast, such a change does not
occur in males (2,3; and Table 1). The adrenal cortex in men
shows substantial decreases in the production of cortisol (4) and
pregnanediol (5). Specific age-related changes of cell activities
have recently been associated with altered levels of hormones, such
as the atrophy of the vaginal and uterine epithelium in humans (6)
and rodents (7) after reproductive senescence. Changes in liver
enzyme regulation observed in aging rodents by this author (8),
by Adelman (9), and others (10) may also be attributed to altered
hormone regulation. Because of the well established effect of
steroid hormones (11), T_3 (12), and pituitary hormones (13) on
cell nuclei, many other changes of cell activities during aging are,
doubtlessly, consequences of changes in hormones.

If changes of cell activities prove to be hormone-related in
general, then many phenomena of aging may be reversible. The
responsiveness of the uterus and vagina to estrogens (6,7) is
an excellent case in point. However, not all aging processes
are controlled by hormones, e.g. the damage of skin by exposure
to sunlight (14) and the tendency of arterial lesions to develop
near points of maximum turbulent blood flow near arterial branch-
ings (15). The origin of changes of hormone regulation during
aging thus is of major importance to elucidating aspects of aging
which may be amenable to control.

A strong argument that the brain controls some hormonal
changes of age can be made from studies of female reproductive

229

TABLE 1

PLASMA TESTOSTERONE, AGING, AND DISEASE IN C57BL/6J MALE MICE

	n	Testosterone (ng/ml plasma) mean ± 95 percentiles		n	Testicular weight (mg) mean ± S.E.
Health Mature Mice (12-mo-old)	23	1.12	(.19–12.28)	15	222 ± 5.4
Healthy Senescent Mice (30-mo-old)	25	1.17	(0–7.31)	23	215 ± 3.1
Diseased Senescent Mice	9	0.22	(.08–0.47)	13	193 ± 4.5

Testerone was determined by radioimmunoassay.

Data from Nelson, Latham, and Finch (38).

senescence in rodents. Shortly after midlife (16-20 mo), rats and
mice commonly show a loss of ovarian cycles (16,17,18). Although
the ovary is known to lose oocytes continually from birth onwards
(19), transplantation of the acyclic rat ovary to young hosts
may cause reinitiation of cycles (17,18). In contrast, young rat
ovaries do not show cycles after transplantation to an old host
(17,18). Thus, there is some failure in regulation at a higher
level in the rat. Corresponding experiments in CBA mice give
differing results, i.e. old ovaries in young hosts do not cycle,
whereas young ovaries in old hosts do (19). Possibly, species and
strain differences in reproductive senescence are involved here
(19). The pituitary in mammals does not appear to lose its capacity
to secrete gonadotropins: on the contrary, reproductive senescence
of rats and women is followed by increased production of gonadotropins (20,21) and the hypothalamic releasing factors (20,22);
although output is increased, cyclic changes so characteristic of
the fertile mammal are absent. Thus, attention may be focused on
the centers of the brain which control or influence the cyclic release of gonadotropins: the hypothalamus, preoptic region, and
amygdala (23).

     Recent experiments suggest that a deficiency of catecholamines
in these or other brain regions may underlie the cessation of cyclic
gonadotropin production. Estrous cycles are reinitiated in a majority of rats by intra-peritoneal injection with L-DOPA, iproniazide,
or epinephrine (24,25): L-DOPA is converted to and increases brain
catecholamines (CA) (26); iproniazide, an inhibitor of monoamine
oxidase, increases brain CA (27); epinephrine is a CA. Although
these drugs could be acting to reinitiate estrous at sites outside
of the brain (e.g. the CA rich female reproductive tract, 28),
we have obtained direct evidence for disturbed CA metabolism in the
brains of aging male mice (discussed below). The relationship of
brain CA to the control of pituitary hormones is still controver-
sial, but it is well established that drugs which disturb CA
levels also alter hormone output by the pituitary: e.g. α-methyl-
p-tyrosine (29), and the phenothiazenes (30). The concentration of
CA stores in the hypothalamus (31) and the response of hypothalamic
tyrosine hydroxylase to thyroidectomy, castration, or adrenalectomy
(32) further supports this role. Finally, dopamine has been directly implicated in the control of the gonadotropin-releasing factors
(33).

     Because of the evidence from the ovarian transplant experi-
ments described above and because of the striking age-related increase of Parkinson's disease (34), which is associated with gross
depletions of brain CA (35,36), we initiated a study of CA metabolism in aging rodents in 1971. Our studies to date have been conducted in male C57BL/6J mice. In this phase of our work, male
animal models are emphasized because they lack short term endocrine

such as estrous and show no change in plasma levels of corticosterone (3,37), testosterone (38, and Table 1), or of four pituitary hormones (39): follicile stimulating hormone, prolactin,
growth hormone, or thyroid stimulating hormone. Thus, changes in
brain CA could not be simply a result of the failure of steroid
production which could influence brain CA metabolism (32). Ad-
ditionally, the health status of these mice is well characterized
so that mice with tumors and other characteristic diseases are
culled out. It is pertinent that, in over 800 necropsies of aging
C57BL/6J male mice, tumors of endocrine glands or in the brain
have not been found (40). The distinction between disease-related
changes of aging (pathogeric changes) and normal changes (eugeric,
64) is often not clear in many published studies which were undertaken on animals or subjects of undefined health status. The importance of this distinction is illustrated by a study of testicular
function in mice from our colony: no age changes in testicle weight
or in plasma testosterone was found in healthy mice 8-28 month-old;
however, mice with major pathologic lesions had smaller testicular
wt. and lower mean plasma testosterone (38, and Table 1).

    Several manifestations of altered CA mechanisms occur in
the hypothalamus of the aging mouse. We have found a decreased
(30-40%) conversion of ^{3}H-L-tyrosine and ^{3}H-L-DOPA to the catecholamines dopamine (DA) and norepinephrine (NE) (12 vs 28-month-old
mice) (40, and Table 2). This decrease cannot be ascribed to a
reduced uptake of these precursors by neural tissue, as was indicated by an absence of age-differences in brain ^{3}H after i.p.
injections (40) and by in vitro studies of uptake by slices (41).
Measurements of turnover with radiolabelled precursors show significant decrease (Table 2A). Total hypothalamic NE levels do not
change with age (40, and Table 1B). (Murine hypothalamic DA was
not measurable with the fluorometric assay available 2 years ago.)
Very recent studies with enzymatic assays have shown variations
of DA and NE within hypothalamic "nuclei" (31). Thus, the assay
employed in our original studies could not detect possible changes
in small cell groups which may be of crucial importance to relating
CA changes to specific endocrine phenomena of aging.

    Another facet of CA mechanisms which may be of importance
to neuroendocrine controls is the selective transport process present in neural membranes. Preparations of pinched off nerve end-
ings "synaptosomes" possess a stereospecific, high affinity DA and
NE transport mechanism which may regulate the duration of CA action
at the synapse (42). For example, interference with this transport mechanism by chlorpromazine will block estrous (27). We have
recently found that DA uptake is reduced by 20% in old hypothalamic
synaptosomes (43, and Table 2C). Strikingly, we detected no age
change in uptake of L-NE, serotonin, or L-tyrosine (43). This
finding specifically implicates the dopamine containing neurones

TABLE 2

CATECHOLAMINE METABOLISM AND AGING IN C57BL/6J MALE MICE

A. Norepinephrine Turnover in the Hypothalamus*

	Half-life (± 95% Confidence Intervals)	
	Experiment 1	Experiment 2
mature	122 ± 82 min	135 ± 74 min
senescent	315 ± 106 min	180 ± 75 min
% change	-60%	-30%

B. Catecholamine Levels** (ng/mg DNA)

	Hypothalamus mean ± S.E.	Neostriatum mean ± S.E.
1. dopamine		
mature		3,215 ± 130
senescent		2,515 ± 80
% change		-20%
2. norepinephrine		
mature	210 ± 14	
senescent	236 ± 9	
% change		

C. Uptake by Hypothalamic Synaptosomes***

	Percent change senescent/mature:	
	n	mean ± S.E.
1. dopamine	8	73.2 ± 1.35
3. tyrosine	8	94 ± 2.0

*Turnover was measured by washout of ^{3}H-NE and ^{3}H-DA derived from ^{3}H-L-DOPA (40).

**Levels were measured in regions of individual mice by fluorometry (40).

***Uptake was measured in crude synaptosomes from regions of individual mice at a concentration of 10^{-8} M ^{3}H-L-DA or ^{3}H-L-tyrosine (43).

of the arcuate 'nucleus' in the hypothalamic: the arcuate neurones
are considered to be of particular importance to the cyclic control of gonadotropins because they are rich in estrogen receptors
(44) and dopamine (45) and because they project to the median
eminance (45), where gonadotropin releasing factors are discharged.
The effect of chlorpromazine in blocking of estrous in young rats
(30) (vide infra) suggests that reduced DA reuptake by hypothalamic
membranes could contribute to the loss of cyclicity in aging female
rodents. It remains to be shown, however, that changes in CA levels,
turnover or reuptake actually occur in the female hypothalamus
during aging. The ability of L-DOPA, iprioniazide, and epinephrine
to reinitiate ovarian cycles of senescent female rats (24,25)
strongly supports the hypothesis of CA depletion in one or more
hypothalamic or limbic loci. At present, the evidence for reduced
CA turnover and synthesis and the evidence for reduced DA reuptake
cannot be readily fitted to a simple model of aging in the hypothalamus. We suspect a complex picture of changes will emerge,
one for example in which aging changes in one neural locus may affect others in turn. It would appear necessary to map age changes
in the known critical cell groups and pathways (basilar amygdala,
stria terminalis, median forebrain bundle, medial preoptic nucleus,
paraventriacular nucleus, arcuate nucleus, median eminance, etc.)
by autoradiographic and histologic studies as well as stereotaxic
implants of CA in various brain regions to localize the altered
cell groups.

Steroid receptors represent another facet of neuroendocrine
control mechanisms which may be crucial to reproductive senescence
as well as to the regulation of other endocrine changes [e.g. ther-
moregulation (8), fat and carbohydrate regulation (46)]. A study
by Roth (47) showed decreasing high affinity cortisol binding
sites in "cerebral hemispheres" of old rats. We have recently
found that there are also significant corticosterone receptor
changes in the old mouse brain (Table 3): high affinity binding

TABLE 3

CORTICOSTERONE BINDING TO BRAIN CYTOSOL AND AGING

Regions	Senescent-matutre/mature
Hippocampus	-20%, -60%
Hypothalamus	+40%, +60%

Binding was characterized as ^{3}H-corticosterone/mg cytosol protein
(100,000 g/60 min supernate retained in the exclusion peak after
passage over Sephadex G-100 (Finch and Latham, 1962). The numbers
refer to separate experiments.

capacity decreases in the hippocampus, whereas it increases in
the hypothalamus. A rationalization of these surprising findings
is suggested by observations that the hippocampus exerts an inhibitory influence on the secretion of ACTH (48). If the hypothalamic homeostat for ACTH and for glucocorticoids is dominant
over the hippocampus and if corticosterone receptors in both loci
are limiting for their homeostat, then the decreased corticosterone
binding in the hippocampus would result in a disinhibition of
the hypothalamic homeostat which, in turn, might be compensated
for by increased corticosterone receptors in the hypothalamus.
At present, information about the effect of age on sex steroid
receptors in the brain is not available.

If changes occur in hormone receptors in the brain, then
an alteration in CA metabolism could result. Hormone levels are
known to influence CA metabolism by altering tyrosine hydroxylase
activity in vivo (32) and in vitro (49) and by influencing the
uptake of CA at membranes (50). Although the molecular basis for
the influence of hormones on CA mechanisms is poorly understood,
the current evidence suggests key links between changes in hormone
levels, brain hormone receptors, and CA influences on the pituitary. The sensitivity of the CA mechanisms in the hypothalamus to
hormones permits construction of some interesting neuroendocrine,
cybernetic models of non-random aging processes. Although it is
premature to propose specific details, a characteristic of such
models is the instability of endocrine states. For example, changing levels of a steroid at maturation could influence CA metabolism,
storage or release in the hypothalamus or some other brain region
which regulated hormone output; in turn, an altered output of
pituitary hormones could then result, leading, in sequence, to
changes in steroids, or other hormones which then could influence
further the CA metabolism in the brain. An attractive feature
of such models is that intrinsic degenerative changes are not
required at any stage: only the transcription of genes coding
for a physiologically unstable system is necessary. Other hormonally sensitive molecules [e.g. glycine N-methyltransferase (51)]
could participate in such regulatory cascades.

Support for the general hypothesis that aging is a neuro-
endocrine cascade beginning possibly early in life is suggested
by observations that some aspects of development and aging are in-
terlocked. For example, in the Hutchinson-Guilford progeria syndrome which affects children, truncated growth and arrested sexual
development generally precede manifestations of premature aging
(52,53). Also, in Warner's progeria syndrome, which affects adults,
body size is usually small and sexual development is subnormal
(54). The possibility of experimental manipulations of postnatal
development and aging is shown by the effect of caloric restriction
on a "balanced diet" in delaying the expression of many diseases
(55-58). In one experiment, Ross extended the maximum lifespan

of rats to 5 years by restricted feeding, almost 2 years longer
than the maximum of libitum fed controls (56,57,58); this finding
may be the record shift of longevity in mammals by nongenetic
manipulation. Although the endocrine status of the rats in McCay's
and Ross' studies is uncharacterized, other studies have shown that
underfeeding of rats (59) and prolonged dieting of women (60) reduce gonadotropin output. The effect of diet on longevity and the
diseases of aging in rats may be restricted to a critical postnatal
period (during the first year of life), since small benefit was
found if the diet was imposed after maturation (57). These results
suggest a striking analogy to the critical period in the sensitivity
of the neonatal rodent hypothalamus to sex steroids (61), as well
as to other critical stages during development.

SUMMARY

        Much evidence indicates the role of age-changes in catechola-
mines in the brain in some endocrine dependent phenomena of aging.
It is possible that regulatory cascades, involving an interplay between hormone levels and brain catecholamines or other hormonally
sensitive molecules, underlie control of the aging process.

REFERENCES

1.   Kaplan, H.-G. and M.M. Hreshchyshen. Amer. J. Obstet. and
      Gynecol. 111:386 (1971)
2.   Vermeulen, A., K. Reubens and L. Verdonck. J. Clin.
      Endocrinol. and Metabol. 34:730 (1972)
3.   Nelson, J., K. Latham and C.E. Finch. In preparation.
4.   Romanoff, L.P., M.N. Baxter, A.W. Thomas and G.B. Ferrechio.
      J. Clin. Endocrinol. and Metabol. 28:819 (1969)
5.   Romanoff, L.P., A.W. Thomas and M.N. Baxter. J. Gerontol.
      25:98 (1970)
6.   Lin, T.J., J.L. So-Bosita, H.K. Brar and B.V. Roblete.
      Obstret. and Gynecol. 41:97 (1973)
7.   Ingraham, D.L. J. Endocrinol. 19:182 (1959)
8.   Finch, C.E., J.R. Foster and A.E. Mirsky. J. Gen. Physiol.
      54:690 (1969)
9.   Adelman, R.C. J. Biol. Chem. 245:1032 (1970)
10.   Adelman, R.C. Nature 228:1095 (1970)
11.   Hamilton, T.H. Science 161:649 (1968)
12.   Samuels, H.H. and J.S. Tsai. Proc. Nat. Acad. Sci. U.S.A.
      70:3488 (1973)
13.   Oravec, M. and A. Korner. J. Mol. Biol. 58:489 (1971)
14.   Cockerell, E.G., R.G. Freeman and J.M. Knox. Arch. Dermatol.
      84:157 (1961)
15.   Blumenthal, H.T., F.P. Handler and J.O. Blache. Amer. J.
      Med. 17:337 (1954)

16. Thung, P.J., L.M. Boot and O. Muhlbock. Acta Endocrinol.
    23:8 (1956)
17. Ascheim, P. Gerontologia 10:65 (1965)
18. peng, M., and H. Huang. Fertil. and Steril. 23:535 (1972)
19. Krohn, P.L. Proc. Roy Soc. (London) B157:128 (1962)
20. Clemens, J.A. and J. Meites. Neuroendocrinol. 7:249 (1971)
21. Tsai, C.C. and S.S.C. Yen. J. Clin. Endocrinol. and Metabol.
    32:766 (1971)
22. Seyler, L.E., Jr. and S. Reichlin. J. Clin. Endocrinol. and
    Metabol. 37:197 (1973)
23. Everett, J.W. Ann. Rev. Physiol. 31:383 (1969)
24. Clemens, J.A., Y. Amenomori, T. Jenkins and J. Meites. Proc.
    Soc. Exp. Biol. Med. 132:561 (1969)
25. Quadri, S.K., G.S. Kledzik and J. Meites. Neuroendocrinol.
    11:248 (1973)
26. Dowson, J.H. and I. Laslo. J. Neurochem. 18:2501 (1971)
27. Spector, S., D. Prockop, P.A. Shore and B.B. Brodie. Science
    127:704 (1957)
28. Falck, B., G. Gardmark and G. Nybell. Endocrinol. 94:1475
    (1974)
29. Kalra, S.P. and S.M. McCann. Endocrinol. 93:356 (1963)
30. deWied, D. Pharmacol. Rev. 19:251 (1967)
31. Palkovits, M., M. Brownstein, J. Assvedra and J. Axelrod.
    Brain Res. 77:137 (1974)
32. Kizer, J.S., M. Palkovits, J. Zivin, M. Brownstein, J.M.
    Saavedra and I.J. Kopin. Endocrinol. 95:799 (1974)
33. Kamberi, I. Prog. Brain Res. 39:276 (1973)
34. Hoehn, M.M. and M.D. Yahr. Neurology 17:427 (1967)
35. Hornykiewicz, O., in Proceedings of the 2nd Symposium of the
    Parkinson's Disease Information and Research Center. (Eds.)
    E. Costa, L.J. Cote and M.D. Yahr, Raven Press, New York (1965)
    p. 171
36. Bernheimer, H., W. Birkmayer, O. Hornykiewicz, K. Jellinger
    and F. Seitelberger. J. Neurol. Sci. 20:415 (1973)
37. Latham, K. and C.E. Finch. In preparation.
38. Nelson, J.F., K. Latham and K. Finch. Acta Endocrinol.
    In press.
39. Finch, C.E., D. Lindsay, R.S. Swerdloff and Y.N. Sinha. In
    preparation.
40. Finch, C.E. Brain Res. 52:261 (1973)
41. Finch, C.E., V. Jonec, G. Hody, J.P. Walker, W. Morton-Smith,
    A. Alper and G.J. Dougher. J. Gerontol. 30:33 (1975).
42. Cooper, J.R., F.E. Bloom and R.H. Roth. The Biochemical Basis
    of Neuropharmacology, Oxford University Press, New York. (1974)
43. Jonec, V. and C.E. Finch. Brain Res. In press.
44. Stumpf, W.E. Science 162:1001 (1968)
45. Jonsson, G., K. Fuxe and T. Hokfelt. Brain Res. 40:271 (1972)
46. Hruza, A. and M. Jelinkova. Gerontologia 8:36 (1963)
47. Roth, G.S. Endocrinology 94:82 (1974)
48. Kawakami, M., K. Seto, E. Terasaw, K. Yoshida, T. Miyamoto,
    M. Sekiguchi and Y. Hattori. Neurocrinology 3:337 (1968)

49. Beattie, C.W. and L.F. Soyka. Endocrinology 93:1453 (1973)
50. Endersby, C.A. and C.A. Wilson. Brain Res. 73:321 (1974)
51. Mays, L.L., E. Borek and C.E. Finch. Nature 243:411 (1973)
52. Thomson, J. and J.O. Forfar. Archives of Diseases of Child-
    hood 25:224 (1950)
53. Cooke, J.V., J. Pediat. 42:26 (1953)
54. Epstein, C.J., G.M. Martin, A.L. Schultz and A.G. Motulsky.
    Medicine 45:177 (1966)
55. McCay, C.M., M.F. Crowell and L.A. Maynard. J. Nutr. 10:63
    (1935)
56. Ross, M.H. J. Nutr. 75:197 (1961)
57. Ross, M.H. and G. Bras. J. Nat. Can. Inst. 47:1095 (1971)
58. Ross, M.H. Amer. J. Clin. Nutr. 25:834 (1972)
59. Howland, B.E. and K.R. Skinner. Canad. J. Physiol. Pharmacol.
    51:759 (1973)
60. Lev-Ran, A. Fertil. and Steril. 25:459 (1974)
61. Harris, G.W. Endocrinol. 5:627 (1964)
62. Finch, C.E. and K.R. Latham. In preparation.
63. Finch, C.E. Exptl. Gerontol. 7:53 (1972)

AGING AND THE DISPOSITION OF GLUCOSE

Reubin Andres and Jordan D. Tobin
The Clinical Physiology Branch, Gerontology Research
Center, National Institute of Child Health and Human
Development, NIH, Baltimore City Hospitals, Baltimore,
MD 21224

I. INTRODUCTION

The rather peculiar title of this paper was chosen to emphasize the interesting historical development of a now burgeoning
field. In a sense the ontogeny of individual workers in this
field has in many cases recapitulated the phylogeny of the entire
endeavor. Interest in carbohydrate metabolism and aging dates
back well over 50 years. Clinicians became fascinated by a new
diagnostic test for diabetes, the glucose tolerance test, and
proceeded to explore all sorts of variables which influenced the
efficiency with which the body could dispose of an oral glucose
load. Age soon reared its head as an annoying complexity in
attempts to standardize the interpretation of performance on this
test. With the discovery and subsequent availability of insulin
to physicians in the early 1920's, the accurate diagnosis of diabetes became important; the hallmark of the disease was the presence of inappropriately elevated levels of glucose in circulating
blood.

It is remarkable to observe the continued production of
manuscripts in the 1920's, 1930's, 1940's and down to the present
day which demonstrate over and over again that with increasing
age the ability to dispose of a glucose load diminishes (Andres,
1971).

We can understand this apparently uncontrollable compulsion
to confirm an over-documented finding, since we also had to prove
to ourselves 10 years ago that aging and poor glucose tolerance
were associated. In the mid-1960's however, a change occurred.
The development of techniques for the accurate assay of insulin

in plasma led to a quantum leap from passive observation of age differences in performance to active efforts to understand the mechanism(s) underlying these differences.

This paper then will summarize (1) the implications (both theoretical and "practical") of the age effects on carbohydrate metabolism and (2) the efforts to understand the underlying mechanisms.

II. IMPLICATIONS OF THE AGE EFFECT

A selection of representative studies, Tables 1-3, was recently published (Andres and Tobin, 1972). The tables demonstrate some facts clearly but omit other important observations. First, it must be emphasized that for each of these three diagnostic tests for diabetes (the oral and intravenous glucose tolerance tests and the intravenous tolbutamide response test) only mean values are presented. For a fuller interpretation of aging effects the range or variance must also be taken into account. Second, middle-aged subjects are omitted. In nearly all cases their values lie between those of the young and old subjects.

The tables illustrate some (but by no means all) of the difficulties involved in decisions concerning the selection of standards of normality. Note that the dose of glucose given, especially in the oral test, varies widely. Note also the definition of "young" and "old" is by no means uniform. The number of subjects examined varies widely (and is sometimes quite small) -- we have attempted to select the most reliable studies. Also omitted from the tables is a description of the populations studied. They vary from carefully controlled randomized samples of large populations, to community surveys, to a variety of specialized groups such as food-handlers, volunteers in studies of aging, residents of aged homes, etc. A number of important technical differences, such as the chemical method for glucose used, also have been omitted.

These three tables do demonstrate (with all their deficiencies) that the effect of aging is always found. True, there are large quantitative differences in the estimates of the magnitude of the effect, and these differences have disturbing effects on efforts to create normative standards. The differences among the studies must be caused by a combination of differences in technical variables in the performance of the test and in the procedures used for subject selection. Discussion of these factors are beyond the scope of this presentation. A report of The Committee on Statistics of the American Diabetes Association (1969) should be consulted for discussion of these variables.

The age effect is so large on each of these three tests that

TABLE I

ORAL GLUCOSE TOLERANCE TEST

(References for this table are given in Andres and Tobin, 1972)

Study	Glucose Dose(g)	Source of Blood [d]	Age (yr) Young	Age (yr) Old	Mean Blood Gluc. [e] (mg%) One Hr Young	One Hr Old	Two Hr Young	Two Hr Old	Age Effect on glucose conc. (mg% per decade life) One Hr	Two Hr
1. U.S. Nat. Center Health Stat., 1964	50	V	18-24	75-79	100	166	--	--	12	--
2. Welborn et al., 1969	50	V	21-29	>70	86	135	--	--	10	--
3. Boyns et al., 1969	50	V	<24	>55	89	125	74	78	9	1
4. Nilsson et al., 1967	(50)[b]	C	20-39	60-79	111	154	--	--	11	--
5. Butterfield, 1966	50	C	20-29	70-79	125	194	86	121	14	7
6. Diabetes Survey Working Party, 1963	50	C	<29	>70	122	186	98	119	13	4
7. Hayner et al., 1965	100	V	16-19	70-79	100	177	--	--	13	--
8. Unger, 1957	100	V	18-29	50-59	--	--	99	131	--	11
9. Studer et al., 1969	100	C	25-34	65-74	--	--	98	127	--	7
10. Gerontology Research Center, 1972	(122)[c]	V	20-29	70-79	144	174	113	145	6	6

[a] In studies 3-6 and 8-10, glucose was ingested in the morning after an overnight fast. In studies 1, 2, and 7 subjects presented themselves for testing at various times of the day and at various time intervals after the last meal.

[b] 30 g glucose per M^2 surface area - 50 g for man of average size

[c] 1.75 g per kg body weight = 122 g per 70 kg man

[d] V = antecubital venous blood; C = capillary blood

[e] It should be stressed that these values should not be taken as the upper limits of normality. They represent mean values. Note that at two hours the mean value for the old subjects is equal to or exceeds 120 mg%, a level commonly taken to be the upper limit of normality.

TABLE II

INTRAVENOUS GLUCOSE TOLERANCE TEST

(References for this table are given in Andres and Tobin, 1972)

Study	Glucose Dose	Age of Subjects[a]		Mean Decay Constant, K[b]		Age Effect on K (percent per decade of life)[c]
		Young	Old	Young	Old	
1. Schneeberg & Finestone, 1952[d]	0.33g/kg	16-39(48)	60-90(39)	1.88	1.14	0.15
2. Conard, 1955	0.33g/kg	20-39(33)	60-88(27)	1.85	1.09	0.19
3. Silverstone et al., 1957	25g	23-37(12)	65-87(11)	1.68	0.98	0.15
4. Streeten et al., 1964	25g	21-32(23)	70-92(15)	2.35	1.16	0.21
5. Dyck & Moorhouse, 1966[e]	50g/1.73m^2	18-39(31)	60-75(13)	2.61	1.48	0.28
6. Cerasi & Luft, 1967[f]	25g	20-39(49)	60-79(14)	1.76	1.45	0.09
7. Gerontology Research Center, 1972	0.375g/kg	20-39(70)	60-79(111)	1.37	1.01	0.09

[a]The number of subjects in each age group is given in parentheses.

[b]The decay constant is computed from the absolute glucose concentration, not from the increment in glucose over the fasting value. K has the dimensions of percent glucose disappearance per minute.

[c]Computed from the difference between mean K of the young and old groups divided by the difference between the mean age of these two groups, multiplied by 10.

[d]K values computed from table of mean glucose concentrations at 30 and 60 minutes.

[e]The higher mean K values in this study are due to the high glucose dose used. The authors consider the limit of normality to be 1.50 with this dose.

[f]The high mean K value in the older subjects in this study is at least partly due to the elimination of subjects with K < 1.00; the authors wished to study "normal" old subjects. The mean is thus arbitrarily raised.

TABLE III

INTRAVENOUS TOLBUTAMIDE RESPONSE TEST[a]

(References for this table are given in Andres and Tobin, 1972)

Study	Age of Subjects		Mean Glucose Conc. at 30 minutes (% of fasting value)		Pre-screening by Oral GTT[b]
	Younger	Older	Young	Old	
1. Unger & Madison, 1958	----	----	----	51	*
2. Vechhio et al., 1965	App 20-58	----	54	---	*
3. Kaplan, 1961	18-59	60+	57	63	*
4. Oberdisse et al., 1962[c]	App 18-45	----	58	---	*
5. Haas, 1964[c]	Young adults		60	---	
6. Swerdloff et al., 1967	20-29	50-81	60	75	
7. Pereira et al., 1962	14-48	---	61	---	
8. Marigo et al., 1962	20-59	60+	63	75	
9. Bronzini et al., 1964	----	64-89	---	65	
10. Mazzi et al., 1964	----	65+	---	78	
11. Ortone, 1964[d]	----	64-86	---	84	

[a]Studies selected for this table have met the following criteria: (1) the age of the subject must be given reasonably clearly, (2) the age range of the younger subjects must not have exceeded 59 years, and (3) the number of subjects in an age group must be at least 19. The Unger and Madison study is included despite uncertainty of the age range since it is the original publication which provides the generally accepted standards for judging performance.

[b]In the studies marked by an asterisk, in order to be included for tolbutamide testing, subjects had to first pass a stringently interpreted oral glucose tolerance screening test. Subjects in these studies therefore represent that fraction of the population which performs superiorly on diabetes testing. This probably explains the lower glucose concentrations (i.e. the better tolbutamide performance) in the 4 studies marked with the asterisks as compared to the 7 done on subjects not preselected in this manner.

[c]These data were computed by us from illustrations, not from tabular data and are therefore subject to minor errors in our readings of the illustrations.

[d]One subject with fasting glucose values of 140 and 122 mg% was included by Ortone but excluded in our computations in the table above.

approximately half of the older subjects would "fail" the test
if standards of normality (for example, the mean + two standard
deviations) were derived from the performance levels of young
adults. It is this disturbing fact which has led to a healthfully
acrimonious debate concerning aging and the diagnosis of diabetes.
In essence two -- or perhaps three -- schools have evolved. One
group favors the concept that age differences in performance with
age are normal (or physiologic or adaptive -- and thus appropriate
or perhaps even beneficial). A contrary view is that these age
differences represent the emergence of ever increasing numbers
of true diabetics and are therefore to be considered as abnormal,
pathologic, harmful. These ideas have been presented in more
detail recently (Andres, 1971; O'Sullivan, 1974). The third view
can almost be characterized as a vigorous pox-on-both houses
attitude (Siperstein, 1974); in this article the glucose tolerance
test is given a vote of no confidence at all as a diagnostic test
for diabetes. This view, by presenting the most extreme extension
of the difficulties of test interpretation, will serve to test
the mettle of workers in this field in coming years.

It is probably fair to characterize the present confused
situation by saying that the consensus has moved in the direction
of admitting some validity to the first viewpoint, that is, that
aging per se influences test performance, but that no clear consensus concerning just what adjustments in normal standards should
be made or at what age adjustments become mandatory.

Two approaches toward a resolution of this dilemma seem
possible. Both approaches are obvious and difficult. One involves
the longitudinal long-term study of large populations who receive
these tests early in life and are repeatedly re-tested and re-
examined for the stigmata of diabetes over many years. In essence
this approach is the same as those actuarial studies that demonstrated the life-shortening effects of elevated blood pressure
and elevated body wt. The question to be answered is: just what
degree of elevation of blood sugar at just what age will carry
with it a shortened life or earlier myocardial infarctions or
the development of specific diabetic microvascular complications?
This long-term study then is a way to test the tests.

III.   STUDIES ON THE MECHANISM OF THE AGE EFFECTS

A second approach to resolving the dilemma is, in essence,
the development of other diagnostic tests which are uninfluenced
by age. A corollary of this approach is the design of studies
which will elucidate the mechanism of the age differences and,
therefore, will differentiate these effects from the (hopefully
different) mechanism of the disease, diabetes. The design of
such studies could be a penetrating discussion question to test
a student's depth of understanding of the physiology of the body's

glucose economy. Where should one start? The disturbed ability
to dispose of a glucose load might be secondary to gastro-intes-
tinal factors, to delayed glucose disposal in a variety of tissues
(liver, adipose tissue, muscle), to a failure to reduce endogenous
glucose production by liver and kidney, or to disturbances in
the kinetics of glucose distribution with age. A "second generation" of questions might involve endocrine responses to hyperglycemia. Is insulin released appropriately, that is, rapidly
enough and in large enough amounts? Is the insulin biologically
effective (is the precursor hormone proinsulin inappropriately
released)? Are tissues normally responsive to the effects of
insulin? Depending upon defects found in such studies, a third
set of questions would arise: Is insulin synthesis in the beta
cell normal? Are there defects in insulin receptors on cell
surfaces?

This list is of course not intended to be exhaustive. It
is a potpourri of possible approaches and demonstrates something
of the complexity and magnitude of the problem. The major effort
to date has been an examination of the role of insulin in the
age differences in handling glucose. A considerable number of
studies have examined the serum insulin response to the administration of glucose orally and intravenously. Interestingly
these studies have been carried out exclusively in man. A summary
of the results in man are given in Tables 4 and 5 and are indeed
bewildering.

Clearly one of the difficulties in interpreting these studies
is that the pancreatic beta cell responds in both tests to the
hyperglycemia induced by the glucose load. Although the glucose
load (by vein or by mouth) may be constant, the stimulus to the
beta cell is clearly different in young and old subjects, since
the poor glucose tolerance in the old group represents, by definition, an increase in the blood glucose concentration. Thus
the older pancreas is, on the average, exposed to a greater
glucose stimulus than is the younger pancreas. There is, in
addition an insulinotropic stimulus from the gut in the oral test,
the so-called gastrointestinal insulin-stimulating hormone(s).
These GI factors deserve investigation with respect to age but
no studies have as yet been reported.

These two difficulties (uncontrolled hyperglycemia and GI
hormones) can both be avoided by the glucose-clamp technique
(Andres et al., 1969). This "glucose-clamp" technique depends
upon: (1) the intravenous infusion of glucose to create a chosen
hyperglycemia plateau; (2) the rapid periodic measurement of the
actual blood glucose concentration achieved; (3) the periodic
servo-correction of the glucose infusion rate using the negative
feed-back principle. A major advantage of this technique is that

TABLE IV

EFFECT OF AGE ON SERUM INSULIN RESPONSE TO ORAL GLUCOSE

Insulin response	Comments
A. Increase	
Chlouverakis et al., 1967	At 60 min., but p < 0.1 only
Hales et al., 1968	At 60 and 90 min.
Boyns et al., 1969	Males only; females no change
Sensi et al., 1972	Increase at 120 min.; decreased at 30 min.
Nolan et al., 1973	At 60 min.
Sandberg et al., 1973	At 60 to 120 min.
B. No change	
Welborn et al., 1966	
Reavan and Miller, 1968	
Boyns et al., 1969	No change in females; males increased
Björntorp et al., 1971	
C. Decrease	
Zhukov, 1965	Rat diaphragm bio-assay for insulin
Sensi et al., 1972	Decrease at 30 min.; increase at 120 min.

a constant exact hyperglycemic stimulus is presented to the pancreatic beta cells of all subjects, regardless of age, obesity, diabetic state, etc. In a series of studies of normal wt. young and old men, hyperglycemic levels of 140, 180, 200, and 300 mg/dl were maintained for two hr periods. The plasma insulin response in both young and old were characteristically biphasic with an initial peak at about four min, a fall to a nadir of 10–15 min, then a gradual progressive increase for the remainder of the study. The time course of the insulin response did not differ with age, but the insulin levels achieved were significantly lower in the old group at the 140, 180, and 220 levels. Insulin responses were the same in young subjects at the 220 and 300 levels; in the old subjects the insulin response continued to increase in this range. Thus at the 300 level, old and young responses were not significantly different. These results can be interpreted as showing no decline in the maximal response of the beta cell with age, but a "shift to the right" (i.e., a decrease) in sensitivity of the beta cell to hyperglycemia.

Very few studies dealing with the question of age differences

TABLE V

EFFECT OF AGE ON SERUM INSULIN RESPONSE TO INTRAVENOUS GLUCOSE

Insulin response	Comments
A. Increase	
Streeten et al., 1965	At 20 min. "Insulin-like activity" assayed by fat-pad
Sensi et al., 1972	Increase at 40 and 60 min; decrease at 3 min.
Schreuder, 1972	Increase for 0-60 min. area
B. No change	
Johansen, 1973	
Palmer and Ensinck, 1974	
C. Decrease	
Crockford et al., 1966	At 6 min.
Barbagallo-Sangiorgi et al., 1970	At 2,5 and 10 min.
Dudl and Ensinck, 1972	At 3 to 5 min.
Sensi et al., 1972	Decrease at 3 min.; increase at 40 and 60 min.

in the effectiveness of insulin at its target organs have been reported. The question can also be posed as one of possible age differences in the sensitivity of the tissues to insulin. The test generally used in clinical medicine to assess tissue sensitivity is the "intravenous insulin tolerance test." In the standard test 0.1 U of insulin per kg body wt. is injected nearly instantaneously. This results in a sudden surge of insulin which greatly exceeds those levels achieved by normal physiological mechanisms. The fall in blood glucose is the measure of sensitivity to insulin. Two aging studies in man (Kalk et al., 1973; Martin et al., 1968) showed no age differences in sensitivity to insulin. There are two difficulties in interpretation of the results of this type of test: (1) Insulin levels are unphysiologic and (2) The fall in blood glucose is a resultant not only of tissue response to insulin but also of the effectiveness of complex neuro-endocrine counter-regulatory responses to hypoglycemia (catecholamines, glucagon, growth hormone, glucocorticoids).

To avoid these problems, we adapted the glucose-clamp technique in order to assess tissue sensitivity to insulin (Tobin et al., 1972). After a priming infusion, insulin was infused continuously at rates of one or two mU/kg body wt./min; steady-state arterial plasma insulin concentrations of 100 or 200 μU/ml were achieved -- well within the physiologic range. Hypoglycemia was prevented by a servo-controlled intravenous glucose infusion. The rate of glucose infused under steady-state conditions is a measure of sensitivity of body tissues to insulin. No differences in sensitivity with age were present in these studies.

The hyperglycemic clamp described above as a technique to evaluate beta cell function also generates data bearing on the question of tissue sensitivity to insulin. During the steady-state of hyperglycemia the rate of infusion of glucose is equal to the rate of metabolism of glucose. Thus the ratio glucose metabolized:insulin concentration is a measure of the effectiveness of the circulating endogenously-released insulin at the tissue level. Here again no age differences in sensitivity to insulin were seen.

IV. CONCLUSIONS

1. Aging is associated with large decrements in performance on variout diagnostic tests for diabetes. The significance of these age differences is in dispute. Long-term studies in large population groups are needed to resolve this dispute.

2. One major factor which contributes to the mechanism of this age effect is a decrease in sensitivity of the pancreatic beta cell to hyperglycemia.

3. The sensitivity of tissues both to endogenously released and to exogenously administered insulin is not altered with age.

REFERENCES

1. Andres, R. Med. Clin. N. Amer. 55:835 (1971).
2. Andres, R. and J. D. Tobin. Proc. 9th Int. Cong. Geront. 1:276 (1972).
3. Andres, R., R. Swerdloff, and J. D. Tobin. Proc. 8th Int. Cong. Geront. 1:36 (1969).
4. Barbagallo-Sangiorgi, G., E. Laudicina, G. D. Bompiani, and F. Durante. J. Am. Geriat. Soc. 18:529 (1970).
5. Bjorntorp, P., P. Berchtold, and G. Tibblin. Diabetes 20: 65 (1971).
6. Boyns, D. R., J. N. Crossley, M. E. Abrams, R. J. Jarrett, and H. Keen. Brit. Med. J. 1:595 (1969).
7. Chlouverakis, C., R. J. Jarrett, and H. Keen. Lancet 1: 806 (1967).

8.   Committee on Statistics of the American Diabetes, Association. Diabetes 18:299 (1969).
9.   Crockford, P. M., R. J. Harbeck, and R. H. Williams. Lancet 1:465 (1966).
10. Dudl, R. J. and J. W. Ensinck. Diabetes 21:357 (1972).
11. Hales, C. N., R. C. Greenwood, F. L. Mitchell, and W. T. Strauss. Diabetologia 4:73 (1968).
12. Johansen, K. Acta Endocrinol. 74:511 (1973).
13. Kalk, W. J., A. I. Vinik, B. L. Pimstone, and W. P. U. Jackson. J. Geront. 28:431 (1973).
14. Martin, F. I. R., M. J. Pearson, and A. E. Stocks. Lancet 1:1285 (1968).
15. Nolan, S., T. Stephan, S. Chae, C. Vidalon, C. Gegick, R. C. Khurana, and T. S. Danowski. J. Am. Geriat. Soc. 21: 106 (1973).
16. O'Sullivan, J. B. Diabetes 23:713 (1974).
17. Palmer, J. P. and J. W. Ensinck. In: Program of the Gerontological Society 27th Annual Scientific Meeting (1974) p. 46.
18. Reaven, G. and R. Miller. Diabetes 17:560 (1968).
19. Sandberg, H., N. Yoshimine, S. Maeda, D. Symons, and J. Zavodnick. J. Am. Geriat. Soc. 21:433 (1973).
20. Schreuder, H. B. Isr. J. Med. Sci. 8:832 (1972).
21. Sensi, S., M. Corotenuto, F. Capani, G. Camilli, P. Caradonna, and D. Policicchio. Gior. Geront. 20:228 (1972).
22. Siperstein, M. D. Advances Internal Med. 20:297 (1974).
23. Streeten, D. H. P., M. M. Gerstein, B. M. Marmor, and R. J. Doisy. Diabetes 14:579 (1965).
24. Tobin, J. D., R. S. Sherwin, J. E. Liljenquist, P. A. Insel, and R. Andres. In: Proceedings of the 9th International Congress of Gerontology. (Eds.) D. F. Chebotarev, V. V. Frolkis, and A. Ya. Mints. Kiev, U.S.S.R., The Congress (1972) Vol. 3, Abstracts, p. 155.
25. Welborn, T. A., A. H. Rubenstein, R. Haslam, and R. Fraser. Lancet 1:280 (1966).
26. Zhukov, N. A. Fed. Proc. 24:T597 (1965).

THE SCIENTIST AND SOCIAL POLICY ON AGING

Elias S. Cohen

Department of Community Medicine

University of Pennsylvania School of Medicine

When I first accepted your invitation and suggested that I would speak about the auto-immunological response of social policy on aging, I had in mind the pursuit of an analogue to the auto-immunological theory of aging. As Walford pointed out many years ago, the theory postulates that a progressively increasing immuno-genetic diversification of the dividing cell populations of vertebrates occurs with increasing age. This gradual diversification leads to loss of recognition patterns between the body cells which loss of is manifested by auto-immune-like reactions. Thus, aging is considered a generalized, mild but prolonged type of auto-immune phenomenon (1). My thought was that I could postulate that the aged are part and parcel of the normal cell structure of society. As societies aged, social values came under pressure and the body politic did not distinguish well between normal cells and deviant cells. Leo Simmons' seminal study of the aged (2) in seventy-one societies noted great variation among them in the treatment of the aged, ranging from the most profound respect and reverence to callous rejection, abandonment and deprivation. It appeared, according to Simmons, that the degree of cultural achievement might be viewed as the independent variable against which one might look at treatment of the elderly. But in all societies there are some elderly and it is fair to say that aging and growing old is viewed as normal among mankind's various cultures.

However, it is also true, so my analogy went, that the body politic makes distinctions about these old cells and treats them as foreign bodies. The degree to which that occurs, according to Simmons, and the relationship to cultural achievement, differs from group to group. A crude generalization that may be drawn from his

251

data, is that prestige of the aged is highest in those societies
falling in the middle range of cultural development. Prestige may
be equated with acceptance, or "fit" within the body politic. In
the most primitive societies where barest subsistence is always a
question, killing and abandonment of the aged is most often found.
On the other hand, those societies which have achieved a level we
regard as "civilized", also show in many cases an attitude of dis-
regard and rejection for the aged, tempered, but only somewhat, by
a sense of obligation with respect to their maintenance and care.

Another element in the analogy I intended to draw had to do
with the developments in the United States. Increasing numbers of
the elderly, i.e. the chronologically, not necessarily biologically elderly, and increasing proportions of the elderly affect societal homeostasis. Societies and communities, like the human body,
tend toward the steady state. There is a kind of inertia that ren-
ders society conservative in the classical sense of the word.
Where the equilibrium is disturbed by virtue of the numbers of the
elderly, their proportion in the population, their consumption of
particular resources with respect to other parts of the population
or shifts in instrumental roles, there is a need to recreate the
equilibrium through the application of external force, realloca-
tion of resources, or in the case of primitive societies, more
drastic measures such as callous rejection, abandonment, deprivation, and killing. The more I pursued the analogy, however, the
deeper I wandered into the bramble bush. Like so many analogies it
was too cute and too precious. To the extent that I pursued the
thought that the elderly were "normal cells" in the body politic,
I might have a shot at suggesting an auto-immune response. On the
other hand, however, one could make out a good argument that society views the elderly as foreign bodies and under that kind of con-
ception the response is not an auto-immune one at all but an immune
response.

In our own society, as in others going all the way back to the
Greeks, old age is viewed as a form of deviance. The classical
Greek view was that aging is an unmitigated misfortune. Rosalie
Rosenfelt in a sharply inciteful article entitled, "The Elderly
Mystique" (3) suggests our modern day counterpart. She points out
that at some point, late in life, a person comes to regard himself
as old. He compares himself in important respects to what he considered himself to be at an earlier time of life. "According to
the mystique, this point marks an unmitigated misfortune which a
series of lugubrious losses, deficits, and declines has forced upon
his attention. Despite his grim determination to 'think young'
destiny has had the last laugh, has forced him to the mat for the
final countdown."

She describes the deviance of the elderly in no uncertain
terms. "Health and vigor it is assumed are gone forever. The

senses have lost their acuity. The memory is kaput. Education
and new learning are out of the question, as one expects to lose
his mental faculties with age. Adventure and creativity are for
the young and courageous. They are ruled out for the old who are
ipso facto timid and lacking in moral stamina. As for the pleasure
of sexual relationships, the very thought of the old person in
such a context brings smiles. Some people are even prone to as-
sociate the sex life of the aged with senile delinquency... As
a worker, (the older person) has become a liability. His rigidity,
his out-of-date training, his proneness to disabling illness, not
to mention his irritability, lowered efficiency and arrogant manner, all militate against the likelihood of his being hired or promoted. Fussdudiness is his special quality. Besides, he is more
than the pension plan ever bargained for."

Goffman points out that the elderly suffer greatly from the
stigma and tend to come together in "huddle together self-help
clubs formed by the divorced, the aged, the obese, the physically
handicapped, the ileostomied and the colostomied" (4). Rose has
suggested that this results in the formation of the sub-culture of
the aging (5), arising from contempt for the inefficacy of the old
which brings about rejection by the young and finally a mutual
closing of the ranks. The elderly mystique suggests that there is
no hope in old age and those who grow old are quite hopeless.

But this is a dangerous course to follow. To be sure, elderly people do differ in important ways. Not only are they differentiated by their chronological age, but they tend to be more
widowed than younger adults; more chronically ill or disabled, but
not always; poorer by half measured in terms of median income;
more poorly housed; more depressed; more often mentally impaired;
more often living alone; and more apt to be female than male. To
say, however, that this represents a deviant population is to come
too close to casting their lot with the criminals, the mentally
ill, the mentally retarded, the flotsam and the jetsam that society has cast aside or carefully stored.

So it is that I will not engage in relentless pursuit of the
analogue that intrigued me when I first received your invitation.
Nevertheless, I do intend to discuss with you some of the factors
which I might have included in that pursuit without putting you
through the torture of convoluted reasoning. Furthermore, I hope
that I can address, if ever so gently, the significance and positive gains to be obtained from improved communication between the
so-called "hard" scientists, like yourselves, and the "soft" scientists whom I represent, although that may be gilding the lily
somewhat.

There are a great many beliefs about social policy and how it

is formed. Some hold that it derives from national consensus
which converges around particular events or a particular time.
Others suggest that it represents a balancing of interest in a
pluralistic society. Still othes feel that it springs full-blown
from the brains of legislative solons, like Venus from the brow of
Zeus. Scientists, hard and soft, would like to believe that social
policy has some roots in data. Others, more cynical, suggest that
data is never relevant to the makers of social policy and that the
political process is necessarily a matter of influence, venal interest, and petty concerns.

In his book The Pursuit of Loneliness (6), Philip Slater suggests that there is "a compulsive American tendency to avoid con-
frontation of chronic social problems: We are, as a people, perturbed by our inability to anticipate the consequences of our acts,
but we still wait optimistically for some magic telegram informing
us that the tangled skein of misery and self-deception into which
we have woven ourselves has vanished in the night." He goes on to
suggest we are besieged by such "telegrams" announcing that the
transportation crisis will be solved by a bigger road, mental illness with a pill, poverty with a war on it, slums with a bulldozer,
and death on the highway with radar. We don't like to wrestle
with persistent social problems, much less make the extensive re-
adjustments required to affect them significantly. We are enamored
of crash programs that will wipe up a problem in quick order, but
it is difficult to point to any that have worked. Our social policy about the aging has arisen from this avoiding tendency which
lies at the root of American character, according to Slater. Being
a large country with a mobile population, we were able to escape to
a new frontier and the hope of a better life. Even today, that is
our approach to the problems of the city - escape to the suburbs.

Slater has some disturbing things to say in connection with
the elderly. He suggests that when some members of our society
cannot care for themselves, America takes the route of institu-
tionalization. He hastens to add that this does not mean insti-
tutionalization is bad, but rather that American society is not
geared to handle in any other way the problems that the aged, the
psychotic, the retarded, and similar groups present. This is
significant, given the current press in legislature and in the
executive branch to provide what are being called "alternatives to
institutional care." One cannot successfully alter one facet of
a social system if everything else is left the same, for the patterns are interdependent and reinforce one another. Slater says,
"In a cooperative stable society, the aged, infirm, or psychotic
person can be absorbed by the local community which knows and un-
derstands him. He presents a difficulty which is familiar and
which can be confronted daily and directly. This condition cannot
be reproduced in our society today. The burden must be carried by
a small, isolated, mobile family unit that is not really equipped

for it". But understanding alone does not permit us to ignore
what we are doing.

Our ideas about "institutionalizing" the aged, psychotic, retarded, and infirm are based on a pattern of thought that Slater
calls the toilet assumption - the notion that unwanted matter, unwanted difficulties, unwanted complexities and obstacles will disappear if they are removed from our immediate field of vision.
The result of our social efforts has been to remove the underlying
problems of our society farther and farther from daily experience
and daily consciousness, and hence to decrease in the mass of the
population the knowledge, skill, resources, and motivation necessary to deal with them.

When the ramifications of these discarded problems rise to the
surface again - a riot, a protest, a nursing home fire - we react
as if a sewer had backed up; shocked, disgusted, and angered, we
call for the emergency plumber - the special commission, the crash
program - to be certain that the problem is once again removed from
consciousness.

I start from the proposition that we do not have a coherent
public policy on aging in the United States. We have a series of
legislative enactments, authorizations, and appropriations designed
to respond to the worst of the problems, hopefully to control them.

Public policy is that accumulation of laws, regulations, guide-
lines, and official pronouncements which have been promulgated on
any particular given topic. It is tangible, it can be measured,
dealt with, clearly modified, ratified or left alone.

Social policy, on the other hand, represents the synthesis of
competing energies to achieve various goals within the framework of
a social philosophy that reflects the salient values of our society.
It is difficult to define or quantify at any given moment. The
measure of social policy is not so much in the words, as it is in
the results. The public policy of the Older Americans Act, setting
forth the goals and the intent of the Congress, would lead us to
believe that the Older Americans Act, the Administration on Aging,
the state units on aging, and the Area Agencies on Aging were the
source of the good society for the elderly, and that is is, indeed,
within our grasp. Social policy, on the other hand, would be better reflected in the fact the elderly comprise a fifth of all those
who are poor in this nation, are obliged to live in sub-standard
housing, have twice the average hospital stay, and occupy 98% of
the long-term care chronic illness beds, and 25-30% of the mental
hospital beds. Borrowing from another field, one might point to
the Full Employment Act of 1948, a statute that has been with us
for over a quarter of a century, and the actuality of employment

for the under-educated, Blacks, Indians, Spanish Americans, and others. The Full Employment Act is <u>public</u> policy; the actuality of employment for these groups represent <u>social</u> policy.

Social policy reflects major value belief clusterings salient in American culture. Some of these have been identified and one might conclude that about half of the value beliefs denigrate the elderly. Let me just list these:

*1.   Activity and work
*2.   Achievement and success
  3.   Moral orientation
  4.   Humanitarianism
*5.   Efficiency and practicality
*6.   Science and secular rationality
*7.   Material comfort
*8.   Progress
  9.   Equality
 10.   Freedom
 11.   Democracy
 12.   External conformity
 13.   Nationalism and patriotism
 14.   Individual personality
*15. Racism and related group superiority

Gross points out that "Running through these complex orientations as still more highly generalized themes is an emphasis on the worth of active mastery rather than a passive acceptance of events ... and a high evaluation of individual personality rather than collective identity and responsibility" (7). If his formulation is correct, the characteristics of the aged in our society exclude them from high value considerations.

Some years ago I suggested that if we are to achieve any success in affecting social policy in aging in a positive way and thereby develop more effective coherent and humane public policy, we would have to do more research on the relationship of the value system, social attitudes, and the aged population (8). I was inclined to agree with Gross that "the systematic explication and analysis of values as causes and consequences of social action is an essential part of the urgent task of purposive, objective diagnosis of societal functioning." While I continue to believe that to be true, I have come to the not too startling conclusion that there is some significance to good, hard data.

Sound social policy on aging and sound public policy that would reflect such social policy requires good data in the hard scientific areas no less than a good social policy on environmental

---

*Value beliefs tending to denigrate the elderly.

pollution, the improvement in the quality of life through peace-
ful uses of the atom, or relief of worldwide famine through improved crop yields. Social planning, if it is to go beyond the
arena of political competition, must provide a systematic method
of selecting choices in resource allocation to achieve given objectives.

Planning, particularly in the public sector, is becoming highly stylized throughout the United States. To the extent that programs in aging, whether involving research, medical care, income
maintenance, nutrition, or that broad group of activities called
social services, are government funded, they will be subjected
to some form of program planning budgeting system, program evaluation review techniques, and similar methods of systematic analysis.
Program Planning Budgeting Systems (PPBS) and Management by Objective approaches have made it very clear that we don't have the
indicators, the social data that are comparable, or the raw materials necessary for making program decisions. The new budgeting
technology would attempt to provide the following kinds of information; none of this should seem strange to you as scientists since
they are simply other ways of suggesting hypothetical formulation:

1. Direct and indirect outcomes likely to result from A, B,
    C, or D types of activity.

2. Certain types, quantities, and qualities of end product
    outputs made possible by A, B, C, or D types of activities.

3. Quantification of input and output measures will permit
    comparison of alternative approaches to problem solving
    on cost-benefit as well as other bases.

Attempting a somewhat more precise technique in planning would
hopefully lead us to some conceptual innovation in social planning
in aging. The following innovative approaches have been suggested.
Again, these should not be strange to you since they may be the
very stuff with which scientists deal with all the time at a conceptual level.

1. Redefining and broadening the approach to a major area
    that has up until now been narrowly defined. An example
    of this might be the examination of poverty among the
    elderly. Redefinition and broadening the approach to
    poverty might include the use of a comparable income with
    the rest of society, rather than the use of a hard dollar
    line. It might include the desirability of conceiving of
    poverty in terms of well-being, economic and cultural.
    More precise measurement of income would include measure-
    ment of assets, services received, as well as income sub-

stitutes (such as food stamps), while the cultural dimensions of poverty might include the aspects of self-
respect, status, and participation in society.

2. Identifying major paradoxes confronting policy makers.
    Among the elderly we often hear the expressed desire for
    more participation, but just as often encounter an unwil-
    lingness to accede to results or accept responsibility.
    Similarly, we note the expressed desire for work by the
    elderly but increasing optional retirement of men at age
    62.

3. Changing some of the traditional parameters in a changing
    situation. For example, neither public nor social policy
    fully recognizes that public education is not limited to
    the youth period, nor need it be limited to the educa-
    tional establishment.

4. Conceptual innovation is required in defining difficult
    areas about which the social scientists write much but
    plan little. What are the indicators of loneliness, self-
    mastery, dignity, aesthetics.

5. In highly defined areas we may raise conceptual issues
    with great but as yet unexplored potentialities for re-
    structuring action. For example, in the highly vaunted
    program of nutrition for the aged currently at a level of
    over $100,000,000, the framing of objectives has been
    fuzzy-minded, emotional, and imprecise. What is the base
    line for measuring the impact of a nutrition program? To
    what extent have we sought out the biochemists and asked
    them the hard question about the impact of giving three
    or five meals a week to individuals who presumably are
    not getting an adequate diet? Is the nutrition program
    the best way to get food in the belly? What is the re-
    lationship between the so-called nutritional part of the
    program and the social component of the program? If we
    want to improve nutrition, what steps would be most ef-
    fective, and then obviously how do we measure it?

6. Examination of basic concepts in emotion-charged areas
    suggesting various paths toward re-construction. Some
    examples of this include the question of filial respon-
    sibility and support laws or the application of laws re-
    lating to the recovery of public assistance payments
    through use of property liens and other recovery measures;
    or the issues of euthanasia, prolongation of life and so
    on.

I would like to suggest that the social scientists and the biologists and biochemists have more to talk about together than they have formerly thought was so. There are some obvious examples. The social scientists for their part must begin to learn something about what the cell biologists and the biochemists are up to. What is the long range impact or potential impact of their researches? Can we translate into language that the social scientists will understand more than the faddish and interesting controversy about whether man's lifespan is governed by the biological clock that limits the extension of life, i.e. the Strehler-Comfort (9) dichotomy, or even exploration of potential life-expectancy changes that inhere in cancer or renal disease research results. To be sure, the Institute of Society, Ethics and the Life Sciences is vigorously engaged in examining the ethical issues and formulation of some policy concerning medical ethics, death, dying, scarce medical resources, transplantation and hemodialysis (10). But even this is far from the scientific knowledge base that ought to lie behind a great deal of public policy on aging. Let me illustrate from the nutrition program.

Currently the appropriations for Title VII of the Older Americans Act the Nutrition program, are at a level of over $100,000,000. I would suggest to you that after three years of the program, by which time we will have spent perhaps three-quarters of a billion dollars on the program, given federal, state, local, public and private resources, we will have absolutely no idea of the nutritional impact of the nutrition program. Social scientists are simply not equipped to think about that impact. Social scientists, who have been concerned with the effects of poverty on the elderly, have not addressed adequately and certainly not scientifically, the issues surrounding the impact of low-income on nutrition except in the most subjective and gross way.

Those of us concerned with nursing home care, long-term institutional care, and particularly mental impairment, have no notion whatsoever about the direction of research concerning organic brain disease, chronic brain syndrome, and so on, which might enable us to affect the allocation of research funds for this purpose. Medical economists must understand, although they seem not to, that the most ubiquitous disabilities among the elderly are those concerned with brain function. How should the social scientist plan for dealing with a mentally impaired population? What will the numbers be? What are the directions of research? What are the promising avenues of inquiry and so on? And for our part, the social scientists must begin to understand where the biochemists can enlarge our horizons. It is high time that we move beyond the popular articles about the elderly of Abkhazia, Hunza, and Vilcabamba (11). It is time for the social scientists to take note of what the biologists and biochemists are up to. But in order for us to do that, the biologists and biochemists may have to do some translating so that we can understand what they are saying. Perhaps together we may undertake some conjectures or hypotheses that will permit some marrying of our respective disciplines to occur.

The social scientists for their part must come to the bio-chemists and biologists and ask them about the programs they are about to launch, whether they are nutrition programs, income main-tenance programs, medical treatment programs, or medical-social programs designed to relieve particular kinds of problems. I would suggest also that what the social scientists have learned about the value system in general, and the value systems of the very old, the newly retired and those facing old age, are important to the biologists and the biochemists. There is a practical kind of politics in this that can and should be useful. And finally and perhaps most difficult, the biochemists, biologists, and social scientists must begin to converse about resource allocation. It is time for mutual exclusivity to diminish.

I am heartened in this respect through the associations I have had via the Gerontological Society. For example, in testimony before Congressional Committees then considering legislation in 1972 to authorize a National Institute on Aging, it was Marrot Sinex, a biochemist, who argued strongly and forcefully for the inclusion of social, economic, and psychological research compo-nents in the new National Institute on Aging, moving well beyond the politically attractive purpose of the National Institute on Aging of prolonging life (12).

What I am suggesting is easier said than done. Social sci-entists and clinicians, medical, social and psychological, have not understood, nor have they wanted to understand, the policy signi-ficance of good biological indices of aging. Biologists and bio-chemists have not helped in this regard. One result, I would sug-gest is the nutrition boondoggle for which we must all share some blame. Similarly, we have ignored discussing mental impairment and the relationship of environment to the elderly mentally impaired organism. If research, treatment methodology and social policy are to move forward systematically and effectively we must produce the forums, topics, and perhaps language that will permit us to start.

The new National Institute on Aging may afford us that oppor-tunity. Let us begin.

And with that let me close with Edna St. Vincent Millay's words (13),

...Upon this gifted age, in its dark hour
Rains from the sky a meteoric shower of

              facts ... they lie unquestioned, uncombined,
          Wisdom enough to teach us of our ill
          Is daily spun, but there exists no loom
          To weave it into fabric.

REFERENCES

1. Walford, R. The Gerontologist 4:195 (1964)
2. Simmons, L. The Role of the Aged in Primitive Societies.
    Yale University Press, Connecticut (1945)
3. Rosenfelt, R. J. of Social Issues XXI:37 (1965)
4. Goffman, E. Stigma, Notes on the Management of Spoiled Iden-
    tity, Prentice Hall, New Jersey (1963)
5. Rose, A. The Gerontologist 2:123 (1962)
6. Slater, P. The Pursuit of Loneliness. Beacon Press, Boston
    (1971)
7. Gross, B. Individual and Group Values, The Annals of the
    American Academy of American Academy of Political and Social
    Science. Vol. 371, May 1967.
8. Cohen, E. Geriatrics 8:337 (1960)
9. Comfort, A. New Scientist 11:549 (1969)
10. See Bibliography of Society, Ethics, and the Life Sciences,
    Hastings-on-Hudson, 1974.
11. Leaf, A. National Geographic 143:93 (1973)
12. Sinex, M. Testimony before the Select Subcommittee on Educa-
    tion, U.S. House of Representatives, March 7, 1972
13. Millay, E. Collected Sonnets. Washington Square Press, New
    York (1959)

CELL TYPES ORIGINATING FROM YOUNG AND OLD MOUSE KIDNEY EXPLANTS

J. LIPETZ and R.E. BOSWELL

Department of Biological Sciences, Drexel University
Philadelphia, Pennsylvania 19104

We have been able to identify two different cell populations
originating from young (4-week-old) and old (8-to-9-month-old)
I.C.R. mouse kidneys explanted and transferred to new organ culture dishes every 24 hr. The explants were bathed in Eagle's
minimal essential medium with Hanks' salts and 10% calf serum,
supplemented with glutamine and antibiotics.

One of these cell types, which we refer to as "A" cells, are
highly cytoplasmic, have undulating borders and generally contain
only one nucleolus. The nucleus has an average diameter of
1.6 ± 0.6 μ, the cells are 6.7 ± 0.4 μ long and 2.4 ± 0.1 μ wide.
These cells made up 80-90% of the cells growing out of young explants during the first 16 days after explanting. When subcultured
on the same medium, these cells were capable of at least seven
doublings and were contact-inhibited.

The second or "B" type cells are predominant from the first
in explants taken from old mouse kidneys. These cells are considerably less cytoplasmic, usually contain more than one nucleolus
in their nuclei and have a more vacuolated cytoplasm. These cells
are 2.9 ± 0.5 μ long and 1.2 ± 0.2 μ wide with a nuclear diameter
of 0.6 ± 0.4 μ. When subcultured on the same medium they appear
capable of only two or three doublings. We have not as yet
been able to grow them to sufficient density to determine
if they are contact-inhibited.

Explants from young mouse kidneys yield more than 50% A-type
cells for about the first twenty days in culture, after this the
percentage of A-type cells decreases dramatically and the percentage of B cells increases rapidly to make up over 80% of the population by the 26th day in culture. In contrast, old mouse kidneys
only produce more than 50% A cells for one transfer, and cease
production of these cells by about the 20th day. In these ex-

plants B-type cells never make up less than 45% of the population
and reach 100% by about the 20th day. At the end of about 32
days no cells grow out of the old kidney, whereas the young kidney continues to produce both A and B cells for at least 42 days
after explanting.

We believe that these data present a new insight into the
well-known phenomenon of latency, and may with further exploration yield further information on the question of cellular and
organismal aging.

ALTERATIONS IN THE GROWTH RATE AND GLUCOSE METABOLISM OF CHINESE

HAMSTER CELLS IN VITRO

J.M. RYAN AND D.M. PACE

The Wistar Institute, Philadelphia, PA, and Univ. of the
Pacific, Dept. of Pharmacology, Stockton, CA

The lifespan of animal cells in culture is characterized
by a period of rapid cell proliferation (Phase II) followed by
a period in which the fraction of cells undergoing division within
the cell population gradually declines (Phase III) and the culture
is lost or transforms to a cell line which can be propagated in-
definitely. This phenomenon has been described for cell cultures
derived from human, mouse, chick, rat kangaroo, rabbit, and tortoise
tissues.

In this study, we show that cell cultures derived from
Chinese hamster (Don) lung tissue (ATCC, CCL16) also undergo a
gradual decline in proliferation (Phase III). In addition, cells
in Phase III utilize approximately 1.2 - 2.2 as much glucose/10^4
cells and produce 1.3 - 2.1 as much lactic acid/10^4 cells than do
Phase II cell cultures during the growth cycle. The amount of
lactic acid produced/µg glucose consumed did not vary significantly
in Phase II and Phase III cultures.

THE CRISTOFALO INDICES OF MUTANT HUMAN CELLS

R.A. VINCENT, JR., AND P.C. HUANG

Dept. of Biochemical and Biophysical Sciences, The John
Hopkins University, School of Hygiene and Public Health,
Baltimore, Maryland 21205

Cristofalo and Sharf [Exp. Cell. Res. 76, 419-27] observed
a linear decrease with increasing population doubling level (PDL)
in the proportion of WI-38 and WI-26 cells able to incorporate
tritiated thymidine during replication. The possibility that this
correlation may exist and reflect cellular aging in other cultures
was investigated in this study which followed their experimental
protocol.

With the exception of the HeLa culture, all cultures were
of fibroblast cells derived from human skin. Cultures were examined from nonaffected donors and from patients with Progeria
(Patient KH), Fanconi's anemia (FA), and Xeroderma pigmentosum
(XP) of genetic complementation groups A, B, C, and D. Progeria
is characterized by premature aging, while both FA and XP are
noted for predispositions to malignancy. The cellular bases for
Progeria, FA, and XP are thought to involve the inability to rejoin DNA strand breaks, the defective repair of cross linkage
damage in DNA, and the deficient removal of thymine dimers from
UV-irradiated DNA, respectively.

The Cristofalo indices (percent labeled cells) were found to
vary with PDL in three different ways. The first way, reflected
by the cultures of nonaffected and XP cells, was represented by
a linear or logarithmic decrease in Cristofalo index with increased
PDL. In this respect, a culture from a 42-year-old nonaffected
donor reached 50% labeled cells at 21 population doublings (PDs),
while a culture of WI-38 fetal lung cells required 48 PDs. These
observations are in agreement with the well-documented inverse
correlation of proliferative capacity with donor age. The six
XP cultures reached 50% labeled cells at 28-33 PDs, as would be
expected from the donor ages 7-28 years. The second way in which
proliferation varied with PDL, characterized by the Progeroid and

FA cultures, was by decreasing sinusoidal fluctuations in Cristofalo index through the entire life span of the culture. The Progeroid and FA cultures reached 50% labeled cells at 13 and 18 PDs, although the donor ages were only 15 and 5 years, respectively. The same cultures reached 50% labeled cells in final waves at 28 and 31 PDs, respectively. The low PDLs at which these cultures reached 50% labeled cells, and their fluctuating Cristofalo indices are indicative of possible proliferative impairment. The third way in which the Cristofalo indices varied with PDL was exemplified by the HeLa culture of a carcinoma of the cervix and a diploid culture established from a benign growth on the lip of an otherwise normal female. These cultures have not reached 50% labeled cells after 246 and 70 PDs, respectively. Apparently, the aberrant, but nonmalignant, nature of the latter cells is associated with an increased life span _in vitro_.

The above observations suggest that the Cristofalo index assay may be useful for comparing the proliferative capacities of normal donors of different ages. The assay was sufficiently sensitive to detect perturbed proliferation in cultures from the Progeroid and FA patients and the benign growth. Furthermore, the results show that the excision-repair deficiency of each XP complementation group does not have a pleiotropic effect on proliferative capacity under stringent growth conditions.

Supported by funds from the National Foundation/March of Dimes, the American Cancer Society/Maryland Division, and the National Institutes of Health.

ALTERED DNA METABOLISM IN AGED AND PROGERIC FIBROBLASTS

J.R. WILLIAMS, J.B. LITTLE, J. EPSTEIN, and W. BROWN

Harvard University School of Public Health

Aspects of DNA metabolism in aged human fibroblasts and fibroblasts from patients with the Hutchinson-Gilford progeria syndrome have been compared to aneuploid and hybrid mammalian cells. We find the dynamics of DNA metabolism as measured by rejoining of radiation-induced DNA breaks and cyclic repair of DNA is decreased in the "old" cells and in certain progeric cells. Aged fibroblasts and strains of progeric fibroblasts EX-441 and AK are more susceptible to cell death as measured by endonucleolytic DNA degradation.

Hybrid mammalian cells evidence an extreme resistance to ionizing radiation as measured by colony formation, rejoin DNA breaks most rapidly and appear most resistant to cell death. Aneuploid cells, tumor cells and early passage (< 10 doublings) diploid fibroblasts appear to be equally sensitive as measured by these endpoints. Middle passage human fibroblasts (10 to 45 population doublings) repair DNA breaks less rapidly. Progeric strains LD and SJ repair still less rapidly than these cells and progeric strains KH and EX-17 are even more deficient. Senescent human cells evidence mixed populations with different repair capabilities.

To develop an animal model system, we have investigated DNA repair characteristics during the in vitro lifespan of Syrian hamster embryo cells. These cells evidence either senescence after 6 to 10 mean population doublings or grow exponentially for over 20 population doublings. These cells evidence reduced DNA repair as measured both by unscheduled DNA synthesis and rejoining of DNA strand breaks as they reach senescence.

Further, we have observed DNA repair capabilities are influenced by co-cultivation with competent cells. EX-17 and EX-441 are progeric strains which evidence different DNA metabolic deficiencies. However, when they are co-cultivated 2-8 hr both deficiencies are ameliorated and DNA metabolic activity returns to that of normal cells.

THE SURVIVAL OF HAPLOID AND DIPLOID VERTEBRATE CELLS AFTER

TREATMENT WITH MUTAGENS

L. MEZGER-FREED

The Institute for Cancer Research, Philadelphia, PA

Lethal recessive mutations should be expressed in diploid cells with a frequency equal to the square of that in haploid cells. According to mutation rates in bacteria, therefore, the proportion of diploid cells which survive mutagen treatment should be at least 10^5 times that of haploid cells. A haploid-diploid comparison should, in fact, be a test for the mutagenic nature of a compound.

This prediction was tested by treating monolayer cultures of three sets of haploid and diploid Rana pipiens cell lines with each of five compounds mutagenic to bacteria. The proportion of cells which survived treatment was determined by extrapolating to zero time the slope of the growth curve once a normal cell doubling time was reestablished. In none of the fifteen comparisons (three sets times five mutagens) was the proportion of survivors in diploid cultures more than ten times greater than that in haploid cultures. Possible explanations include: (1) the lethality of the five compounds, which are mutagenic to bacteria, is not primarily due to mutagenesis; (2) vertebrate cells have evolved ways of preventing the expression of gene mutation (i.e., by multiple gene copies per haploid set, more efficient DNA repair).

(Supported by grants CA-05959, CA-06927 and RR-05539 from the National Institutes of Health, contract AT(11-1) 3110 with the AEC, and an appropriation from the Commonwealth of Pennsylvania.

CAPACITY OF CULTURED FIBROBLASTS FROM DIFFERENT MAMMALIAN SPECIES TO METABOLIZE 7,12-DIMETHYLBENZ(A)ANTHRACENE TO MUTAGENIC METABOLITES: A CORRELATION WITH LIFESPAN

A. SCHWARTZ

Fels Research Institute and Department of Microbiology
Temple University School of Medicine
Philadelphia, Pennsylvania 19140

Much evidence suggests that the majority of chemical carcinogens are metabolized to their mutagenic and carcinogenic forms. It is possible to determine the capacity of cultured fibroblasts to metabolize 7,12-DMBA to its mutagenic form by measuring the rate of 8-azaguanine-resistant mutants produced in a test strain exposed to 7,12-DMBA which has been activated by the cultured fibroblasts. Using cultured fibroblasts from several different mammalian species, there was a good correlation between lifespan and the capacity of these cells to activate 7,12-DMBA to its mutagenic form. These preliminary data are consistent with the hypothesis that mutagenesis by substances which undergo metabolic activation may contribute to aging in mammals.

EXTENSION OF THE IN VITRO LIFESPAN OF HUMAN WI-38 CELLS IN CULTURE BY VITAMIN E

L. PACKER and J.R. SMITH

Dept. of Physiology-Anatomy, Univ. of Calif., and Energy and Environment Div., Lawrence Berkeley Lab., Berkeley, 94720, and Physiology Res., Veterans Administration Hospital, Martinez, Calif. 94553

Normal human cells in culture exhibit a finite capacity for cell proliferation. It has been proposed that this may be an expression of aging at the cellular level. We are investigating the possibility that accumulated oxidative damage may be a major cause of cell senescence and death in vitro. WI-38 cells grown in the presence of 10 or 100 µg dl-α-tocopherol (the major natural membrane antioxidant) per ml medium (added without organic solvents) have a lifespan increased from 50 ± 10 to > 100 population doublings. In tocopherol-treated cells at the 97th passage level, about 95% of the cells are capable of synthesizing DNA, which suggests that these cells are capable of many more population doublings. Tocopherol-treated cells do not accumulate fluorescence damage products, and have morphology and karyotype characteristic of young cells. In acute experiments where cells were subjected to environmental stress by visible light and high oxygen toxicity, tocopherol also protected against the increased rate of cell death. These results suggest that vitamin E may slow the occurrence and accumulation of oxidative damage such that the growth potential and survival of human fibroblasts in vitro is enhanced. These findings have broad implications for the use of human cells in somatic cell genetics and transformation studies, cell culture in general, and may be relevant to mechanisms of cell aging.

DIMINISHED INOTROPIC RESPONSE TO CATECHOLAMINES

IN THE AGED MYOCARDIUM

E.G. LAKATTA, G. GERSTENBLITH, C.S. ANGELL, N.W. SCHOCK,
AND M.L. WEISFELDT

Gerontology Research Center, Natl. Inst. of Child Health
and Human Development, Natl. Institutes of Health, PHS,
U.S. Dept. of Health, Education & Welfare, Bethesda, and
the Baltimore City Hospitals, Baltimore, Maryland 21224

It is known that the cardiovascular response to stress in
both intact animals and in man diminishes with advancing age.
In order to define the role of the myocardium in these age associated changes, the direct inotropic response to left ventricular traveculae carneae from young adult (6 mo) and aged (24 mo)
rats was examined during exposure to catecholamines. The muscles
were stimulated to contract isometrically at 24 beats per min
at 29°C in Krebs-Ringer bicarbonate solution, modified by lowering
the Ca^{++} to 1.0mM, the Mg^{++} to 0.6mM, and by adding glucose to a
concentration of 16mM. At control, active tension (AT), maximum
rate of tension development (dT/dt) and contraction duration (CD),
measured as the interval from the onset of tension development to
the time tension fell to one-half of its maximum value were:

Age	N	AT (g/mm^2)	dT/dt $(g/mm^2/sec)$	CD (msec)
6	19	2.92 ± .25	33.7 ± 3.06	255.8 ± 7.4
25	15	3.31 ± .31	34.5 ± 3.88	300.3 ± 9.2

AT and dT/dt were not age related, but CD was prolonged in the
aged group (P<.001). Some of these muscles were exposed to increasing concentrations of Norepinephrine (NE) and others to Isoproterenol at a single concentration of $1x10^{-6}$ M. At a NE concentration of $1x10^{-5}$ M, the response of dT/dt and AT (Fig. 1A and
B) was greater in the young, while CD was shortened proportionate-

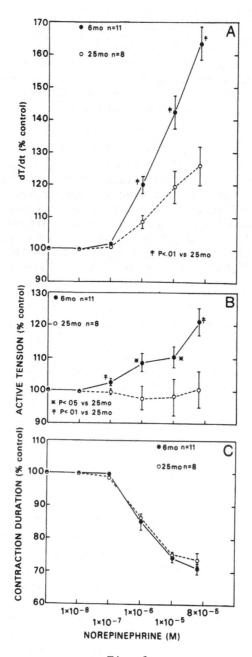

Fig. 1

ly in each age group (Fig 1C). Similar results were obtained
after Isoproterenol. The diminished cardiovascular response
to stress which occurs with advanced age results at least in part
then from a diminished intrinsic inotropic response of aged myocardium to catecholamines. The response to increasing concentrations of Ca^{++} was measured over a Ca^{++} range of 0.5mM to 2.5mM,
that concentration at which maximal response occurs. In contrast
to the response of catecholamines, no age differences in AT or
dT/dt were found at any Ca^{++} concentration.

Since the inotropic response to Ca^{++} is preserved in aged
myocardium, it appears that the age difference in response to
catecholamines resides in the mechanism whereby catecholamines
increases the amount of Ca^{++} available to the myofilaments.
Also it is of interest that in aged rat myocardium, under the
conditions employed in this study, the dual actions of catecholamines can be dissociated, i.e., in aged myocardium the duration
of active state (CD) is shortened equally as well as in young muscles, but the active state intensity (dT/dt) is enhanced less,
resulting in no significant change in AT in the aged muscles.

STUDIES IN AGE-RELATED ION METABOLISM IN RAT MYOCARDIUM

S.I. BASKIN, P.B. GOLDBERG and J. ROBERTS

The role cardiac ionic movements play with respect to age was studied to characterize some of the underlying causes of declining heart function observed senescence. Stimulated and quiescent left atria of Fisher 344 rats of 1, 3, 6, 12, 24 and 28 months were analyzed for the following parameters: Total tissue water, inulin space (I), sodium space, intracellular sodium (Na) and Potassium (K) concentrations, Na and K influxes and effluxes and ion accumulation. Although there was no appreciable change in muscle cell water with age, I increased from 0.248 ± 0.05 ml/g in the 3 month animal to 0.378 ± 0.03 ml/g in the 24 month rat but increased in the 24 month rat to 21.0%. The Na influx markedly decreased in the 24 month animal (0.967 ± 0.006 min^{-1}) when compared to younger animals (i.e. 3 months; 0.105 ± 0.009 min^{-1}). At least 2 rate components (K_1 and K_2) were obtained in Na efflux studies. A progressive age-dependent decrease in both K_1 and K_2 were observed between 1 and 24 month rats. The Na influx rate constants for resting muscles are greater than for stimulated muscles at all ages. The reverse is true for Na efflux (K_2) constants. No significant differences were found in the K influx rate constants. However, K efflux rate constants decreased with age. Na accumulation was found to change with age. The 12 month muscle binds only 59.7% of Na that is bound in 1 month muscle. At all ages the resting muscle binds more Na than the stimulated muscle. These data suggest that the age-related ionic membrane changes could account for the electrophysiological alterations observed with aging. (Supported in part by USPHS HD 06267 and Heart Assoc. of S.E. Penna.)

THE EFFECTS OF ISOPROTERENOL STRESS ON THE HEARTS OF OLD AND YOUNG RATS

M. VENUS, W.J. DiBATTISTA and G. KALDOR

The Dept. of Physiology and Biophysics, The Medical
College of Pennsylvania, Philadelphia, PA 19129

In pharmacological doses isoproterenol, a typical beta agonist, produces a positive inotropic and chronotropic cardiac effect. On the other hand in even large doses isoproterenol has a negative inotropic effect, may produce various cardiac arrhythmias and, also, necrosis in the cardiac tissue. Rona et al. (1) discovered that isoproterenol inflicted serious damage on the hearts of old rats, whereas, younger animals were relatively more resistant to the toxic effects of this drug. The results of our own experiments are summarized in Table 1. After a single intraperitoneal injection of isoproterenol (70 mg/kg) approximately 80% of the older rats became very sick and after the second injection (1 injection/day), 50% of the rats died within two hours. On the other hand, only 10% of the younger animals became sick and died under otherwise similar experimental conditions. Propranolol (4 mg/kg) decreased and aminophylline (50 mg/kg) increased the effects of isoproterenol. These results led us to believe that the isoproterenol stress may serve as a useful tool in uncovering biochemical differences, if any, between the hearts of old and young rats.

Experiments on intact animals and with isoproterenol on Langendorf preparations have shown that a slightly positive chronotropic and inotropic effect on 3-month-old rats as compared to 12-month-old rats. In Langendorf preparations 2.5 mg/ml aminophylline plus 0.7 mg/ml isoproterenol reduced the survival time of the 12-month-old rat hearts from 98.7 to 19.8 min. Quazodine was found to be a 10 times more potent inhibitor of the cardiac phosphodiesterase than aminophylline (2) and in a dose of 0.25 mg/kg, also, reduced the survival time of the rat hearts in the presence of 0.7 mg/kg isoproterenol. For this reason we became interested in certain aspects of the cyclic

TABLE 1

EFFECT OF ISOPROTERENOL AND AMINOPHYLLINE ON RATS

Drug Injected	3 Month Old Rats			12 Month Old Rats			24 Month Old Rats		
	No. of Rats	No. of Sick Rats After Injection	No. of Dead Rats 48 Hours After Injection	No. of Rats	No. of Sick Rats	No. of Dead Rats	No. of Rats	No. of Sick Rats	No. of Dead Rats
4 mg/kg propranolol + 70 mg/kg isoproterenol	16	-	1	16	-	7	-	-	-
70 mg/kg isoproterenol	30	3-5	3	30	20-25	15	5	5	5
30 mg/kg isoproterenol	15	0	1	16	4-6	3	-	-	-
30 mg/kg isoproterenol + 50 mg/kg aminophylline	-	-	-	17	17	14	-	-	-

AMP metabolism in the hearts of old and young rats. The results obtained so far are summarized in Table 2. It may be seen that we found no age related change in the cardiac phosphodiesterase activity of these rats, whereas, there was a 24% decrease in protein kinase activity in the hearts of old animals. The protein kinase activity was reduced by 72% in the epididymis of the old rats. The significance of these results with regard to the aging process is being studied at the present time in our laboratory.

Supported by NIH Grants HD 06267 and NB 06157.

References:

1) Rona, G., Chappel, C.I., Balazs, T. & Gaudry, R. (1959) J. Gerontol. 14, 169.

2) Amer, M.S. (1971) Proc. Soc. Exp. Biol. Med. 136, 750.

3) Weiss, B., Lehne, R. & Strada, S. (1973) Anal. Biochem. 45, 222.

4) Li, H. Ch. & Felmly, D.A. (1973) Anal. Biochem. 52, 300.

TABLE 2

PHOSPHODIESTERASE AND PROTEIN KINASE ACTIVITIES IN HEART MUSCLE OF AGING RATS

(1) Phosphodiesterase Activity

AGE	Luminescence Biometer Reading – 2 mg tissue
3 months old No. of Rats 3	2.85×10^8 1.43×10^8 2.50×10^8
6 months old No. of Rats 2	4.38×10^8 1.52×10^8
12 months old No. of Rats 3	3.40×10^8 5.66×10^8 4.63×10^8
24 months old No. of Rats 2	2.86×10^8 2.55×10^8
28 months old No. of Rats 2	2.71×10^8 3.82×10^8

(2) Protein Kinase Activity

AGE	Heart CPM/mg tissue	S.E.M.	Epididymis wt. mg. CPM/mg tissue	S.E.M.	Head Section of Epididymis CPM/mg tissue	S.E.M.	Tail Section of Epididymis CPM/mg tissue	S.E.M.
6 months old No. of Rats	888	± 42 5	446	± 6 4	425	± 93 4	540	± 58 4
12 months old No. of Rats	892	± 100 6	382	± 24 4	332	± 51 4	390	± 97 4
24 months old No. of Rats	–		169	± 20 8	115	± 11 4	141	± 39 4
28 months old No. of Rats	675	± 31 5						

(1) For method see reference 3.
(2) For method see reference 4.
(3) S.E.M. Standard error of the mean.

THE EFFECT OF AGE AND FASTING ON SERUM CHOLESTEROL LEVELS AND

CHOLESTEROL ESTERIFICATION IN THE RAT

A.G. LACKO, K.G. VARMA, T.S.K. DAVID and L.A. SOLOFF

From the Lipid Research Laboratory, Dept. of Medicine
Temple University Health Sciences Center
Philadelphia, Pennsylvania 19140

Free and total serum cholesterol levels and the in vitro rate of cholesterol esterification were measured in rats of age 2, 12 and 24 months. Free and total cholesterol increased with age in animals fed ad Libitum and decreased as the result of a one day fast in the two older groups. Prolonged fastings (up to six days) resulted in further decreases of serum cholesterol levels particularly in the 24 month-old-group.

The rate of cholesterol esterification did not change substantially between ages of 2 months and 12 months, but decreased significantly by 24 months. If the esterification is expressed as the fractional rate (% esterification per time) and thus corrected for the individual variation in serum free cholesterol then the differences become much more pronounced.

These findings will be discussed and compared to the known changes in cholesterol metabolism with age in man.

LIPID METABOLISM IN AGING RATS

J.A. STORY, S.A. TEPPER and D. KRITCHEVSKY

The Wistar Institute of Anatomy and Biology
Philadelphia, Pennsylvania 19104

Studies in Sprague-Dawley and Wistar rats have shown that
with age the following lipid changes generally take place: serum
cholesterol and triglyceride levels and liver cholesterol levels
rise; hepatic cholesterogenesis falls; and cholesterol adsorption
(measured by fecal excretion of administered cholesterol) decreases.
We studied serum and liver lipids in Fisher 344 rats. In the
first experiment we used 6 rats each at ages 2, 6, 12, 18 and 24
months. Body wt. (avg.) was 230 g at 2 months, 276 g at 6
months and 430 g in the older rats regardless of age. Liver wt.
rose with age but was not increased in proportion to body wt.
Serum cholesterol was 46.2 mg/dl at 2 months and rose sharply only
at 24 months (76.8 mg/dl). Liver cholesterol was only 9% higher
at 24 than at 2 months. Serum triglyceride levels were about
125 mg/dl until 18 months when they rose to 186 mg/dl and at 24
months they were 251 mg/dl. Liver triglycerides rose from 142
mg/100g at two months to 211 mg/100g at 6 months and 267 mg/100g
at 18 months. In a second experiment using rats of 2, 9, 12 and
24 months similar results were obtained.

Cholesterol biosynthesis was measured using liver slices and
$[1-^{14}C]$ acetate as substrate. Incorporation of acetate into
cholesterol at 9 months was 72% of the 2 month level and in the
older rats it was about 50% of that seen at 2 months.

In contrast, conversion of acetate to liver fatty acids was
lowest in the 2-month-old rats (by 10-50%). Another measure of
cholesterol biosynthesis, the activity of 3-hydroxy-3-methylglutaryl
CoA reductase (HMG-CoA reductase) showed activity of this enzyme
in livers of 9-, 12- and 24-month-old rats to be lower than that
observed in 2-month-old rats by 50, 54 and 51%, respectively.

Several aspects of bile acid synthesis were also measured.
In Wistar rats aged 18 months, the oxidation of $[26-^{14}C]$ cho-

lesterol to $[^{14}CO_2]$ by liver mitochondria was 30% that of preparations from 2-month-old Wistar rats. The activity of liver
cholesterol 7 α hydroxylase in 2-month-old Wistar rats was 147%
higher than that in 18-month-old rats. Hepatic cholesterol
7 α hydroxylase in Fisher 344 rats hardly changes with age, however. The activity of this enzyme at 6, 12, 18 and 24 months
was 98, 81, 86 and 91% of that found in 2-month-old rats.

The cholesterol biosynthesis and degradation data reflect
the serum and liver cholesterol levels of Fisher 344 rats.
Whether these differences between aging Fisher rats and other
strains are related to wt. gain or to other physiological
factors is under investigation. (Supported, in part, by USPHS
grant HL-03299 and Research Career Award HL-0734 and by a grant-
in-aid from the National Live Stock and Meat Board.)

EXERCISE, THYROID SECRETION RATE AND LIPID METABOLISM
IN RATS

J.A. STORY and D.R. GRIFFITH

Iowa State University, Ames, Iowa

The effects of exercise on the thyroid hormone secretion rate (TSR) and lipid metabolism on young (2 months) and old (9 months) Sprague-Dawley rats were measured. TSR was effectively increased by exercise in both young and old animals. In the young TSR was increased by exercise, and in the old exercise negated the normal decline in TSR observed with advancing age. Serum cholesterol and serum and liver triglycerides (TG) were significantly higher in the older rats. Exercise lowered serum and liver TG in both age groups and lowered serum and liver cholesterol in the old animals and liver cholesterol in the young. All lipid levels studied were inversely correlated with TSR.

ACCELERATED AGING OF THE BRAIN: NEUROENDOCRINE STUDIES IN

HUNTINGDON'S DISEASE

S. PODOLSKY and N.A. LEOPOLD

Boston VA Outpatient Clinic and
Boston Univ. School of Medicine, Boston, Mass.

Neuropathological studies of Huntingdon's disease reveal
neuronal atrophy, lipofucsin accumulation and other findings
characteristic of the aged brain. The pathology is limited to
specific areas such as the caudate nucleus, cerebral cortex and
hypothalamus.

Nine of 17 patients with documented Huntingdon's disease
had impaired carbohydrate tolerance, according to the criteria of
Fajans and Conn, although none had fasting hyperglycemia. Mean
plasma glucose level 2 hr after 100 g oral glucose administration
was 96.9 ± 5.5 mg/100 ml (mean $\pm$ SEM) for those with normal GTT and
146.2 ± 7.1 mg/100 ml for those with abnormal GTT. Insulin and
growth hormone (GH) measurements have been completed on ten
patients. Four with normal GTT had normal insulin responses (2 hr
level of 35.8 ± 8.4 µU/ml) and six with abnormal GTT had exaggerated
insulin responses (2 hr level of 197.5 ± 41.8 µU/ml). There was
failure of suppression of growth hormone during the GTT, with a
rise to abnormally high levels at 5 hr (18.6 ± 5.6 ng/ml). When
the GTT was repeated after three days of L-dopa priming, including
0.5 g administered 30 min prior to the test, there was a complete
suppression of their elevated basal GH levels (fasting = $17.9 \pm
2.3$ ng/ml; 1 hr = 3.1 ± 0.7 ng/ml), although 15 control subjects
had a GH rise under these conditions (fasting = 6.4 ± 1.3 ng/ml;
1 hr = 14.5 ± 2.9 ng/ml). In patients with a normal GTT, arginine
infusion in a dose of 0.5 g/kg resulted in normal insulin response,
with a peak insulin at 30 min of 44.0 ± 6.1 µU/ml. In those with
a diabetic GTT, arginine infusion resulted in an elevated insulin
response, with a peak insulin at 30 min of 96.3 ± 21.3 µU/ml.
Arginine infusion also resulted in an exaggerated GH response in the
majority of patients, with a peak GH level at 60 min of $28.3 \pm
3.7$ ng/ml, compared to a peak level of 17.6 ± 2.7 ng/ml at this time
for 20 control subjects.

The observations that patients with hereditary chorea have markedly elevated insulin responses to the administration of glucose or arginine, exaggerated growth hormone responses to falling glucose levels or arginine, and a paradoxical suppression of .growth hormone after L-dopa plus glucose, may be a result of hypothalamic neuronal degeneration or possible increased sensitivity to intracerebral dopamine in this disease.

CHANGES IN BRAIN ADENOSINE - 3'5' - MONOPHOSPHATE IN THE AGING RAT

I.D. ZIMMERMAN and A.P. BERG

The Medical College of Pennsylvania
Philadelphia, Pennsylvania 19129

Even in subjects selected as clinically healthy and free
of the usual pathologies of the aged, deficits in both verbal
and motor performance may be revealed by careful measurements
under mild stresses such as the imposition of time limits or the
introduction of new and unfamiliar material or unusual testing
situations. If we accept these observations as indicative, then
it would appear that the aging nervous system is likely to be
most sensitively deviant in those elements which are critically
involved in the dynamic responses necessary to adaptation and
that the most fruitful lines of research are those which probe
these elements rather than those mainly indicative of the steady
state. Out of the plethora of possibilities admitted by this
approach we have chosen to study the cyclic-AMP levels of the
cerebral cortex of the rat. The cortex, because it appears to
be involved in those higher functions which are the first to be
slowed by advancing age; and the cyclic-AMP system, because it
occupies a central position as a carrier information from the outside of the cell to its interior and has been implicated in the
mediation of the metabolic response of the cell to an adaptive
demand.

When cortical CAMP was assayed in various aged rats concentrations averaging 20 pmoles/mg protein were found in 1, 2,
and 3 month old animals, whereas at 6, 12 and 24 months of age
the average was only 5 pmoles/mg. That is, between the 3rd and
6th month of life there is a four-fold decrease in cyclic-AMP
levels, with little overlap between the groups apparent.

With this difference between the younger and older animals
in hand we turned to experiments designed to determine why cyclic-
AMP levels declined. One of the simplest explanations, hence a
logical first choice to test, was that 6-, 12- and 24-month-old
animals have less adenyl-cyclase, the cyclic-AMP synthesizing

enzyme, than 1-, 2- and 3-month-old rats and therefore less cyclic-AMP. Cyclase measurements were carried out by quantitating the rat of incorporation of radioactive ATP into cyclic-AMP in freshly homogenized cerebral cortices. Incubations including labeled ATP at various concentrations were carried out at 37°C for 10 min. Following incubation the cyclic-AMP was purified chromatographically and its radioactivity determined. No significant difference in adenyl-cyclase activity was observed by this method in any of the animals. The activities are essentially identical for the 1-, 2- and 3- as well as the 6-, 12- and 24-month-old groups.

An alternative explanation for the change in cyclic-AMP values seen as these rats age, is that the older cortices contain more phosphodiesterase, the cyclic-AMP degrading enzyme, and therefore lower values of cyclic-AMP. Phosphodiesterase assays were performed on cortical samples, homogenized in 0.32 molar sucrose and diluted before assay to approximately 1 µg protein/ml. The phosphodiesterase in these samples was used to catalyze hydrolysis of added cyclic-AMP to 5'-AMP which by coupled reaction was converted to ATP. The ATP produced was quantitated via the firefly luciferenase reaction.

It was seen that the action of phosphodiesterase as assayed on cortex obtained from the 1-, 2- and 3-month-old and the 6-, 12- and 24-month-old animals did not differ remarkably nor in such a manner as to explain the observed decreases in CAMP between these two groups. Thus it seems clear that neither adenyl-cyclase nor phosphodiesterase activity can account for the four-fold drop in endogeneous cyclic-AMP levels occurring between the 3rd and 6th month. Clues to the mechanism of this decrease have to be sought elsewhere. One of the possibilities that presents itself is that the levels and effects of the known modifiers of adenyl-cyclase and phosphodiesterase change with age even though the levels of the enzymes themselves remain the same.

Data from the following two experiments support this hypothesis. In this work the cerebral cortex was subjected to stimulation by either norepinephrine or electrical pulses in vivo. Both these treatments are known to potently stimulate cyclic-AMP accumulation. Rats were injected with alpha-chlorolose, I.P. (110 mg/kg) and after reaching surgical depth a small portion of the parietal cortex was exposed by removing both the overlying bone and dura mater. Although anesthetized animals generally showed lower absolute levels of cyclic-AMP, the shape of the function with age remains the same, with the younger animals clearly showing higher levels of cyclic-AMP than the older. Freshly prepared norepinephrine was dissolved in physiological saline at a final concentration of 1 mM, was applied to a cotton wick positioned in contact with the exposed cortex. After 5 min exposure the animals were sacrificed and the cyclic-AMP determined. There

is a strong age-dependence in the observed values with stimulated
levels at one through three months averaging 25 to 30 pmoles/mg
while those from animals six months and older averaged only 10
pmoles/mg. The stimulation by epinephrine is consistently two
to three times the control values regardless of age although
in the older animals since their levels are low to begin with,
this results in a smaller total accumulation.

In a different set of experiments the cortex was subjected
to stimulation by electrical pulses. These were applied directly
to the exposed cortex via a concentric electrode at a frequency
of 100 cycles/sec for a total of 10 sec. The pattern of response
differs from that seen in the norepinephrine stimulated animals.
The electrically stimulated cyclic-AMP level change relatively
little with age. The one through three month values averaged
20 pmoles/ml. The six through 24 month values averaged only
25% less at 15 pmoles/mg. It is obvious that relatively high
levels of cyclic-AMP can be obtained in the older cortices when
they are driven electrically. If the primary change in the adenyl-
cyclase-cyclic-AMP system was a change in the levels of either
adenyl-cyclase or phosphodiesterase this should not be possible.
However, if the primary change is in the regulatory modification
of these enzyme activities, then the differential results between
stimulation with norepinephrine and electrical pulses is explica-
ble. Further the differential results from the two conditions
imply that the age related change in modifier action is itself
a differential one and not merely a change in modifiability in
general. Work currently in progress is concerned with attempting
to determine which of a large number of likely modifiers of the
adenyl-cyclase-cyclic-AMP system change with age in such a way
as to account either singly or jointly for the present findings.

EVIDENCE RELATING THE AMOUNT OF ALBUMIN mRNA TO THE INCREASED

ALBUMIN SYNTHETIC ACTIVITY OBSERVED IN OLD RATS

M.F. OBENRADER, A.I. LANSING and P. OVE

The recent finding (Chen et al., BBA, 312, 598, 1973), that albumin synthesis is 50% higher in isolated old rat liver microsomes than in young rat liver microsomes, has led us to investigate the mechanism responsible for this age-related change. Purified polysomes were isolated from young and old rat livers and their sedimentation patterns were analyzed. The polysome profiles obtained for the young and old preparations were almost identical. Differences in the relative amounts of albumin-synthesizing polysomes in the young and old polysome fractions were detected in two ways. (1) The extent of specific binding of ^{125}I-anti-rat serum albumin to those polysomes synthesizing albumin was measured. It was found that more ^{125}I-anti-rat serum albumin bound to old rat liver polysomes than to equal amounts of young rat liver polysomes. (2) Albumin-synthesizing polysomes were directly precipitated from both young and old total polysome population using two different immunological procedures. The results showed that more albumin-synthesizing polysomes were precipitated from old rat liver polysomes than from equal amounts of young rat liver polysomes. This evidence suggests that there is an increased amount of messenger RNA coding for albumin in the total polysome fraction of old rats when compared to young rats. This concept has been further supported by preliminary experiments which involve the isolation of specific messenger RNA (mRNA) populations by the use of immunological procedures and poly (dT) cellulose chromatography. Labeled mRNA populations (poly A-containing material) were isolated from young and old rat liver polysomes which had been obtained from rats that were pulsed with ^{3}H-orotate for 10 min prior to polysome isolation. The specific mRNA populations were: (1) total mRNA; (2) albumin mRNA; (3) total mRNA population from which the albumin mRNA had been removed. It was found that more labeled poly A-containing material (mRNA) was isolated from the total labeled polysomal RNA of old rats than from young rats. This difference appeared to be due entirely to the amount of label incorporated into the poly A-containing material isolated from albumin-synthesizing polysomes, since, when this fraction of material was removed no difference was observed in the amount of label incorporated into the remaining poly A-containing material when young and old rats were compared. Our data indicate that albumin mRNA is synthesized faster in old rats than in young rats, while the total mRNA fraction from which the albumin mRNA has been removed is synthesized at the same rate in both young and old rats.

PROPERTIES OF CATALASE MOLECULES IN RATS OF DIFFERENT AGES[1]

J.A. ZIMMERMAN[2], H.V. SAMIS, M.B. BAIRD and H.R. MASSIE

Masonic Medical Research Laboratory, Utica, N.Y. 13503

The error accumulation theory of aging as proposed by Orgel suggests that senescence results from the time dependent accumulation of altered molecules. Such molecules are envisioned as consequent to a primary error in the synthesis of a single molecule of an enzyme which in itself is involved in macromolecular synthesis. The theoretical prediction that senescence be accompanied by altered populations of molecules has been partially substantiated by the immunological identification of missynthesized isocitrate lyase and fructose 1,6-diphosphate aldolase in aging nematodes. Similar studies in mammals have demonstrated altered populations of liver aldolase and possibly of skeletal muscle aldolase in old mice.

The hypothesis, as presently stated, requires the random appearance of missynthesized proteins - that is, evidence of molecular missynthesis should not be confined to just a few enzymes, but should be ubiquitous. However, several studies have failed to reveal evidence of accumulated aberrant muscle LDH or brain acetylcholinesterase during aging. Furthermore, an examination of the literature reveals that the activity of many enzymes does not decline, but an ever increasing proportion of molecules is missynthesized (which may result in inactive or partially active molecules), then there should be a net gain in protein in the organ in question - a phenomenon which has not been observed.

We have chosen to study catalase in our examination of altered molecule theories because this enzyme may be classed as a cellular luxury - that is, studies with acatalasemic Drosophila suggests that the presence of the enzyme does not seem to be of importance in survival of the organism. Hence, the "error catastrophe" predicted by Orgel would not be expected to be lethal to the cell since a critical enzyme is not involved. Thus, missynthesized molecules would be expected to accumulate to greater levels than found in more critical enzyme populations.

Initially, liver and kidney homogenates and red cell ly-
sates from male CFN rats 190 and 1002 days of age were incubated
at 48°C for up to 60 min. Production of altered catalase molecules
would be expected to change the thermostability of the molecular
population but inactivation curves were identical in both age
groups. A biphasic thermal inactivation curve was observed in
all samples and was believed due to denaturation of the protein
and disaggregation of the tetrameric catalase molecule.

Antisera to crude preparations of hepatic catalase from
young and old rats were raised in rabbits. The anti-old catalase
sera were used to eliminate the possibility that missynthesis
resulted in new antigenic determinants rather than antigenic de-
letion. These antisera were unable to differentiate between
catalase from young and old rats in both quantitative precipitin
and Ouchterloney gel diffusion tests.

In light of these data and in consideration of the wealth
of data both pro and con, we feel that a reappraisal of the error
theory as applied to in vitro aging is warranted. As it presently
stands the theory is too narrowly drawn and cannot accomodate data
such as those presented herein.

1. These investigations were supported by the Masonic Foundation
    for Medical Research.

2. Olsen Memorial Postdoctoral Fellow.

THERMAL DENATURATION OF BIOMOLECULES AT NORMAL BODY TEMPERATURE

H.A. JOHNSON, M.D.

Dept. of Pathology, Indiana Univ. School of Medicine

According to the laws of chemical kinetics, all organisms must suffer some degree of thermal injury even at normal body temperature. The important question is whether the slow thermal denaturation of proteins and nucleic acids at 37°C is trivial or whether it may account for a significant loss of essential biological information during the life of a cell or an organism and may thus be a factor in determining its lifespan.

The loss of proliferative capacity of hamster fibroblasts in vitro due to elevated temperatures (41–46°C) has the thermodynamic characteristics of a denaturation reaction. The rates of cell loss from the proliferative pool due to thermal denaturation at elevated temperatures can be extrapolated to 37°C, giving an expected loss of 0.2% of cells per hour due to thermal denaturation reactions at physiological temperature.

That such a rate of loss from the proliferative pool does in fact occur at physiological temperature can be shown by comparing cell generation time with population doubling time. The slow thermal denaturation of essential biomolecules at 37°C accounts for nearly all of the spontaneous loss of proliferative function in these cells in vitro, and it may' be a primary factor in the time dependent loss of function of cells in vivo.

References:

1) Johnson, H.A. & Pavelec, M. (1972) Am. J. Pathol. **66**, 557.

2) Johnson, H.A. & Pavelec, M. (1972) Am. J. Pathol. **69**, 119.

3) Johnson, H.A. (1974) Am. J. Pathol. **75**, 13.

PARTICIPANTS

Absher, Marlene, University of Vermont College of Medicine,
    Burlington, VT 05401

Adelman, R.C., Fels Research Institute, Temple University,
    Philadelphia, PA 19140

Angell, C.S., John Hopkins University, Baltimore, MD 21218

Andres, Reubin, Gerontology Research Center, Baltimore, MD 21224

Baird, M.B., Masonic Medical Research Laboratory, Utica, NY 13501

Baird, William M., The Wistar Institute, Philadelphia, PA 19104

Balin, Arthur, The Wistar Institute, Philadelphia, PA 19104

Baskin, S.I., Medical College of Pennsylvania, Philadelphia, PA
    19129

Berg, A., Medical College of Pennsylvania, Philadelphia, PA 19129

Berger, Henry J.

Bergey, James L., Temple University, Philadelphia, PA 19122

Blank, Michael S.

Blose, S.H., University of Pennsylvania, Philadelphia, PA 19174

Boswell, R.E., Drexel University, Philadelphia, PA 19174

Britton, Gary W., Fels Research Institute, Temple University,
    Philadelphia, PA 19140

Britton, Venera J. Fels Research Institute, Temple University,
    Philadelphia, PA 19140

Brown, T., Harvard University, Cambridge, MA 02138

Buchanan, James, University of Pennsylvania, Philadelphia, PA
    19174

Burney, Spencer W., Veterans Administration Normative Aging Study,
    Boston, MA 02108

Ceci, Louis, Fels Research Institute, Temple University,
    Philadelphia, PA 19174

Chacko, Samuel F., University of Pennsylvania, Philadelphia, PA
    19174

Chase, Anita A.

Cohen, Elias S., University of Pennsylvania, Philadelphia, PA
    19174

Cristofalo, V.J., The Wistar Institute, Philadelphia, PA 19104

Daniel, C.W., University of California, Santa Cruz, CA 95060

David, T.S.K., Temple University, Philadelphia, PA 19122

Davidson, L., The Wistar Institute, Philadelphia, PA 19104

Davies, Howard E.F., Gerontology Research Center, Baltimore, MD
    21224

Davis, Robert, Veterans Administration Center, Bay Pines, FL
    33504

Dell'Orco, Robert, The Samuel Roberts Noble Foundation, Ardmore,
    OK 73401

DiBattista, W., Medical College of Pennsylvania, Philadelphia, PA
    19129

Dietrich, Karen, Chestnut Hill College, Chestnut Hill, PA 19118

Denny, Paul C., University of Southern California, Los Angeles,
    CA 90007

Epstein, J., Harvard University, Cambridge, MA 02138

Fand, Irwin, Creedmoor Institute, Adelphi University, Garden City,
    NY 11530

Finch, C.E., Ethel Percy Andrus Gerontology Center, Los Angeles,
    CA 90007

Florini, J.R., Syracuse University, Syracuse, NY 13210

Freedman, Bernice, McNeil Laboratories, Fort Washington, PA 19034

Freeman, Colette, Fels Research Institute, Temple University,
    Philadelphia, PA 19140

Garwal, A., Institute for Cancer Research, Philadelphia, PA 19111

Geary, S., Syracuse University, Syracuse, NY 13210

Gerstenblith, Gary, Gerontology Research Center, Baltimore, MD
    21224

Goldberg, P.B., Medical College of Pennsylvania, Philadelphia, PA
    19129

Grant, Norman, Wyeth Laboratories, Philadelphia, PA 19101

Griffith, D.R., Iowa State University, Ames, IO 50010

Grove, Gary Lee, The Wistar Institute, Philadelphia, PA 19104

Hadley, Evan, The Wistar Institute, Philadelphia, PA 19104

Han, Seong S., University of Michigan School of Dentistry, Ann
    Arbor, MI 48104

Hagopian, Arpi, Merck Institute, Rahway, NJ 07065

Hayflick, Leonard, Stanford University School of Medicine,
    Stanford, CA 94305

Hrebeniak, Irene N.

Huang, P.C., John Hopkins University, Baltimore, MD 21205

Iyengar, Raja M., University of Pennsylvania, Philadelphia, PA
    19174

Johnson, Horton A., Indiana University, Indianapolis, IN 46205

Kaldor, G., Medical College of Pennsylvania, Philadelphia, PA
    19129

Karoly, Karen, Fels Research Institute, Temple University,
    Philadelphia, PA 19140

Kelliher, Gerald, The Medical College of Pennsylvania,
    Philadelphia, PA 19129

Kim, Sangduk, Fels Research Institute, Temple University,
    Philadelphia, PA 19140

Kleiner, Arthur I., Fels Research Institute, Temple University,
    Philadelphia, PA 19140

Klug, Thomas L., Fels Research Institute, Temple University,
    Philadelphia, PA 19140

Kniskern, Peter J., Merck Institute, Rahway, NJ 07065

Kovacs-Szuts, Maria

Kritchevsky, David, The Wistar Institute, Philadelphia, PA 19104

Lakatta, E.G., John Hopkins University, Baltimore, MD 21218

Lacko, Andras Gyorgy, Temple University Medical School,
    Philadelphia, PA 19140

Lansing, A. Ingram, University of Pittsburgh School of Medicine,
    Pittsburgh, PA 15213

Leathem, J. Hain, Rutgers University, New Brunswick, NJ 08903

Leopold, Norman A., Hahnemann Medical College, Philadelphia, PA
    19102

Lett, John Terrence, Colorado State University, Fort Collins, CO
    80521

Lipetz, Jacques, Drexel University, Philadelphia, PA 19104

Little, John Bertram, Harvard School of Public Health, Boston,
    MA 02115

Lynch, Sister Eva Marie, Chestnut Hill College, Philadelphia, PA
    19118

Maciag, Thomas, University of Pennsylvania, Philadelphia, PA
    19174

Makinodan, T., Gerontology Research Center, Baltimore City
    Hospitals, Baltimore, MD 21224

Malhotra, S., The Wistar Institute, Philadelphia, PA 19104

Manowitz, E.J., Syracuse University, Syracuse, NY 13210

Markofsky, Jules, Orentriech Foundation, New York, NY 10021

Martin, G., University of Washington, Seattle, WA 98105

Masoro, E.J., University of Texas, San Antonio, TX 78284

Massie, H., Masonic Medical Research Laboratory, Utica, NY 13501

McKnight, William

Meek, T.J.

Mezger-Freez, Liselotte, Institute for Cancer Research,
    Philadelphia, PA 19111

Miller, Dennis, Sinai Hospital of Baltimore, Baltimore, MD 21215

Moment, Gairdner Bostwick, Goucher College, Baltimore, MD 21204

Moynihan, Jeremiah

Obenrader, Mark, University of Pittsburgh, Pittsburgh, PA 15213

Ogbuen, Charles, University of Washington, Seattle, WA 98105

Opalik, Allen, Medical College of Pennsylvania, Philadelphia, PA
    19129

Ove, Peter, University of Pittsburgh, Pittsburgh, PA 15213

Pace, D.M., University of the Pacific, Stockton, CA 95202

Packer, Lester, University of California at Berkeley, Berkeley, CA
    94720

Paik, Woon Ki, Temple University, Fels Research Institute,
    Philadelphia, PA 19140

Plaut, G.W.E., Temple University School of Medicine, Philadelphia,
    PA 19140

Podolsky, S., Boston Veterans Administration Outpatient Clinic,
    Boston, MA 02108

Rednor, Ronald, Temple University School of Medicine, Philadelphia,
    PA 19140

Roberts, J., The Medical College of Pennsylvania, Philadelphia, PA 19129

Rotenberg, Samuel, Fels Research Institute, Temple University, Philadelphia, PA 19140

Roth, G., Gerontology Research Center, Baltimore City Hospitals, Baltimore, MD 21224

Ryan, J.M., The Wistar Institute, Philadelphia, PA 19104

Saito, Y., Syracuse University, Syracuse, NY 13210

Samis, H.V., Masonic Medical Research, Utica, NY 13501

Schwartz, Arthur G., Fels Research Institute, Temple University, Philadelphia, PA 19140

Sheppard, Herbert, Hoffman La Roche, Inc., West Orange, NJ 07052

Shock, Nathan W., Gerontology Research Center, Baltimore City Hospitals, Baltimore, MD 21224

Smith, J.R., University of California at Berkeley, Berkeley, CA 94720

Smith, Lester, National Institute Child Health and Human Development, Bethesda, MD 21224

Soloff, L.A., Temple University, Philadelphia, PA 19140

Sorrentino, R.S., Syracuse University, Syracuse, NY 13210

Spitzer, Judy A., Hahnemann Medical College and Hospital, Philadelphia, PA 19102

Spurgeon, H., Gerontology Research Center, National Institute Child Health and Human Development, Bethesda, MD 21224

Sridhara, Vishala, Temple University, Philadelphia, PA 19140

Starkey, R.J., Drexel University, Philadelphia, PA 19174

Stevens, Ralph, Temple University, Philadelphia, PA 19140

Stoltzner, Gordon, Gerontology Research Center, Baltimore City Hospitals, Baltimore, MD 21224

Story, J., The Wistar Institute, Philadelphia, PA 19104

Szuzepaniak, John P., Haverford State Hospital, Haverford, PA
    19041

Tepper, S., The Wistar Institute, Philadelphia, PA 19104

Tobin, Jordon D., Gerontology Research Center, Baltimore City
    Hospitals, Baltimore, MD 21224

Toyshima, Kuji, Medical College of Pennsylvania, Philadelphia, PA
    19129

Varma, K.G., Medical College of Pennsylvania, Philadelphia, PA
    19129

Venus, M., Medical College of Pennsylvania, Philadelphia, PA 19129

Viceps, Dace, The Wistar Institute, Philadelphia, PA 19104

Vincent, Russell A., John Hopkins University, Baltimore, MD 21218

Weisfeldt, M.L., John Hopkins University, Baltimore, MD 21218

Weymouth, Lisa, University of Pennsylvania, Philadelphia, PA 19174
    and Institute of Cancer Research, Philadelphia, PA 19111

Williams, Jerry R., Harvard University, Cambridge, MA 02138

Wolosewick, John

Wright, Woodring, Stanford University School of Medicine, Stanford,
    CA 94305

Yang, Da-Ping, Wyeth Laboratories, Inc., Philadelphia, PA
    19101

Yaros, Michael, Temple University, Philadelphia, PA 19140

Zimmerman, Irwin D., Medical College of Pennsylvania, Philadelphia,
    PA 19129

Zimmerman, Jay A., Masonic Medical Research Laboratory, Utica, NY
    13501

Zuckerman, Bert M., University of Massachusetts, East Wareham, MA
    02538

SUBJECT INDEX

Acetylcholine, 201
Acetylcholinesterase, 203
Acid phosphatase, 57
ACTH, 202, 210, 211, 214-216,
    218, 223-226, 235
Actinomycin D, 151
Action potential, 135, 137, 139,
    142-146
Adenyl cyclase,
    norepinephrine-stimulated,
    85
    adipocyte, 202
Adipocytes, 85, 93, 184, 191,
    202, 206
    plasma membranes, 85
Aldosterone, 69
Alkaline phosphatase, 89
Amino acids,
    extracellular, 156, 157,
    159
    intracellular, 156, 157,
    159
    precursors of in protein,
    157, 159, 161
Amphipathic lipids, 84
Amygdala, 231
Androgen, 201
Anemic W/W^v, 3
Antibody, 4
Antiarrhythmic effects, 144,
    145
Anucleate cytoplasms, 40, 41,
    43, 45
Aorta, 169, 173, 176, 178, 182,
    190

Arcuate neurones, 234
Arrhythmias, 119, 139, 143,
    145
Arteriosclerosis, 163-165
Atherogenesis,
    theory of, 189
Atherosclerosis, 164, 165,
    169, 172, 173, 190
ATPase,
    CA^{++} and Mg^{++}, 92
    Na^{++} and K^{++}, 92
Autoradiography, 9, 59
AV block, 126, 127, 129, 142

Barrier function,
    of membranes, 81, 84, 85
Basal lamina, 168
Biological membranes, 93
Blood vessels, 163
Bone marrow, 30, 34

Calcium, 114, 115, 117
Calcium transport, 90, 93
    ATP-dependent, oxalate
    promoted, 92
Cap cells, 14
Cardiac function, 96
Cardiac hypertrophy,
    induction of, 152
Cardiac membranes, 120, 145,
    146

Cardiac muscle, 149, 155
Cardiac output, 96
Cardiac tissue, 119, 125, 134
    electrophysiological behav-
    ior of, 119, 134, 145
Catecholamine, 111, 117, 202,
    231, 232, 236, 247
    depletion, 234
    levels, 234
    mechanisms, 235
    metabolism, 231, 232, 235
Cells,
    WI, 26, 58
    WI38, 39, 40, 44, 53, 58,
    67, 69, 73
Cell division, 1, 10, 12
Cell proliferation, 14
Cerebral hemispheres, 201, 206
Chalone, 171
Chemical sympathectomy, 133, 146
Chlorpromazine, 232, 234
Cholesterol, 168, 169
Cholinoreceptor, 201
Chromatin, 197, 203
Circadian activity, 224, 225
Cloning efficiencies, 176, 180
Clonal selection, 172
Clonal senescence, 170, 172, 174,
    190, 191
    theory of atherogenesis,
    189
Coronary artery atherosclerosis,
    165
Coronary flow, 97, 98
Corticoid binding proteins, 202
Corticosterone, 210–218, 220,
    221, 223–226, 232
    receptors, 234, 235
Cortisol, 57, 68, 198, 202, 204
    binding sites, 234
Cortisone, 70, 75
Cortol, 71
Cyclic AMP, 34
Cyclic GMP, 34
Cycloheximide, 151
Cytochalasin B, 41, 43
Cytoplasmic receptors, 197, 203
Cytoplasts, 40, 43, 44, 47, 48,
    50, 54

Cytosyl arabinoside, 61, 63

Dexamethasone, 69, 71, 198
Diabetes, 165, 168, 239, 240,
    244, 246, 248
Differentiation, 28, 32, 34,
    36
Dimethylaminoethanol, 86
DNA, 60
DNA synthesis, 7, 60, 64, 66,
    67, 70, 71, 75, 203
Donor age, 11
L-DOPA, 231, 234
^{3}H-L DOPA, 232
Dopamine, 232, 234

Elastase, 174, 176, 180, 181,
    190
Electrical activity, 134, 137,
    139, 142
Electrical refractory period,
    114
End bud, 12, 14
Endoplasmic reticulum, 81
Endothelial cells, 182, 189
Endothelial injury, 172
Enucleation, 41
11-epicortisol, 70
Epinephrine, 202, 231, 234
Errors, 39, 54
Error catastrophe theory of
    Orgel, 189
Erythrocytes, 90, 93
Estradiol receptors, 203
Estrogen, 201, 206, 229
Estrogen receptors, 234
Estrous cycles, 231, 234

Fat cell homogenates, 85
Feed back inhibition, 170
Fibroblast, 39, 54, 184, 190
Fibrocytes, 14
^{14}C-fluorodinitrobenzene, 151

Follicle stimulating hormone, 232
Fusion, 40, 41, 43-46, 49, 52, 53

Glucagon, 202, 225, 247
Glucagon receptors, 202, 203
Glucocorticoids, 225, 247
    (also see individual)
Glucocorticoid binding, 201, 203, 206
Glucorticoid receptors, 203, 206
Glucokinase, 209, 210, 224, 225
Glucose-6-phosphate dehydro-genase, 171, 189
Glucose tolerance, 239, 240, 244, 245
β glucuronidase, 57
Glutamine synthetase, 75
Gompertz function, 168
Gonadotropins, 231, 234
Golgi complex, 81
Growth hormone, 232, 247
Growth regulation, 10

Hemolysis, 90
Hemopoeitic cell transplants, 3
Hepatocytes, 89, 93
Heteroplasmons, 40, 44, 48, 50
Hippocampus, 201, 206, 235
Homocystinuria, 172
Hormonal regulation, 229
Hormonal responses, 197
Hormonal stimuli, 195
Hormones, 195, 197, 202
Hormone receptors, 206, 235
Human fibroblasts, 39, 54
Hutchinson-Guilford progeria syndrome, 235
Hybrids, 40, 49, 50, 53
Hydrocortisone, 57, 58, 60, 62-69, 71-73, 75, 77

18-hydroxycorticosterone, 69
6-hydroxydopamine, 133, 134, 142, 146
Hypertension, 95, 155, 165, 169
Hypotension, 155
Hypothalamus, 231, 234-236
Hypothalamic homeostat, 235
Hypothalamic norepinephrine levels, 232

Immune response, 83
Immunocompetent unit, 32, 36
Information transfer, 83
Insulin, 89, 202, 210, 225, 226, 239, 245-248
Intimal proliferation, 168, 172
Iproniazide, 231, 234
Isoproterenol, 203

Lag period, 153
Left ventricular function, 105
Left ventricular hypertrophy, 101
Left ventricular volume, 101
Leucine,
    intracellular, 151, 159
Leucine pool, 151, 158
Leucyl-t-RNA, 160
Lipid bilayer, 84
Lipid depositions, 168
Lipid peroxidation, 84
Lipid phosphorous, 91
Lipoprotein subclasses, 90
Liver, 199, 202
Lymphocyte, 21, 29, 30, 34, 36, 206
Lymphoid cells, 203
Lysosomes, 81

Macrophages, 31, 36
Maltase, 89

Mammary epithelium, 1, 4, 7, 12, 14
Mammary transplant system, 4, 5
Medial calcinosis, 164, 168
Membrane, 81-85, 87, 90, 93
    biology, 87
    bound phosphorylated intermediate, 92
    lipids, 84
    proteins, 84
    responsiveness, 139, 144, 146
    structure, 84, 85, 86
Membrane organelles, 81
Mesothelial cells, 182, 191
Metabolic regulation, 81
Metabolic time, 10
C57B1/6 mice, 150, 210, 217, 220
Microangiopathy, 168
Microsomal fraction, 87
Microsomes, 87, 90
Mitochondria, 81
Mitochondrial membranes, 83
Mitochondrial preparations, 87
Mitogens, 169
Molecular architecture of membranes, 83, 84
Monckeberg's sclerosis, 164, 168
Muscle cells, 206
Muscle relaxation, 90
Mutations, 169, 171
Myocardium, 119
Myointimal cells, 170

Nephrosclerosis, 165
Neuroendocrine controls, 232, 234
Neurons, 206
Norepinephrine, 85, 232
Nuclear control,
    of cell aging, 52

Organoid culture, 182, 190

Ovarian cycles, 231
Ovaries, 201
Overshoot, 136, 137, 139, 144
Oviduct, 201
Oxygen extraction, 97

Pacemaker activity, 125, 142
Parkinson's disease, 231
Perfused heart, 149, 154, 155, 161
Perfusion of mouse hearts, 150, 154
Pharmacological agents, 123, 145
Phenylalanine, 160, 161
Phosphatidylcholine, 86, 91
Phosphatidylethanolamine, 85, 91
Phosphatidylinositol, 91
Phosphatidylserine, 91
Phosphodiesterase, 89
Phospholipids, 85, 91
Phospholipid to protein ratio, 87, 91
Phytohemagglutin, 34
Pituitary, 231, 235
    hormones, 229, 231
Plasma membrane, 81-83, 85, 87, 93, 202
Platelets, 172
Polyunsaturated fatty acids, 84
Potential cell doublings, 10
Prednisolone, 69, 71
Preoptic region, 231
Progeria, 235
Progeroid syndromes, 169
Progesterone receptors, 201, 206
Prolactin, 232
Proliferation, 21, 32, 34, 36
Proliferative potential, 6, 10, 11
Prostate gland, 201
Protein synthesis, 149, 151, 153-155, 157, 160, 161

Quinidine, 129–131, 139, 140,
    144, 146

Rate of rise, 135, 139, 142,
    143, 144, 146
Reactivity, 119, 140
Receptor, 83, 206, 207
Red cells, 90
Replicative potential, 169,
    175, 181, 184, 189, 190
    (see also proliferation)
Repolarization, 136, 137, 142,
    144, 146
Resting potential, 136, 137,
    139
Restricted feeding, 236

Salivary gland, 203
Sarcoplasmic reticulum, 90, 92,
    93
Saturation density, 58
Scatchard Analyses, 197, 204
Selective transport process,
    232
Sendai virus, 43–46, 53
Serial transplantation, 5, 6, 17
Skeletal muscle, 91, 201
Skin tests, 35
Skin transplantation, 2
Smooth muscle, 189–191
Sodium transport, 92
Spleen, 28, 30, 32, 34
Splenic leukocyte, 203, 206
Sprague–Dawley rats, 209, 210,
    212, 213, 215–218, 220,
    223–226
Static phase, 10
Stem cell, 14, 26, 29, 32, 169,
    175, 179, 190
Steroid hormones, 197, 202, 229
    (see also individual)
Steroid receptors, 234

Testicle weight, 232
Testosterone, 69, 232
5α-dihydrotestosterone, 201
Thymic hormones, 33
Thymidine, 60, 61, 75
^{3}H-thymidine autoradiography,
    182
Thymidine kinase, 59, 62–66
^{3}H-thymidine uptake, 60, 62,
    63
Thyroid stimulating hormone,
    232
Thyroxine, 152, 154, 155
Transplanted cells,
    identification of, 2
Transport, 81
Triamcinolone, 69, 71
^{3}H-L-tyrosine, 232
Tyrosine aminotransferase,
    202, 210, 212, 215, 220,
    223, 225, 226
Tyrosine hydroxylase activity,
    235

Uterus, 201

Varicose veins, 168
Vascular disease, 163, 168, 190
Vascular smooth muscle, 169

Werner's syndrome, 67, 235

Printed in the United States
by Baker & Taylor Publisher Services